DIFFERENTIAL DIAGNOSIS IN PRIMARY CARE

DIFFERENTIAL DIAGNOSIS IN PRIMARY CARE

Second Edition

R. DOUGLAS COLLINS, M.D., F.A.C.P.

Medical Director of the Collins Specialty Care Center
Banning, California

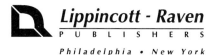
Lippincott - Raven
P U B L I S H E R S
Philadelphia • New York

Acquistions Editor: Stuart Freeman
Sponsoring Editor: Sanford Robinson
Manuscript Editor: Marjory I. Fraser
Indexer: Darbara Littlewood
Art Director: Tracy Baldwin
Designer: Arlene Putterman
Production Manager: Kathleen P. Dunn
Production Coordinators: Caren Erlichman and George V. Gordon
Compositor: Bi-Comp, Inc.
Printer/Binder: R.R. Donnelley & Sons Company

Printed in the United States of America

9 8

Library of Congress Cataloging-in-Publication Data
Collins, R. Douglas
    Differential diagnosis in primary care.

    Rev. ed. of: Dynamic differential diagnosis.
1981.
    Includes index.
    1. Diagnosis, Differential.   I. Collins, R. Douglas.
Dynamic differential diagnosis.   II. Title. [DNLM:
1. Diagnosis, Differential   WB 141.5 C712d]
RC71.5.C62   1987   616.07'5   86-27365
ISBN 0-397-50816-6
for Library of Congress

This work is dedicated to
Stuart Freeman, Medical Editor,
who has been a guiding force
in producing my medical books for over 20 years.

Preface

The most significant change in the new edition of this book on differential diagnosis is the title: *Differential Diagnosis in Primary Care*. The book is directed to the *primary care physician* because he is the one who must be an expert in the differential diagnosis. If he misses the diagnosis, the patient may be referred to the wrong specialist and may find himself out on a limb of the diagnostic tree at the point of no return! Unhappily, a recent case illustrates this untoward side effect of misdiagnosis.

A 23-year-old white woman developed right lower quadrant pain and was examined by her primary care physician. Because of a negative urine pregnancy test and a slight elevation of the white blood cells, the patient was referred to a surgeon who quickly operated on a normal appendix. The next day a serum test for pregnancy was positive but was overlooked. When the patient developed colicky right lower quadrant pain a few weeks later, she was referred to a urologist instead of a gynecologist. The urologist did not find a stone. Nothing further was done for the patient until one night she experienced severe lower abdominal pain and shock. At last she was operated on by the appropriate specialist. The gynecologist found a ruptured ectopic pregnancy. Obviously, the patient's agony and brush with death could have been avoided if the *correct diagnosis* and *correct referral* had been made in the first place!

The latest laboratory, x-ray, and special diagnostic procedures have been included in this edition. Magnetic resonance imaging (MRI) is one of these important advances. It has provided a definitive diagnosis when all else fails, especially in diseases of the nervous system.

The publisher and his staff deserve an honorable mention for the quality of the first edition. I have received no letters or reviews pointing out typographical errors for the first time in my writing career. It is fitting then that this edition be dedicated to Stuart Freeman, Editor, Medical Books at J. B. Lippincott Company for this accomplishment as well as the tremendous part he has played in the publication of all my other books on diagnosis.

R. DOUGLAS COLLINS, M.D., F.A.C.P.

Preface To First Edition

This is not just another reference book on differential diagnosis. The primary purpose of this book is twofold: first, to teach differential diagnosis, and second, to provide a quick reference for the busy physician to use in the office or in the hospital ward before, during, or after examination of the patient. For the past five years the author has been teaching a course in differential diagnosis, possibly the only one of its kind in the United States, first at the Medical University of South Carolina and later at the University of Florida College of Medicine. This book has developed out of the methods applied in this course.

It has been the author's experience that even the most astute clinician, when confronted with a patient complaining of a given symptom, often blindly dives into taking a thorough history and subsequent physical without considering the diagnostic possibilities he's really looking for. After gathering all this information (as much as one or two hours later), he pauses a few minutes to think and then writes down the one or two common disorders that may best explain the patient's complaint and leaves it at that. He proceeds to write his orders for a workup and prescribes

treatment on the basis of those one or two disorders. How many times does he find himself up a blind alley with this method? Too often, in my opinion. The reader of this book will learn how to arrive at a list of perhaps ten to twenty conditions that may explain the patient's complaint in a few seconds, before he initiates the history and physical examination or writes his orders for a workup. Then, with the differential in mind, he can proceed to take a meaningful history and perform a meaningful physical and workup. His history will be more sound because he will ask questions to include or exclude diseases he already has in mind. His physical will be more sound because he will go beyond a routine physical and do special examinations to pinpoint or rule out the diseases he's thinking of. His laboratory workup will be more accurate because it will include tests for all the most likely diseases in the differential.

This book can be used as a quick reference to formulate a differential diagnosis of the problem at hand. A symptom index is provided to assist the clinician in this task. Turning to a particular symptom, the reader will find an illustration of the most common causes, often accompanied by a table providing a more comprehensive list. These features make this little handbook useful to carry wherever one may go.

Of the many people who have assisted in the preparation of this handbook, I would especially like to thank Susan Brenman, the expert illustrator, and Glenda Dehnert and Gillian Ford for the excellent job of typing from my left-handed scribbling. As usual Stuart Freeman, Editor-in-Chief of the J. B. Lippincott Company, and his staff have assisted me immensely throughout the stages of preparation and have made many contributions to the organization and presentation of the material.

R. Douglas Collins, M.D., F.A.C.P.

Introduction

The basic premise of teaching differential diagnosis is that the causes of each symptom can be analyzed by one or more of the basic sciences of anatomy, histology, physiology, and biochemistry. The first step is to group all the symptoms into one or more of the following categories:

1. Pain
2. Mass
3. Bloody discharge
4. Nonbloody discharge
5. Functional change

The remaining symptoms may be grouped under "miscellaneous" for the purpose of this book. The reader will note that the table of contents is based on these categories.

Each of the categories of symptoms may now be analyzed for diagnostic possibilities by applying one or more of the basic sciences:

1. Pain: anatomy and histology
2. Mass: anatomy and histology
3. Bloody discharge: anatomy and biochemistry
4. Nonbloody discharge: anatomy

5. Functional change: pathophysiology and biochemistry

Take, as an instance, **pain.**

A 37-year-old white woman complains of acute right upper quadrant pain of 2 hours' duration. Applying **anatomy,** the physician visualizes the organs of the right upper quadrant. He sees the liver, the gallbladder, the right colon, the duodenum, the head of the pancreas, the right kidney and adrenal gland, the ribs, and the vertebral column and peripheral nerves. Applying the knowledge from the etiological discussion in step two (see below), the student can make an initial differential list including

1. **Inflammation** of the liver (hepatitis), the gallbladder (cholecystitis), the duodenum (duodenitis or ulcer), the colon (colitis), the pancreas (pancreatitis), the nerves (neuritis), the kidney (pyelonephritis)
2. **Obstructive disease** of the liver (cholangitis), gallbladder (gallstones), pancreas (pancreatic duct stone), or duodenum
3. **Vascular disease of the liver** (Budd–Chiari disease, pyelophlebitis, or hemorrhage)

4. **Vascular disease of the kidney** (*e.g.*, embolism or thrombosis)

If he applies *histology*, he will divide the liver into a capsule (parietal and visceral) the parenchyma, supporting tissue, ducts, veins, and arteries. Thus he can apply the various categories learned in step two to each of these tissues. For example, inflammation of the capsule suggests subdiaphragmatic abscess, while inflammation of the supporting tissue suggests collagen disease, and inflammation of the ducts, cholangitis. In the general discussion of each section, the application of the basic sciences will be dealt with in more detail.

Utilizing the basic sciences will enable the physician to develop a list of diagnostic possibilities more meaningful than those derived from the rather haphazard fashion of simply associating certain diseases with particular symptoms. Even so, the list will not be all-inclusive. Therefore, a second step must be taken. All symptoms can be analyzed according to etiological categories, such as vascular, inflammatory, neoplastic, and degenerative. To keep these categories fixed in mind, a mnemonic is extremely helpful. One simple mnemonic is **MINT,** which applies as follows:

M — Malformation
 I — Inflammation and Intoxication
N — Neoplasm
T — Trauma

(Note, however, that this mnemonic leaves out vascular, degenerative, and allergic disorders.)

A more useful and inclusive mnemonic is **VINDICATE,** which includes almost all etiological categories. It is this mnemonic that will be utilized most in the various tables accompanying each symptom in this book.

V — Vascular
I — Inflammatory

N — Neoplastic
D — Degenerative
I — Intoxication
C — Congenital
A — Allergic and Autoimmune
T — Traumatic
E — Endocrine and Metabolic

The physician may wish to develop his own mnemonic with these principles in mind.

Certainly a symptom could be developed from the etiological categories above. For example, if the chief complaint is headache, the **V—Vascular** conditions immediately suggested are migraine and temporal arteritis. Move on to **I—Inflammation** and sinusitis, dental abscess, meningitis, and brain abscess come to mind. **N—Neoplastic** diseases are brain tumors, metastatic carcinomas, and nasal polyps, for example. **D—Degenerative** conditions are rarely associated with headache, but cervical spondylosis should come to mind. **I—Intoxication** suggest a ''hangover'' headache, lead intoxication, chronic ingestion of aspirin and other drugs, and anoxia in chronic emphysema and poor working conditions. **C—Congenital** disorders also infrequently present with headache, but aneurysms and platybasia should not be overlooked. **A—Autoimmune** and allergic diseases like lupus and periarteritis nodosa may present with headache but more common is allergic rhinitis and sinusitis. **T—Trauma** makes one think of concussion and post-concussion headache, epidural and subdural hematomas, skull or cervical spine fractures, and herniated discs. Finally, **E—Endocrine** and metabolic disorders such as pituitary adenomas, acromegaly, and hyperparathyroidism may present with headache, as will metabolic conditions such as porphyria, hepatic precoma, and uremia.

One can readily see that by using the mnemonic **VINDICATE,** one may easily be "vindicated" in a CPC. I hope, however, that the reader will apply both the basic science and the etiological method in developing a list of diagnostic possibilities and that he will see how easily this can be accomplished by using the illustrations and charts in this book.

There is another, more scientific method of developing and recalling etiological categories. This is simply to think of what can happen to each tissue or structure. For example:

The Liver

1. The capsule can become inflamed (subdiaphragmatic abscess), it can become swollen (hepatic vein obstruction), it can become neoplastic.
2. The parenchyma can become inflamed (hepatitis), intoxicated (toxic hepatitis), neoplastic or degenerative, or it can become necrotic (infarct) or replaced by fibrosis (cirrhosis).
3. The ducts can become inflamed (cholangitis), obstructed (ductal stones and extrinsic neoplasms), chronically obstructed on an idiopathic basis (biliary cirrhosis), or neoplastic (cholangiocarcinoma).
4. The supporting tissue can become inflamed (lupoid hepatitis) or it can multiply (sarcoma and cirrhosis).
5. The portal vein can become obstructed by thrombosis or thrombophlebitis (pyelophlebitis). The hepatic vein can also become obstructed by a clot (Budd–Chiari syndrome) or by heart failure. The arteries may be inflamed by periarteritis nodosa or obstructed by occlusive vascular disease.

What happens to the tissue layers of each organ can be related one to another as follows:

Meningitis = pleuritis = peritonitis = pericarditis = perinephric abscess = subdiaphragmatic abscess

Inflammatory disease needs to be broken down further into idiopathic, collagenous, and infectious types. Recall the infections by starting with the smallest etiological agent and building to the largest:

1. Virus
2. Rickettsiae
3. Bacteria
4. Spirochete
5. Parasite
6. Fungus

All of the aforementioned concepts will be developed throughout this book. The **third step** in differential diagnosis is to utilize the history and physical examination to rule in or rule out various possibilities on the list developed by steps one and two. For instance, a family history of headache would suggest migraine or the occupational history of a painter might suggest lead intoxication.

Now the history becomes more meaningful. The clinician knows what questions to ask because he already knows from the presenting complaint what condition to look for. The physical examination becomes more meaningful because the clinician already knows what signs to examine for with a differential diagnosis in mind.

As other symptoms and signs are gleaned from the history and physical, groups of signs and symptoms suggest one diagnosis over another.

Finally, the list of possibilities that remain after the history and physical examination are completed is a useful guide in ordering laboratory, roentgenographic, and other diagnostic tests. Appendices I and II may be consulted for these tests. If the clinician orders on the basis of only the one diagnosis he considers most likely, he may run up a blind alley and waste valuable time in ordering additional diagnostic tests. With a broad differential, he can order appropriate tests early and save time and often money.

Contents

Chapter 3
BLOODY DISCHARGE
180

Chapter 4
NONBLOODY DISCHARGE
207

Chapter 5
FUNCTIONAL CHANGES
227

Chapter 6
MISCELLANEOUS SYMPTOMS AND SIGNS

414

Appendix I
THE LABORATORY WORKUP OF SYMPTOMS

457

DIFFERENTIAL DIAGNOSIS IN PRIMARY CARE

PAIN

Chapter 1

GENERAL DISCUSSION

Developing a list of causes of pain anywhere in the body is achieved best by visualizing the anatomy of the area. If, for example, a patient complains of chest pain, the physician simply visualizes the organs in the chest and the components of the chest wall to get a useful list of possibilities. The heart makes one think of a myocardial infarction, the lungs suggest pulmonary infarction or pleurisy, the esophagus, esophagitis, and so on.

To make the differential more extensive one needs to take a second step, to think of the various etiologies that may affect each organ or structure. Any mnemonic will do, but the best is **VINDICATE.** Apply **VINDICATE** to chest pain and, assuming that pain may be coming from the heart, see what diagnoses might be suggested.

V—Vascular suggests myocardial infarction and coronary insufficiency.
I—Inflammatory suggests pericarditis.
N—Neoplasm suggests mainly direct extension of a carcinoma of the lung (or elsewhere) to the pericardium because rhabdomyosarcomas are rare.
D—Degenerative disease does not cause pain in the chest as a rule, however,
I—Intoxication suggests uremic pericarditis.
C—Congenital anomalies are not usually associated with pain in the chest either.
A—Autoimmune would bring to mind lupus pericarditis.
T—Trauma to the heart can cause a painful hemopericardium.
E—Endocrinopathies do not generally cause chest pain.

This, then, is the system. With practice it will take only a few seconds to apply. Then, as the clinician takes the history and does the physical examination he can rule out many of the diseases suggested by this anatomical–etiological analysis by the presence or absence of other symptoms and signs. For example, chest pain and marked diaphoresis suggest a myocardial infarction, whereas chest pain with hemoptysis suggests a pulmonary infarction.

It is helpful in diagnosing the cause of pain to understand the pathophysiology. Pain is produced by one or more of the following methods:

1. Direct stimulation of sensory nerve endings by an external physical force, an ingested toxin, a toxin released by an infectious agent, or a ruptured or necrotic body cell in the area of the pain.
2. Swelling of an organ because of increased air, extracellular fluid, pus, or blood.
3. Sudden obstruction of the arterial blood supply to an organ so that the cells of the organ die and release toxins that stimulate the nerve endings as mentioned above.
4. Obstruction of the venous drainage from an organ or area, causing swelling of that area with extracellular fluid or blood.
5. Obstruction of a duct that drains fluid from an organ, causing swelling of the organ.

It follows that of the various etiologies suggested by the mnemonic **VINDICATE, vascular disease** is often associated with pain because of mechanisms three and four above; **infectious** or **autoimmune—allergic** and **inflammation** is often associated with pain because of mechanisms one and two above, while **intoxication** is associated with pain only when it has a direct toxic effect on the sensory nerve or when it destroys a significant

number of cells in a certain area, releasing large amounts of intracellular toxins that stimulate the nerve endings. **Trauma** is often associated with pain because of mechanism two. **Degenerative diseases, neoplasms, congenital anomalies,** and **endocrinopathies** are infrequently associated with pain for obvious reasons. (Degenerative diseases do not usually cause an organ to swell and only a few cells die at a time so very few toxins are released.) **Neoplastic diseases** grow slowly as a rule so other structures can move out of the way or the organ may swell slowly. If, however, the neoplasm causes a hemorrhage into the area or acute necrosis (*i.e.,* ovarian carcinomas) there may be pain. Furthermore, pain may develop from a superimposed infection or from a neoplastic obstruction of a duct or blood vessel of the organ (mechanisms three, four, and five). Partial obstruction causes a more severe and colicky pain than complete obstruction.

Congenital anomalies may occasionally lead to duct obstruction or to infection of an area causing pain, but generally they are silent. Likewise endocrinopathies are usually due to atrophy or slow growing tumors in the endocrine gland involved and, with rare exceptions, do not cause pain. The important exceptions are acromegaly (headache), subacute thyroiditis, and orchitis.

The preceding discussion of the pathophysiology of pain will, I hope, assist the recall process even more. After taking the above steps, the physician is ready for the laboratory workup of pain.

Appendix I provides lists of tests frequently used in the workup of different types of pain. Ordering from this "menu" of tests should be done "à la carte" according to the most likely diagnosis in the individual case. In fact, if the clinician has narrowed the list to only a few diagnoses, he might consider using Appendix II, which lists the laboratory and x-ray film tests for each specific disease.

ABDOMINAL PAIN

Abdominal Pain, Generalized

The **gastrointestinal tract** is the only "organ" that really covers the abdomen from one end to the other. Anything that causes an irritation of all or a large portion of this "tube" may cause generalized abdominal pain. Thus gastritis, viral and bacterial gastroenteritis, irritable bowel syndrome, ulcerative colitis, and amebic colitis fall into this category. The remainder of the causes of generalized abdominal pain can be developed by using the mnemonic **ROS** with the anatomy of the entire abdomen.

When faced with a patient with diffuse abdominal pain, think of **R** for **ruptured viscus.** Now take each organ and consider the possibility of its having ruptured. Thus, the stomach and duodenum suggest a ruptured peptic ulcer; the pancreas, an acute hemorrhagic pancreatitis; the gallbladder, a ruptured appendix. The liver and spleen usually rupture from trauma, whereas the fallopian tube may rupture from an ectopic pregnancy. The colon ruptures from a diverticulitis, an ulcerative colitis, or a carcinoma. What is the one thing that should make the physician suspect a ruptured viscus? Rebound tenderness is the answer. In addition, one or both testicles may be drawn up (Collins' sign). If only the right testicle is drawn up, suspect a ruptured appendix or peptic ulcer. If only the left is drawn up, suspect a ruptured diverticulum. If both are drawn up, suspect pancreatitis or a generalized peritonitis.

Now take the letter **O.** This signifies intestinal **obstruction.** Think of adhesions, hernias, volvulus, paralytic ileus, intussusception, fecal impactions, carcinomas, mesenteric infarctions, regional ileitis, and malrotation. The best way to recall all these is with the mnemonic **VINDICATE.**

Next take the letter **S.** This signifies the **systemic** diseases that may irritate the intestines, the peritoneum, or both. Once again the mnemonic **VINDICATE** will remind one to recall the important offenders.

V—Vascular suggests the anemias, congestive heart failure, coagulation disorders, and mesenteric artery occlusion, embolism, or thrombosis.

I—Inflammatory includes tuberculous, gonococcal and pneumococcal peritonitis, and trichinosis.

N—Neoplasms should suggest leukemia, and metastatic carcinoma.

D—Deficiency might suggest the gastroenteritis of pellagra.

I—Intoxication reminds one of lead colic, uremia, and the venom of a black widow spider bite.

C—Congenital suggests porphyria and sickle cell disease.

A—Autoimmune brings to mind periarteritis nodosa, rheumatic fever, Schönlein–Henoch purpura, and dermatomyositis.

T—Trauma would suggest the paralytic ileus of trauma anywhere, the crush syndrome, and hemoperitoneum.

E—Endocrine disease suggests diabetic ketoacidosis, addisonian crisis, and hypocalcemia.

Approach to the Diagnosis

Because of the urgency of the situation in most cases, the history is taken while the patient is examined. The importance of rebound tenderness cannot be stressed enough. Board-like rigidity, lack of bowel sounds, and drawn-up testicles are other signs of peritoneal irritation. Diaphoresis and shock with nausea and vomiting are confirmatory signs and emphasize the need for immediate attention. Hyperactive bowel sounds of a high-pitched tinkling character with distention

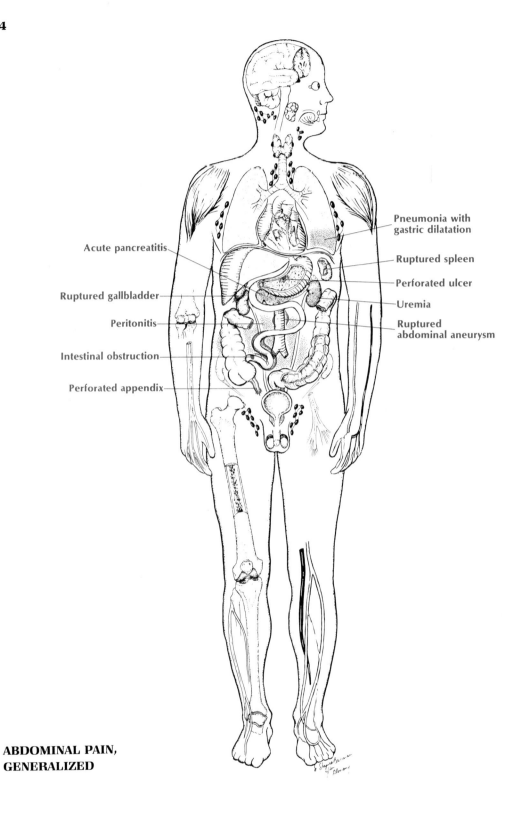

Pneumonia with
gastric dilatation

Acute pancreatitis

Ruptured spleen

Perforated ulcer

Ruptured gallbladder

Uremia

Peritonitis

Ruptured
abdominal aneurysm

Intestinal obstruction

Perforated appendix

**ABDOMINAL PAIN,
GENERALIZED**

and minimal rebound suggest obstruction. The presence of bowel sounds, very little distention, good vital signs, and minimal tenderness suggests a viral gastroenteritis or some other diffuse irritation of the bowel.

In the acute case a nasogastric tube is passed and a flat plate and upright of the abdomen, a chest x-ray, a complete blood count (cbc), fasting blood sugar (FBS), electrolytes, urinalysis, and serum amylase and lipase are ordered. A 2-hour urinary amylase may be desirable, if the serum amylase is normal. Gall bladder ultrasonography may be useful. If these are normal but the vital signs begin to deteriorate, exploratory laparotomy should not be delayed. Special diagnostic procedures that may be worthwhile in the borderline case are a four-quadrant peritoneal tap, repeated amylases, double enemas, stool analysis for occult blood, and urine porphobilinogen. Frequent vital signs and repeated evaluation of the patient with flat plates and cbc's are often necessary if the surgeon chooses to be conservative. Once the acute stage is passed, a more complete workup may be done to get a definitive diagnosis before surgery. The tests that are useful in this stage are listed in Appendix I.

Right Upper Quadrant Pain

The patient is complaining of right upper quadrant (RUQ) pain and you cannot just give him a bag of pills and send him home. His condition may be serious. But you are in a hurry to get out of the office because you have another important appointment. What do you do? The key is to visualize the **anatomy.** Imagine the liver, gallbladder, bile ducts, hepatic flexure of the colon, duodenum, and the head of the pancreas. Surrounding this are the skin, fascia, ribs, and the thoracic and lumbar spine, with the intercostal nerves and arteries and abdominal muscle.

Pain is usually from **inflammation, trauma,** or **infarction.** The patient gives no history of trauma, but he could have a contusion of the muscle from coughing hard. That is not likely, however, unless he has other symptoms of the respiratory tract.

The possible sources of inflammation should be narrowed down first. The **liver** can be inflamed from hepatitis (most likely viral), the **gallbladder** from **cholecystitis** (most likely induced by stones and bacteria), or the **bile ducts** from cholangitis. The **colon** may be involved with diverticulitis, a segment of granulomatous colitis, or perhaps there is a retrocaecal appendix. The **duodenum,** of course, would most likely have a peptic ulcer which could cause an obstruction or a perforation if the patient is vomiting, or pallor and shock if he is bleeding. The **pancreas** could be inflamed with pancreatitis, especially if the patient drinks alcohol.

These are the most important intraabdominal considerations, but if the mnemonic **VINDICATE** in Table 1-1 were applied one might not forget the Budd–Chiari syndrome (thrombosis of the hepatic veins), portal vein thrombosis, or pyelophlebitis; these are rare. In addition, toxic hepatitis from isoniazid, thorazine, and erythromycin estolate (Ilosone), for example, can be painful. Collagen diseases affecting the liver are another possibility.

Now let us round out the differential with extra-abdominal disorders. The **skin** may be involved with herpes zoster or cellulitis. A **fascial rent** may cause a hernia, particularly if there was previous upper abdominal surgery. Compression of the **nerve roots** by a herniated disc, thoracic spondylosis, or a spinal cord tumor is possible but unlikely. Systemic conditions such as lead colic and porphyria and involvement of another organ, such as the kidney, must be considered (pyelonephritis or renal colic).

(*Text continues on p. 8*)

TABLE 1-1. RIGHT UPPER QUADRANT PAIN

	V Vascular	I Inflammatory	N Neoplasm	D Degenerative
Skin		Herpes zoster Cellulitis		
Muscle and Fascia		Diaphragmatic abscess Trichinosis		
Liver	Infarct Pyelophlebitis	Hepatitis Hepatic abscess	Carcinoma	
Gallbladder		Cholecystitis Cholangitis	Cholangioma	
Duodenum	Mesenteric thrombosis	Ulcer Duodenitis		
Colon		Diverticulitis Colitis		
Pancreas		Pancreatitis	Pancreatic carcinoma	
Lymph Nodes		Mesenteric adenitis	Hodgkin's disease Lymphosarcoma	
Adrenal Gland	Adrenal infarcts	Waterhouse–Friderichsen syndrome Tuberculosis	Neuroblastoma Adrenal carcinoma	
Kidney	Occlusions Embolism Renal vein thrombosis	Pyelonephritis		
Thoracic Spine		Tuberculosis Osteomyelitis	Primary, metastatic, multiple myeloma	Osteoarthritis
Referred	See Table 1-5			

Handwritten annotations: "40 fat ♀" near Cholecystitis; "Gastric Carcinoma" in Duodenum/Neoplasm area; "(CA)" near Mesenteric adenitis; "degen disk" near Osteoarthritis.

I Intoxication Idiopathic	C Congenital or Acquired Anomaly	A Autoimmune Allergic	T Trauma	E Endocrine	Foreign Body
	Ventral hernia Incisional hernia AGE		Contusion Cough Hemorrhage		
Alcoholic hepatitis			Contusion Laceration		
			Traumatic rup- ture		Calculi
Ulcer	Diverticulum Obstruction				
	Diverticulum Obstruction				
	Cyst				Calculus
				addison cushing	
Gout Spune liver	Hydronephrosis		Contusion Laceration	Hyperparathy- roidism	Calculi
	Rheumatoid spon- dylitis		Herniated disc Fracture		

Approach to the Diagnosis

Now ask the appropriate questions and do the best physical examination to diagnose the case. Is the pain intermittent (renal colic) or steady (cholecystitis, pancreatitis)? Has it been continuing for 2 or 3 hours (peptic ulcer), most of the day (cholecystitis), or a few days (pancreatitis)? Is there vomiting (chole-cystitis), or is the pain relieved by food (peptic ulcer)? Is there jaundice (hepatitis, cholecystitis) or tender hepatomegaly and jaundice (hepatitis and stone in the common bile duct)? Is there an RUQ mass other than the liver (diverticular abscess, ruptured retrocaecal appendix, hernia, or enlarged gallbladder of advanced cholecystitis)? A few more questions are necessary and it becomes clear

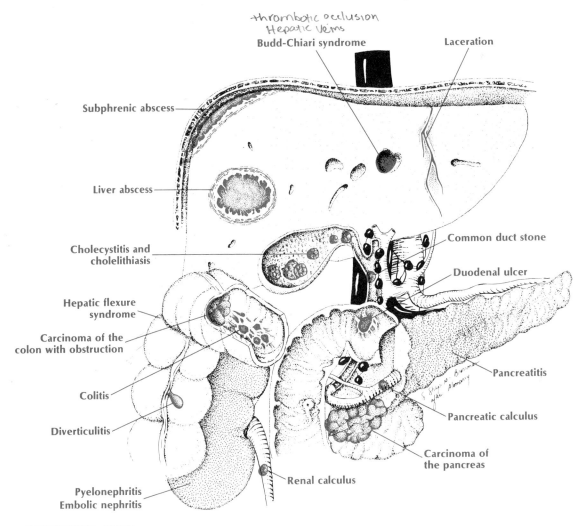

thrombotic occlusion Hepatic Veins

Budd-Chiari syndrome

Laceration

Subphrenic abscess

Liver abscess

Cholecystitis and cholelithiasis

Common duct stone

Duodenal ulcer

Hepatic flexure syndrome

Carcinoma of the colon with obstruction

Colitis

Diverticulitis

Pancreatitis

Pancreatic calculus

Carcinoma of the pancreas

Renal calculus

Pyelonephritis
Embolic nephritis

**ABDOMINAL PAIN,
RUQ**

which orders to write to finish the diagnosis in the hospital or on an outpatient basis, if the patient is not in acute distress and if someone else responsible can watch him carefully. A more extensive list of diagnostic tests is provided in Appendix I to help complete the workup.

Left Upper Quadrant Pain

For all abdominal pain, **anatomy** is the key to recalling the many causes of pain in the left upper quadrant (LUQ) by visualizing the structures layer by layer. In the first layer are the skin, abdominal wall, and ribs; in the sec-

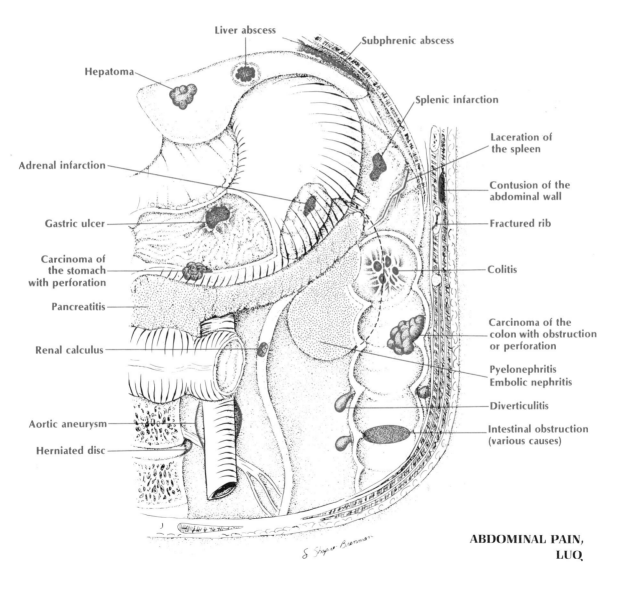

Liver abscess

Subphrenic abscess

Hepatoma

Splenic infarction

Adrenal infarction

Laceration of the spleen

Contusion of the abdominal wall

Gastric ulcer

Fractured rib

Carcinoma of the stomach with perforation

Colitis

Pancreatitis

Renal calculus

Carcinoma of the colon with obstruction or perforation

Pyelonephritis Embolic nephritis

Diverticulitis

Aortic aneurysm

Intestinal obstruction (various causes)

Herniated disc

ABDOMINAL PAIN, LUQ

ond layer, the spleen, colon, and stomach; and in the third layer, the pancreas, adrenal gland, kidney, aorta, and spine. Now it is possible to cross-index the organs with the various etiologies contained in the mnemonic **VINDICATE** (Table 1-2). The following discussion emphasizes the most important of these.

1. **Abdominal wall and ribs.** Pain will occur most commonly from herpes zoster, contusions, hernias, rib fractures, or metastatic tumors.
2. **Spleen.** Painful splenic infarcts are not unusual in subacute bacterial endocarditis, polycythemia, sickle cell anemia, leukemia, periarteritis nodosa, and other autoim-

TABLE 1-2.   LEFT UPPER QUADRANT PAIN

	V Vascular	I Inflammatory	N Neoplasm	D Degenerative and Deficiency
Abdominal Wall	Ruptured vein	Cellulitis	Metastatic carcinoma of ribs	
Spleen	Infarct Aneurysm	Infectious mono- nucleosis Subacute bacterial endocarditis	Leukemia Hodgkin's disease	
Stomach		Gastritis Gastric ulcer	Gastric carcinoma	
Colon	Mesenteric thrombosis *infarct*	Diverticulitis Mucous colitis Parasites	Colon carcinoma	
Pancreas		Pancreatitis	Pancreatic carcinoma Pancreatic cyst	
Adrenal Gland	Infarct		Malignancy with infarction *neuroblastoma*	
Kidney	Embolism Infarction	Pyelonephritis Perinephric abscess	Hypernephroma *renal carcinoma*	
Aorta	Atherosclerotic aneurysm			Medionecrosis with dis- secting aneurysms
Spine		Tuberculosis of the spine Tabes dorsalis *osteomyelitis*	Myeloma Metastatic carcinoma Spinal cord tumors	Osteoarthritis

mune disorders. A ruptured spleen is an important consideration in abdominal injuries, particularly those in children and in patients with infectious mononucleosis.

3. **Stomach.** Acute gaseous distention of the stomach in gastritis, pneumonia, and pyloric obstruction is a common cause of LUQ pain. A gastric carcinoma that ex-

tends beyond the wall of the stomach may cause pain. Episodic obstruction of the stomach in the "cascade stomach" should be considered in the differential diagnosis. Herniation of the stomach through the diaphragm occasionally causes LUQ pain.

4. **Colon.** An inflamed diverticulum or an inflamed splenic flexure from granuloma-

I Intoxication	C Congenital	A Autoimmune Allergic	T Trauma	E Endocrine
			Contusion Hernia	
		Periarteritis nodosa	Ruptured spleen	
Gastric dilatation in pneumonia	Cascade stomach Hiatal hernia		Ruptured stomach	
	Diverticulum obstruction	Granulomatous colitis Crohns	Ruptured colon	
				Waterhouse–Friderichsen syndrome
	Nephroptosis		Renal calculus	
		Fracture Ruptured disc	Osteoporosis	

tous colitis may cause pain in the LUQ. Less commonly the colon develops a perforating or constricting carcinoma in this area, which obstructs the bowel. A mesenteric infarct of the colon, as well as gas or impacted feces in the splenic flexure, may also cause LUQ pain.

5. **Pancreas.** Acute pancreatitis, pancreatic pseudocysts, and carcinoma of the pancreas may cause LUQ pain.
6. **Adrenal gland.** Adrenal infarction from emboli or Waterhouse–Friderichsen syndrome may cause pain, but neoplasms rarely do until they have become massive.
7. **Kidney.** Renal infarcts, renal calculi, acute pyelonephritis, and nephroptosis with a Dietl's crisis may cause LUQ pain. Perinephric abscesses must also be considered.
8. **Aorta.** Dissecting or atherosclerotic aneurysms of the aorta may cause LUQ pain, especially when they occlude a feeding artery to one of the structures there.
9. **Spine.** Herniated disc, tuberculosis, multiple myeloma, osteoarthritis, tabes dorsalis, spinal cord tumors, and anything else that may compress or irritate the intercostal nerve roots can cause LUQ pain.

Approach to the Diagnosis

The presence or absence of other symptoms and signs will be most helpful in the diagnosis. In acute cases, a flat plate of the abdomen, cbc, urinalysis, and perhaps a serum amylase should be done. Gastroscopy and colonoscopy may be desirable before other roentgenograms are done. In chronic cases, however, an upper gastrointestinal (GI) series and barium enema will be indicated, as well as a stool examination for blood, ova, and parasites. Other tests for the workup of abdominal pain are listed in Appendix I.

Right Lower Quadrant Pain

Most cases of acute right lower quadrant (RLQ) pain are considered appendicitis until proven otherwise, but every physician has been wronged by this axiom more times than he would like to remember. For this reason, the astute clinician will want to have a good list of possibilities in mind. For all abdominal pain, **anatomy** is the key to recalling an inclusive list of causes of RLQ pain. Visualizing the structures, layer by layer, one finds the skin and abdominal wall in the first layer; the terminal ileum, caecum, appendix, and Meckel's diverticulum in the second layer; the ureters, tubes, and ovaries (in females) in the third layer; and the muscles, spine, and terminal aorta in the fourth layer. Now the organs can be cross-indexed with the various etiologies that may be encountered by using the mnemonic **VINDICATE** (Table 1-3). The following discussion emphasizes the most important diseases in the differential diagnosis.

1. **Skin and abdominal wall.** Herpes zoster, cellulitis, contusion, and especially inguinal or femoral hernias are significant causes of RLQ pain.
2. **Appendix.** Appendicitis is a major cause of RLQ pain.
3. **Terminal ileum.** Regional ileitis, tuberculosis, or typhoid and intussusceptions may involve the ileum, causing severe pain. Mesenteric adenitis and infarcts may also affect the ileum.
4. **Caecum.** Diverticulitis, colitis (*e.g.,* granulomatous or amebic), and colon carcinoma are the culprits that may cause RLQ pain originating in the caecum. Impacted feces are also a possible cause.
5. **Meckel's diverticulum.** This may become obstructed and inflamed, develop a pancreatitis or a perforated peptic ulcer, or communicate with a periumbilical cellulitis. All of these may cause RLQ pain.

6. **Ureters.** Renal calculi and hydronephrosis may cause RLQ pain.
7. **Ovary and tubes.** A mumps oophoritis may cause pain in the RLQ. Ovarian cysts may twist on their pedicles or rupture, causing pain, as may the rupture of a small graafian follicle in the normal cycle (mittelschmerz). Three significant lesions may involve the tube: salpingitis, endometriosis, and ectopic pregnancy. All three are painful.

8. **Aorta.** Dissecting aneurysms or emboli of the terminal aorta and its branches may seize the patient with acute pain.
9. **Pelvis and spine.** Osteoarthritis, ruptured disc, metastatic carcinomas, Pott's disease, and rheumatoid spondylitis should be considered here.
10. **Miscellaneous structures.** A ruptured peptic ulcer or inflamed gallbladder may leak fluid into the right colic gutter and cause RLQ pain. Any of the numerous

(*Text continues on p. 16*)

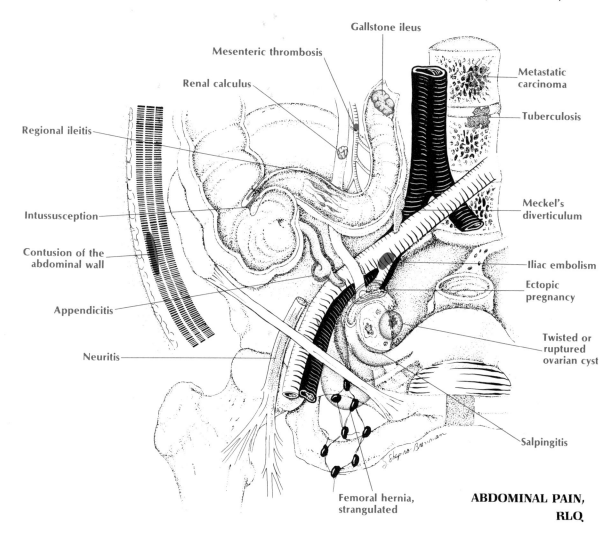

Gallstone ileus

Mesenteric thrombosis

Renal calculus

Metastatic carcinoma

Tuberculosis

Regional ileitis

Intussusception

Meckel's diverticulum

Contusion of the abdominal wall

Iliac embolism

Ectopic pregnancy

Appendicitis

Neuritis

Twisted or ruptured ovarian cyst

Salpingitis

Femoral hernia, strangulated

ABDOMINAL PAIN, RLQ

TABLE 1-3. RIGHT LOWER QUADRANT PAIN

	V Vascular	I Inflammatory	N Neoplasm	D Degenerative and Deficiency
Skin and Abdominal Wall		Herpes zoster Cellulitis		
Terminal Ileum	Mesenteric infarct	Tuberculosis Typhoid Mesenteric adenitis *CrOHNS*		
Caecum		Diverticulitis Amebic colitis Shigella Ascaris	Colon carcinoma	
Appendix		Appendicitis Enterobiasis	Carcinoid	
Meckel's Diverticulum		Meckel's diverticu- litis Cellulitis		
Ureter		Ureteritis *Calculi*		
Ovary and Tubes		*OOph.* Mumps Oophoritis Salpingitis *OrChiti*	Ovarian cyst Neoplasms Endometriosis	
Aorta	Dissecting aneurysm Embolism			
Spine and Pelvis	Pott's disease	Metastatic car- cinoma Myeloma Hodgkin's disease	Osteoarthritis	

acquired

I Intoxication	C Congenital	A Autoimmune Allergic	T Trauma	E Endocrine
	Intussuception Inguinal hernia Femoral hernia		Contusions Incisional hernias	
	Intussusception *obstruction*	Regional ileitis Whipple's disease *Chrons*	*adhesions*	
Toxic megacolon	Diverticulum *obstruction*	Granulomatous colitis	Impacted fece Ruptured bowel *adhesions*	
			Fecalith	
	Ectopic gastric and pancreatic tissue			
	Aberrant blood vessel or congenital band			Ureteral calculi
	Ectopic pregnancy			Ruptured graafian fol- icle (mittelschmerz)
		Rheumatoid spondy- litis Ileitis	Fracture Ruptured disc	

causes of intestinal obstruction (e.g., adhesions or volvulus) may cause pain. Omental infarcts are another miscellaneous cause. Referred pain from pneumonia or pulmonary infarcts has encouraged some surgeons to insist on a chest x-ray film prior to surgery.

Approach to the Diagnosis

Surprisingly, patients may get to the operating room (OR) without a rectal or vaginal examination. In acute cases a flat plate of the abdomen, cbc, urinalysis and amylase are essential before exploration. A pregnancy test is done in women of child-bearing age. In the chronic cases, upper GI series with a progress meal, a barium enema, an intravenous pyelogram (IVP), and even a colonoscopy, cystoscopy, and culdoscopy or laparoscopy may be indicated before surgery. Stool cultures and checking for blood, ova, and parasites are valuable in cases associated with diarrhea.

Left Lower Quadrant Pain

The anatomy of the left lower quadrant (LLQ), like that of the right lower quadrant, will provide a basis for recalling the causes of pain. There are fewer structures to deal with, thus the differential diagnosis is not difficult. Visualizing the structures layer by layer, there are the skin and abdominal wall in the first layer; the sigmoid colon, omentum, and portions of small intestine in the second layer; the ureter, tubes, and ovaries (in women) in the third layer; and the aorta, pelvis, and spine beneath all these structures. Now, by using the mnemonic **VINDICATE,** the organs can be cross-indexed with the various etiologies that may cause pain in this area (Table 1-4). The following discussion emphasizes the most important diseases that must be considered in the differential diagnosis.

1. **Skin and abdominal wall.** Herpes zoster, cellulitis, contusions, and especially inguinal or femoral hernias are significant causes of LLQ pain.
2. **Small intestine.** Regional ileitis, intussusception, adhesions, volvulus, and other conditions that cause intestinal obstruction should be considered here.
3. **Sigmoid colon.** Diverticulitis, ischemic colitis, mesenteric adenitis and infarct, and granulomatous colitis are important causes. Carcinoma of the sigmoid may induce pain by perforating or obstructing the colon.
4. **Ureters.** Ureteral colic must be considered in the differential diagnosis of LLQ pain.
5. **Ovary and tubes.** A mumps oophoritis, ovarian cysts that twist on their pedicles or rupture, and small graafian follicles of the normal cycle that rupture are all included in the differential diagnosis of LLQ pain. The tubes may cause pain if there is an ectopic pregnancy, or if they are inflamed by a salpingitis, or if they are infiltrated by endometriosis.
6. **Aorta.** Dissecting aneurysms and emboli of the terminal aorta may cause acute lower quadrant pain.
7. **Pelvis and spine.** Osteoarthritis, a ruptured disc, metastatic carcinomas, Pott's disease, and rheumatoid spondylitis should be considered here.
8. **Miscellaneous.** Occasionally pain in the bladder, prostate, or uterus is referred to the LLQ. A fibroid of the uterus may twist and cause pain. Impacted feces may cause severe pain. Referred pain from pneumonia, pleurisy, and myocardial infarction is uncommon but must be considered. Metabolic conditions that cause generalized abdominal pain and should be remembered are listed on page 3.

Approach to the Diagnosis

There is no doubt about the value of a good history and physical examination, including both the rectal and pelvic areas. After this the signs and symptoms should be summarized and grouped together; in many cases, this will pinpoint the diagnosis.

The laboratory workup can now proceed. In acute cases the physician should order a flat plate of the abdomen, cbc, urinalysis (and examine it himself), and serum amylase prior to exploratory surgery. A pregnancy test is ordered in women of child-bearing age. In chronic cases, sigmoidoscopy and barium enema, upper GI series, small bowel follow-

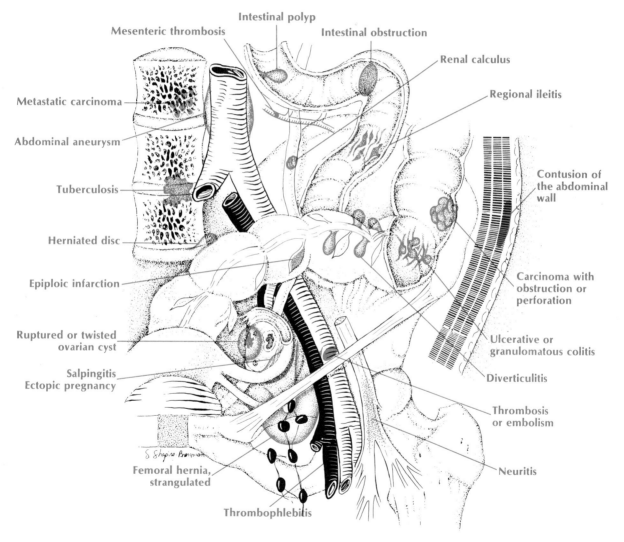

Mesenteric thrombosis

Intestinal polyp

Intestinal obstruction

Renal calculus

Metastatic carcinoma

Abdominal aneurysm

Regional ileitis

Tuberculosis

Contusion of the abdominal wall

Herniated disc

Epiploic infarction

Carcinoma with obstruction or perforation

Ruptured or twisted ovarian cyst

Ulcerative or granulomatous colitis

Salpingitis
Ectopic pregnancy

Diverticulitis

Thrombosis or embolism

S Shapiro Brinman

Neuritis

Femoral hernia, strangulated

Thrombophlebitis

ABDOMINAL PAIN,
LLQ

TABLE 1-4.   LEFT LOWER QUADRANT PAIN

	V Vascular	I Inflammatory	N Neoplasm	D Degenerative and Deficiency
Skin and Abdominal Wall		Herpes zoster Cellulitis		
Small Intestine	Mesenteric thrombosis	Parasites	Polyps with intussus- ception Carcinomas Leiomyomas	
Sigmoid Colon	Ischemic colitis Mesenteric infarct	Diverticulitis Mesenteric adenitis	Carcinoma of the sigmoid	
Ureters		Ureteritis	Papilloma	
Ovary and Tubes		Mumps Oophoritis Salpingitis	Benign and metastatic ovarian tumors Endometriosis	
Aorta	Dissecting aneurysm Emboli			
Spine and Pelvis		Pott's disease	Metastatic carcinoma Myeloma	Osteoarthritis

through and stools for blood, ova, and parasites need to be done before culdoscopy, peritoneoscopy, or colonoscopy is contemplated. An exploratory laparotomy remains a useful diagnostic tool even in chronic cases of LLQ pain. Other laboratory tests that may be worthwhile are listed in Appendix I.

Epigastric Pain

By mental dissection of the epigastrium layer by layer from the skin to the thoracolumbar spine, one encounters all the important or-gans that are the sites of origin of epigastric pain (Table 1-5). **Anatomy,** therefore, is the basic science used to develop this differential diagnosis.

The **skin** may be the site of the pain in herpes zoster, as it is in other types of pain, although it is less likely to be midline. Cellulitis and other lesions of the skin will be readily apparent. Muscle and fascial conditions may be missed, however, if one does not specifically think of this layer. Thus, epigastric hernia, a hiatal hernia, or a contusion of the muscle will be missed, as will diaphragmatic abscesses and trichinosis of the diaphragm.

Acquired

I Intoxication	C Congenital	A Autoimmune Allergic	T Trauma	E Endocrine
	Inguinal and femoral hernias		Contusions Hernias	
Uremia Lead colic	Intussusception Porphyria Congenital polyposis *Obstruction*	Regional ileitis *Crohns*	Rupture Hematoma Adhesions	Diabetic ketosis
		Granulomatous colitis	Contusion Perforation Adhesions	
	Congenital band ureter- ocele			Ureteral calculi
	Ovarian cysts Ectopic pregnancy		Contusion Rupture	Ruptured graafian folli- cle (mittelschmerz)
	Spondylolisthesis	Rheumatoid spondylitis	Fracture Ruptured disc	

The **stomach** and **duodenum** are the next organs encountered; both are prominent causes of epigastric pain. Ulcers, especially perforated ulcers, cause severe pain. Gastritis (syphilitic, toxic, or atrophic) causes a milder form of pain. Pyloric stenosis (from whatever cause), cascade stomach, diverticula, and carcinomas or sarcomas round out the differential diagnosis here. Good collateral circulation makes vascular occlusion a less likely cause.

The **colon** and small **intestines** lie just below the stomach, so one must not forget ileitis, colitis (ulcerative or granulomatous), appendicitis, diverticulitis, Meckel's diverticulum, and transverse colon carcinomas that ulcerate through the wall. Intestinal parasites and mesenteric thrombosis are additional causes that originate here. The various forms of intestinal obstruction are more important than parasites and mesenteric thrombosis.

The **pancreas** sits at the next layer, and acute pancreatitis is a particularly severe form of epigastric pain. Chronic pancreatitis, carcinoma, cysts of the pancreas, and mucoviscoidosis cause less severe forms of epigastric pain. The **lymph nodes** may be involved by Hodgkin's disease and lymphosarcoma, lead-

(*Text continues on p. 22*)

TABLE 1-5. EPIGASTRIC PAIN

	V **Vascular**	**I** **Inflammatory**	**N** **Neoplasm**	**D** **Degenerative** **and Deficiency**
Skin		Herpes zoster Cellulitis		
Muscle and **Fascia**		Diaphragmatic abscess Trichinosis		
Stomach		Gastritis Ulcer Syphilis	Carcinoma Sarcoma	Atrophic gastritis
Duodenum		Ulcer		
Intestines	Mesenteric throm- bosis	starts Appendicitis Ileitis or Colitis Parasites	Polyps Carcinomas Sarcomas	
Pancreas		Pancreatitis	Pancreatic Carcinoma	
Lymph Nodes		Mesenteric adenitis	Hodgkin's disease Lymphosarcoma	
Blood Vessels	Aortic aneurysm Abdominal angina			
Nerves		Herpes zoster		
Thoracic Spine		Tuberculosis Osteomyelitis	mm Primary tumor or metastasis	Osteoporosis Arthritis
Local Referred	Coronary insuffi- ciency Myocardial infarc- tion Congestive heart failure	Hepatitis Cholecystitis Pyelonephritis	Hepatic carcinoma	
Systemic **Referred**	Pulmonary embolism	Pneumonia Epididymitis	Endometriosis Peritoneal car- cinomatosis	Epilepsy Migraine Electrolyte imbalance

I Intoxication Idiopathic	C Congenital Acquired Anomaly	A Autoimmune Allergic	T Trauma	E Endocrine
	Epigastric hernia Hiatal hernia		Contusion Cough hemorrhage	
Gastritis Ulcer	Cascade stomach Pyloric stenosis			Zollinger–Ellison syndrome
Ulcer	Diverticulitis			Zollinger–Ellison syndrome
Dumping syndrome	Meckel's and colon diverticulum Intestinal obstruction			Adrenal insufficiency
Pancreatitis	Mucoviscoidosis Pancreatic cyst			
		Periarteritis nodosa		
Lead colic Porphyria Arachnidism				
		Rheumatoid spondy- litis	Fracture Herniated disc	
		Rheumatic fever	Fractured ribs	Diabetes

ing to intestinal obstruction, but mesenteric adenitis is a much more likely cause. When the retroperitoneal nodes are involved by neoplasms (*e.g.,* sarcoma) the pain is usually referred to the back.

The **blood vessels** are contained in the next layer, and one is reminded of aortic aneurysms, abdominal angina, periarteritis nodosa, and other forms of vasculitis. The sympathetic and parasympathetic nerves are involved by lead colic, porphyria, and black widow spider venom. Conditions of the **thoracic spine** are present in the final layer. Cord tumors, tuberculosis, herniated discs, osteoarthritis, and rheumatoid spondylitis can all lead to midepigastric pain.

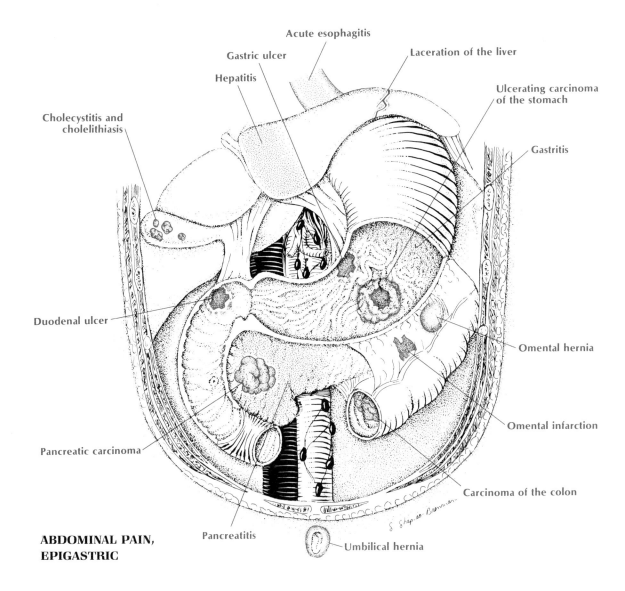

ABDOMINAL PAIN, EPIGASTRIC

Omission of the systemic diseases and diseases of other abdominal organs that sometimes cause epigastric pain is inexcusable. Pneumonia, myocardial infarction, (inferior wall, particularly), rheumatic fever, epilepsy, and migraine are just a few systemic conditions that are associated with epigastric or generalized abdominal pain.

Cholecystitis, hepatitis, and pyelonephritis are some local diseases that also produce midepigastric or generalized abdominal pain. That is why the target system has a useful application here. The center circle of the target is the stomach, the pancreas, and other organs in Table 1-5. The next circle covers the liver, kidney, gallbladder, heart, and ovaries. A further circle covers the brain and the testicles.

Approach to the Diagnosis

The approach to the diagnosis of midepigastric pain is identical to that for generalized abdominal pain (see p. 3).

Hypogastric Pain

Anatomy is the basic science that will open the door to this differential diagnosis. Visualizing the structures in the hypogastrium, one sees the abdominal wall, the bladder and urinary tract, the female genital tract, the sigmoid colon and rectum, the iliac vessels, the aorta and vena cava, and the lumbosacral spine. Occasionally other organs fall into the hypogastrium, thus they must be considered too. A pelvic kidney, visceroptosis of the transverse colon, and a pelvic appendix all may occur.

Now that one has the organs in mind it is necessary only to apply the mnemonic **MINT** to recall the causes of hypogastric pain.

In the **abdominal wall,**

M—Malformations bring to mind the ventral hernias and urachal cysts or sinuses with associated cellulitis.

I—Inflammation includes cellulitis, carbuncles, and other skin infections.

N—Neoplasms of the abdominal wall do not usually present with pain.

T—Trauma suggests contusion of the rectus abdominus muscles or stab wounds.

In the **urinary tract,** one recalls

M—Malformations such as diverticula, cystoceles, ureteroceles, bladder neck obstruction from strictures and calculi, and phimosis and paraphimosis.

I—Inflammation suggests cystitis, prostatitis and urethritis, and Hunner's ulcers.

N—Neoplasms suggest transitional cell papillomas and carcinoma and prostatic carcinoma.

T—Trauma recalls ruptured bladder.

In the **female genital tract,**

M—Malformations that may cause pain include a retroverted uterus, an ectopic pregnancy, and various congenital cysts (*e.g.,* hydatid cyst of Morgagni) that may twist on their pedicles.

I—Inflammation of the vagina and cervix is not usually painful except on intercourse, but endometritis and tubo-ovarian abscesses are associated with pain and fever.

N—Neoplasms like carcinoma of the cervix and uterus do not cause pain unless they extend beyond the uterus or obstruct the menstrual flow, but fibroids often cause dysmenorrhea and severe pain if they twist on their pedicles and endometriosis may spread throughout the pelvis and cause chronic or acute pain.

T—Trauma such as perforation of the uterus during a dilatation and curettage (D & C), delivery, or by the introduction of a foreign body during sexual relations may cause abdominal pain.

The **sigmoid colon** and **rectum** may be the site of pain in

M—Malformations such as diverticulitis

I—Inflammations such as ulcerative colitis with perforation, granulomatous colitis with perforation, amebic colitis, and ischemic colitis

N—Neoplasms that spread beyond the lumen of the bowel or cause obstruction

T—Trauma from introduction of instruments or foreign bodies

Pain in the hypogastrium may also be caused by a dissecting aneurysm of the **aorta** or phlebitis of the **iliac veins** or the inferior **vona cava**. The **lumbosacral spine** may be the site of pain in

M—Malformations such as spondylolisthesis and scoliosis, but these are usually associated with back pain.

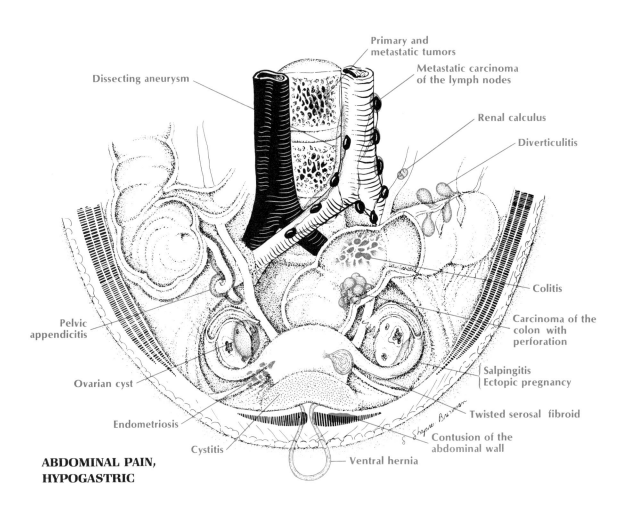

Dissecting aneurysm

Primary and metastatic tumors

Metastatic carcinoma of the lymph nodes

Renal calculus

Diverticulitis

Colitis

Carcinoma of the colon with perforation

Salpingitis
Ectopic pregnancy

Twisted serosal fibroid

Contusion of the abdominal wall

Ventral hernia

Cystitis

Endometriosis

Ovarian cyst

Pelvic appendicitis

ABDOMINAL PAIN, HYPOGASTRIC

I—**Inflammatory** conditions of the spine such as tuberculosis and rheumatoid spondylitis are much more likely to cause hypogastric pain.

N—**Neoplasms,** particularly metastatic carcinomas, multiple myeloma, and Hodgkin's disease may cause hypogastric pain.

T—**Trauma** of the spine may cause a herniated disc fracture or hematoma of the spine and surrounding muscles, producing hypogastric pain from a distended bladder or paralytic ileus, among other things.

The appendix and small intestine may occasionally end up in the pelvis so appendicitis and regional ileitis should not be forgotten as possible causes of hypogastric pain.

Approach to the Diagnosis

The approach to the diagnosis involves a good pelvic and rectal examination as well as urine examination, smear, and culture. Stool examination for blood and parasites is important. A flat plate of the abdomen and a cbc are important in the acute case, but if the urinalysis is negative and all the aforementioned studies are inconclusive, exploration may be necessary. Any question of disease of the urinary tract would prompt an IVP or cystoscopy, whereas a question of a gynecologic problem may warrant culdoscopy or peritoneoscopy prior to exploration. Barium enema and sigmoidoscopy can be done unless there is the possibility of bowel perforation.

ARM PAIN

An **anatomical** breakdown of the arm into its components is the key to a sound differential diagnosis in arm pain. Pain may be referred from more proximal portions of the extremity

such as the shoulder (*e.g.,* bursitis) or brachial plexus (*e.g.,* cervical rib), so these areas must also be examined.

Beginning with the **skin** and **subcutaneous tissue,** one recalls herpes zoster, cellulitis, contusions, and a variety of dermatological conditions that should be obvious. Weber–Christian disease, which usually affects the thighs, is more obscure. Rheumatoid and rheumatic nodules may occur on the skin and are, of course, painful. Beneath the skin the **muscles, fascia,** and **bursae** are frequent sites of inflammation and trauma. Contusions, rupture of the ligaments, and bursitis (particularly tennis elbow) are common acute traumatic conditions (bursitis, however, is more likely the result of chronic strain). Inflammatory lesions of the muscles include epidemic myalgia, trichinosis, nonarticular rheumatism, and dermatomyositis. Muscle cramping from hypocalcemia or other electrolyte disturbances must be considered in the differential diagnosis of arm pain.

The superficial and deep **veins** are the site of thrombophlebitis and hemorrhage, both prominent causes of arm pain. The **arteries** may be involved by emboli (from auricular fibrillation, myocardial infarction, and subacute bacterial endocarditis), thrombosis (especially in Buerger's disease and blood dyscrasias like sickle cell anemia), and vasculitis (periarteritis nodosa is one example). Acute trauma to the artery may cause pain. When one moves centrally along the arterial pathways, additional causes of pain come to mind. For example, dissecting aneurysms or acute subclavian steal syndrome may cause severe pain down the arm, but pain is referred to the arm from a myocardial infarct as well. When superficial or deep infections of the arm spread to the lymphatics, lymphangitis may develop and cause arm pain.

The **nerves** may be a source of pain, both centrally and locally. Buerger's disease, cellulitis, and osteomyelitis may involve the nerve

(*Text continues on p. 28*)

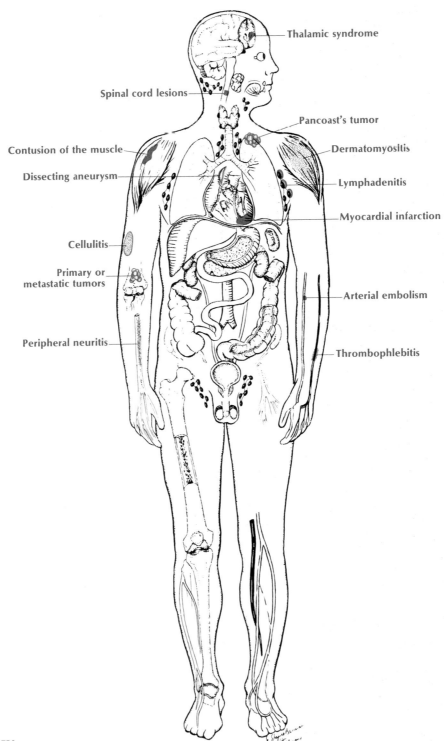

Thalamic syndrome

Spinal cord lesions

Pancoast's tumor

Contusion of the muscle

Dermatomyoslitis

Dissecting aneurysm

Lymphadenitis

Myocardial infarction

Cellulitis

Primary or metastatic tumors

Arterial embolism

Peripheral neuritis

Thrombophlebitis

ARM PAIN

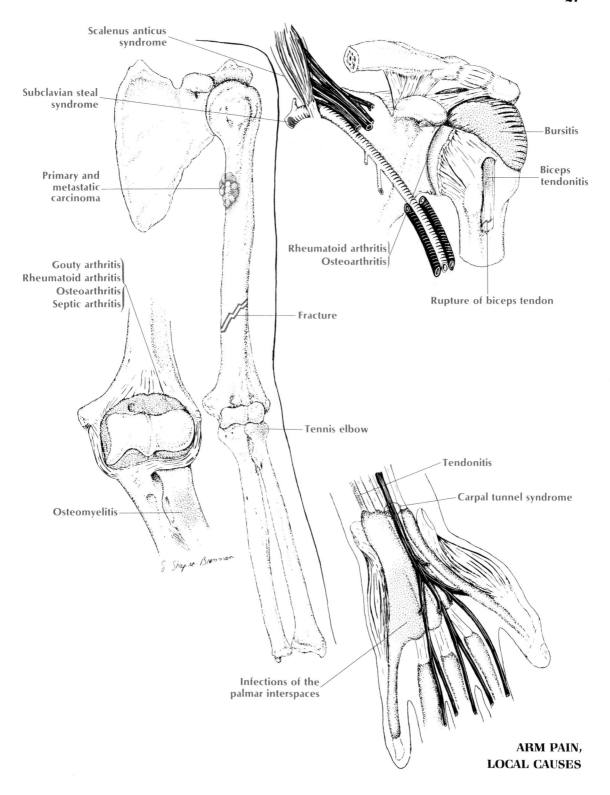

Scalenus anticus syndrome

Subclavian steal syndrome

Primary and metastatic carcinoma

Gouty arthritis
Rheumatoid arthritis
Osteoarthritis
Septic arthritis

Osteomyelitis

Bursitis

Biceps tendonitis

Rheumatoid arthritis
Osteoarthritis

Rupture of biceps tendon

Fracture

Tennis elbow

Tendonitis

Carpal tunnel syndrome

Infections of the palmar interspaces

S. Shapiro Brennan

**ARM PAIN,
LOCAL CAUSES**

locally. Neuromas may cause focal pain in the distribution of the involved peripheral nerve. The carpal tunnel syndrome, which may be caused by rheumatoid arthritis, amyloidosis, acromegaly, hypothyroidism, or multiple myeloma, may compress the median nerve (and occasionally the ulnar nerve) to cause pain in the hand and even up the arm. Moving up the nerve pathways, another frequent spot for nerve compression is the brachial plexus. Pancoast's tumors, cervical ribs, and the scalenus anticus syndrome may be the cause of arm pain originating the plexus.

The **cervical nerve roots** may be compressed by diseases of the spine and spinal cord. A herniated disc, cervical spondylosis, metastatic carcinoma, tuberculosis of the spine, multiple myeloma, and cord tumors (*e.g.*, meningiomas, neurofibromas, and ependymomas) are the most notable. Syringomyelia and tabes dorsalis are other sources of arm pain which originate in the spinal cord. Moving up the cord to the **brain stem,** one recalls the thalamic syndrome (usually caused by occlusion of the thalamogeniculate artery) as a cause of pain in the arm.

The **bone** and **joints** are deeper in the arm. They prompt the diagnosis of osteomyelitis, primary and metastatic bone tumors, and diseases of the joints such as osteoarthritis, rheumatoid arthritis, gout, gonococcal arthritis, and Reiter's syndrome. A more extensive discussion of joint disorders can be found on page 64. Systemic diseases that cause arm pain from peripheral nerve involvement include diabetes mellitus (with ischemic neuropathy), periarteritis nodosa, and macroglobulinemia. Sickle cell anemia may also cause an ischemic neuropathy.

Approach to the Diagnosis

The association of other symptoms and signs found on a good history and physical examination is most important in pinpointing the diagnosis. Thus arm pain with tenderness and limitation of motion at the elbow suggests tennis elbow, gout, or rheumatoid arthritis. Arm pain with loss of sensation in the distribution of the median nerve suggests a carpal tunnel syndrome.

The laboratory workup should include x-rays of the involved area and of the cervical spine, especially if there is a radicular distribution of the pain. At least a cervical rib will not be missed in this way. An electrocardiogram (ECG) and myocardial enzymes may be necessary to exclude a myocardial infarct, and an exercise tolerance test will help exclude coronary insufficiency. Arteriography, phlebography, lymphangiography, electromyogram (EMG) with nerve conduction studies, myelography, and nerve blocks will be necessary in specific cases. These and other useful tests are listed in Appendix I.

BREAST PAIN

Division of the breast anatomically into various components is interesting but not worthwhile in the differential diagnosis of breast pain. It is rather more instructive and practical to use **VINDICATE** in developing a list of causes of this symptom.

V—Vascular infarction in this area is rare, although a pulmonary or myocardial infarction may refer pain to the breast, and congestive heart failure may distend the veins of the breast sufficiently to cause a mastitis.

I—Inflammation in the form of acute bacterial mastitis is not unknown in breast-feeding mothers, but it is infrequent. Under other circumstances chronic cystic mastitis is a common cause of unilateral or bilateral breast pain. A breast abscess may develop during lactation. Herpes zoster may affect the skin and nerve roots supplying the breast.

N—Neoplasms of the breast, like neoplasms elsewhere, are an unlikely cause of breast pain, but if they infiltrate the skin (*i.e.*, in Paget's disease, axillary nerves, or obstruct the ducts) they may cause pain.

D—Degenerative conditions are rarely a cause of breast pain.

I—Intoxication. A number of drugs (*e.g.*, chlorpromazine and alpha-methyldopa) may cause gynecomastia and pain. Alcoholism, estrogen, and birth control pills are probably more frequent causes.

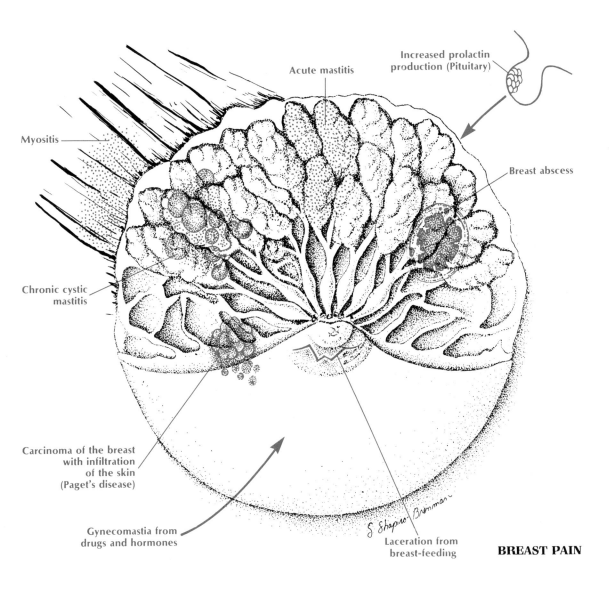

BREAST PAIN

C—Congenital anomalies are not a significant cause of breast pain.

A—Allergic—autoimmune conditions are also unlikely causes of breast pain.

T—Trauma from a bite on the breast by a feeding infant is a common cause of acute mastitis and pain. Frequent sexual relations and masturbation of the breasts may induce pain, although some women are reluctant to admit that their breasts have been traumatized this way.

E—Endocrine causes of breast pain are numerous. Menstruation, menarche, pregnancy, and menopause all are associated with bilateral swollen and painful breasts. Hyperestrinemia from endogenous or exogenous sources is also a frequent cause. Estrogen from birth control pills, estrogen therapy for menopause, the increase of blood estrogen in chronic liver disease, and ovarian tumors are a few of the etiologies in this group. Any pituitary condition associated with an increased output of prolactin may cause swollen, painful, and, of course, lactating breasts. The Chiari-Frommel syndrome is one of these.

Approach to the Diagnosis

The diagnosis of a painful breast is usually made by taking a careful history. What drugs is the patient taking? Associated symptoms and signs (bloody discharge, p. 209 and swelling, p. 115) are also important. A culture of the discharge, mammography, and serum, estrogen, and prolactin levels may be important, but referral to an endrocrinologist is wise when the history does not provide a simple solution, especially when the pain is bilateral. Biopsy (frozen section) is necessary when tumor is suspected and mammography is equivocal, because faith in mammography has declined somewhat in recent years.

CHEST PAIN

Hardly a day goes by in a busy practitioner's office that he is not confronted with a patient complaining of chest pain. His main concern, of course, is to exclude an acute myocardial infarction, which is not an easy task in many cases. He frequently admits the patient for observation, which is the safe thing to do when there is any doubt. With a list of virtually all the diagnostic possibilities in mind, however, fewer patients will require admission for observation. **Anatomy** forms the basis for formulating such a list.

Visualizing the organs of the chest and cross-indexing them with the various etiologies (Table 1-6), one finds that at least 30 or 40 conditions must be considered.

Proceeding from the superficial to the deep structures, one encounters the **skin,** one considers herpes zoster, and one looks for a rash. Next, there is **muscle;** a trichinosis, dermatomyositis, and contusions of the muscle must be considered. Cough-induced contusions should not be forgotten. In the same layer, the **ribs** and **cartilage** remind one of rib fractures, Tietze's syndrome, and metastatic carcinoma and multiple myeloma. Other rarer conditions of the rib are shown in Table 1-6.

Many causes of chest pain arise from the **pleura.** Pneumonia with pleurisy, empyema, pulmonary infarction, and neoplasms of the pleura must be considered. Tuberculous pleurisy and other infectious agents are not uncommon. On the other hand, conditions of the lung are less likely to cause chest pain unless they involve the pleura: this is certainly true of pneumonia and neoplasms. A pneumothorax, however, is a very common cause of chest pain, especially in young adults.

Visualize the **heart** and the **pericardium** comes to mind. This is a source of chest pain in acute idiopathic pericarditis, rheumatic

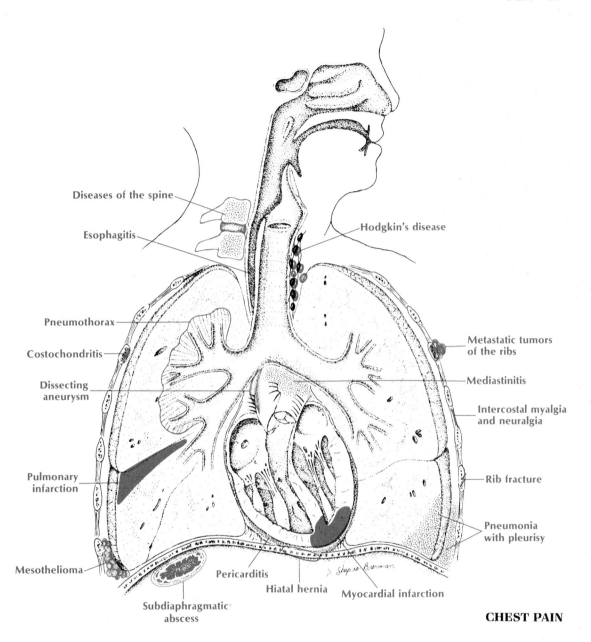

Diseases of the spine

Esophagitis

Hodgkin's disease

Pneumothorax

Costochondritis

Dissecting aneurysm

Pulmonary infarction

Mesothelioma

Subdiaphragmatic abscess

Pericarditis

Hiatal hernia

Myocardial infarction

Metastatic tumors of the ribs

Mediastinitis

Intercostal myalgia and neuralgia

Rib fracture

Pneumonia with pleurisy

CHEST PAIN

carditis, tuberculous and neoplastic pericarditis. The **myocardium** is the source of the most serious form of chest pain, myocardial infarction, but here again the pain is more severe if the pericardium is involved. Angina pectoris and chronic coronary insufficiency are common causes of chest pain arising from the myocardium. Myocarditis (*e.g.,* viral)

(*Text continues on p. 34*)

TABLE 1-6. CHEST PAIN

	V Vascular	I Inflammatory	N Neoplasm	D Degenerative and Deficiency
Skin		Herpes zoster		
Muscles		Epidemic pleurodynia Trichinosis Diaphragmatic abscess		
Ribs and *Cartilages*		Osteomyelitis Tietze's syndrome	Metastatic carcinoma Multiple myeloma sarcoma	Osteitis deformans
Pleura	Pulmonary infarction	Pleurisy Tuberculosis Fungus Empyema	Metastatic carcinoma Mesenthelioma	
Lung		Pneumonia	Carcinoma (primary and metastatic)	
Pericardium		Viral pericarditis Rheumatic fever Tuberculosis	Metastatic carcinoma	
Myocardium	Myocardial infarct Coronary insufficiency	Myocarditis		
Aorta	Aneurysm	Aortitis		Medionecrosis
Esophagus		Ulcer Esophagitis	Esophageal carcinoma	
Mediastinum		Mediastinitis	Dermoid cyst Hodgkin's disease	
Thoracic *Vertebrae*		Osteomyelitis Pott's disease	Metastatic carcinoma	Osteoporosis Osteoarthritis
Spinal Cord		Syphilis Tuberculosis Neuralgia	Tumor	

I Intoxication Idiopathic	C Congenital	A Autoimmune Allergic	T Trauma	E Endocrine
Intercostal neuralgia		Dermatomyositis	Contusion Cough induced hemor- rhage into muscle	
			Fracture contusion	Osteitis fibrosa cystica
Pneumothorax		Pneumothorax		
Uremia				
		Postinfarction syn- drome	Post-commissurotomy syndrome Contusion	
			Ruptured aorta	
Lye erosion, *e.g.*	Diverticulum Hiatal hernia		Ruptured esophagus	
				Substernal thyroiditis
		Rheumatoid spon- dylitis	Fracture Herniated disc	Osteoporosis Osteomalacia
		Transverse myelitis	Hematomyelia	

causes less severe pain, but inflammation of the myocardium from postinfarction syndrome or postcommissurotomy syndrome can be extremely painful.

Now visualize the other central structures: the **esophagus** reminds one of reflux esophagitis and hiatal hernia, the **mediastinum** suggests mediastinitis and substernal thyroiditis or Hodgkin's disease (usually not too painful), the **aorta** suggests dissecting aneurysms, and the **thoracic spine** suggests spinal cord tumors, osteoarthritis, Pott's disease, fractures, and herniated discs, as well as the other conditions listed in Table 1-6.

This chapter would not be complete unless referred pain to the chest were considered. Thus abdominal conditions such as cholecystitis, pancreatitis, and splenic flexure syndrome may present with chest pain. Conditions of the neck that press the cervical nerves may also cause chest pain, particularly scalenus anticus syndrome, cervical ribs, and herniated discs of the cervical spine.

Neurocirculatory asthenia is associated with atypical chest pain; a psychiatric evaluation will assist in this diagnosis.

Approach to the Diagnosis

The approach to the diagnosis of chest pain requires one to rule out systematically each of the above conditions, especially if the pain is atypical and an ECG and chest roentgenogram are negative. In young adults, tenderness of the costochondral junctions with relief on lidocaine injection strongly suggests Tietze's syndrome (costochondritis). Pain on deep breathing without focal chest wall tenderness suggests pleurisy, pulmonary infarction, or esophagitis. Esophagitis pain may be relieved by swallowing lidocaine (Xylocaine) viscus and aggravated or induced by a Bernstein test (see p. 64). Examination of the extremities for thrombophlebitis is essential but it does not rule out pulmonary embolism. Arterial blood gases (ABG) and a perfusion scan will in most cases. Careful examination of the abdomen is axiomatic; admission for observation and continuous cardiac monitoring is essential in most cases. A graded exercise tolerance (GXT) test and thallium scan should be done when chronic coronary insufficiency is suspected.

DYSMENORRHEA

Visualizing the parts of the female reproductive system on page 35, one can systematically formulate a differential diagnosis of this common malady.

At the **cervix,** stenosis, cervical polyps, and other neoplasms may obstruct the egress of blood and induce dysmenorrhea. In the **uterus,** polyps, fibroids, adenomyosis, and deformities such as anteflexion, retroflexion, anteversion, or retroversion may be the cause. Pelvic congestion syndrome is a possibility. The **tubes** may be involved by endometriosis, abscess, or ectopic pregnancy. The **ovaries** may be involved by the same processes as the tubes, but they should suggest the most common cause of dysmenorrhea: hormonal. Thus any condition—thyroid, pituitary or ovarian—that might disturb the cyclical output of estrogen and progesterone in the proper sequence may induce dysmenorrhea. Psychogenic disturbances are especially significant.

Approach to the Diagnosis

The clinical approach to dysmenorrhea is simply to rule out significant organic disease by a thorough pelvic and rectal examination. A smear and culture for gonococcus and chlamydia should be done. A course of contraceptives or progesterone in adequate doses may then be tried. Diuretics may be indicated if

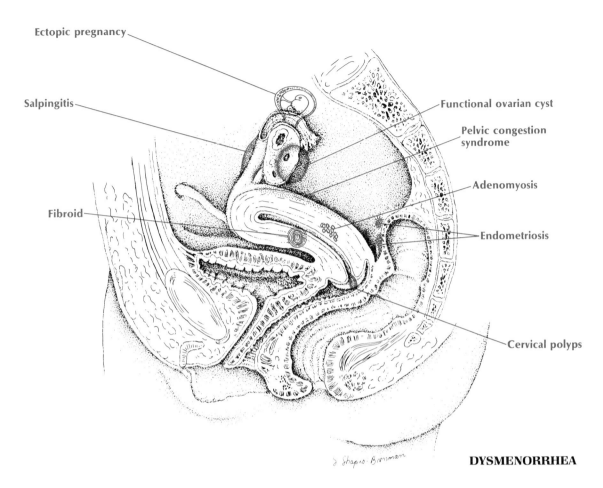

Ectopic pregnancy

Salpingitis

Fibroid

Functional ovarian cyst

Pelvic congestion syndrome

Adenomyosis

Endometriosis

Cervical polyps

J. Shapiro-Brennan

DYSMENORRHEA

examination suggests pelvic congestion. When the aforementioned measures fail, a D & C may be indicated. A gynecologist may decide to do a culdoscopy, a peritoneoscopy, or an exploratory laparotomy.

DYSPAREUNIA

Painful introduction of the male organ or pain during intercourse are both considered under this title. The mnemonic to use here is **MINT.** This can then be applied to the anatomical structures as we explore the genital tract. Of course, psychological disturbances are probably the most common causes of this disorder. They are discussed after the anatomical causes.

M—Malformations include a disproportionately large or deformed male organ (not amusing to the man in this predicament), an unruptured or thick hymen, vaginal stenosis, a retroverted uterus, and prolapsed ovaries.

I—Inflammatory disorders include vulvitis and bartholinitis (often related to gonorrhea), various forms of vaginitis (bacterial, trichomoniasis, and moniliasis) and salpingo-oophoritis. (Note that an inflamed uterus and cervix are only infrequently associated with dyspareunia.) Inflammatory lesions of nearby structures are important. Thus a urethral carbuncle, urethritis, cystitis, hemorrhoids, and anal fissures can cause dyspareunia.

N—Neoplasms causing dyspareunia are leukoplakia vulvitis, kraurosis vulvae, carcinoma of the vulva and vagina, ovarian cysts, and carcinoma. When uterine and cervical carcinomas extend beyond the genital tract, dyspareunia is present. Any neoplasm of the bladder and rectum that has extended into the genital tract will undoubtedly cause dyspareunia.

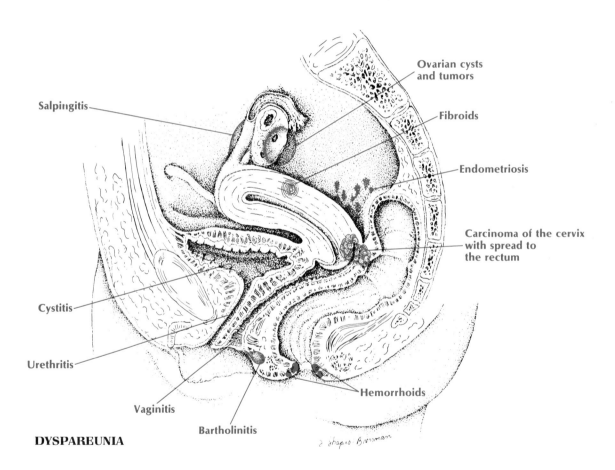

DYSPAREUNIA

T—Traumatic disorders include too frequent intercourse and masturbation. Introduction of the male organ before adequate foreplay has created a lubricated vagina is another cause. The male should be instructed in the gentle introduction of the organ.

Women in menopause may require lubricants to prevent local trauma, as the vagina remains dry even after sexual excitement because of lack of hormonal secretion.

Discovery of psychogenic causes often requires thorough psychoanalysis. Incest, guilt from masturbation, and latent homosexuality are a few of the problems that may be encountered.

Approach to the Diagnosis

The approach to this diagnosis includes an examination of both male and female genital organs and counseling by an understanding physician if these examinations are negative. Appendix I provides other diagnostic tests that may be indicated.

DYSURIA ■

Dysuria is difficult or painful micturition. One could cover most of the causes simply by considering the **inflammatory** lesions of the genitourinary tract in ascending order. Thus, there may be a urethritis or urethral carbuncle, a trigonitis or prostatitis, a cystitis or pyelonephritis with associated cystitis.

This would not, however, cover the disorders that frequently cause associated inflammation of the urinary tract or are associated with difficulty in voiding. To recall these, it is necessary to apply the mnemonic **MINT.**

M—Malformations would bring to mind meatal stricture, bladder neck obstruction by prostatic hypertrophy, median bar, and urethral strictures. Bladder and ureteral calculi should also be considered here.

I—Inflammatory conditions have already been considered.

N—Neoplasms of the prostate and bladder may cause difficulty in voiding or painful urination when secondary infection sets in.

T—Trauma suggests the cystitis and trigonitis (honeymoon cystitis) caused by frequent or traumatic intercourse or by introduction of foreign bodies into the bladder, such as catheters.

The "**N**" may also stand for neurologic conditions; one must not forget multiple sclerosis, poliomyelitis, diabetic neuropathy, and tumors of the spinal cord in the differential diagnosis of dysuria. These are also covered under Incontinence, p. 336.

Approach to the Diagnosis

The approach to the diagnosis includes a urinalysis, urine cultures, smear and culture of any discharge, an intravenous pyelogram, voiding cystogram and cystoscopy, and cystometric examination. In females with "negative" cultures, chlamydia urethritis must be considered and treated. In males with negative cultures, prostatic examination, massage, and evaluation of discharge are done.

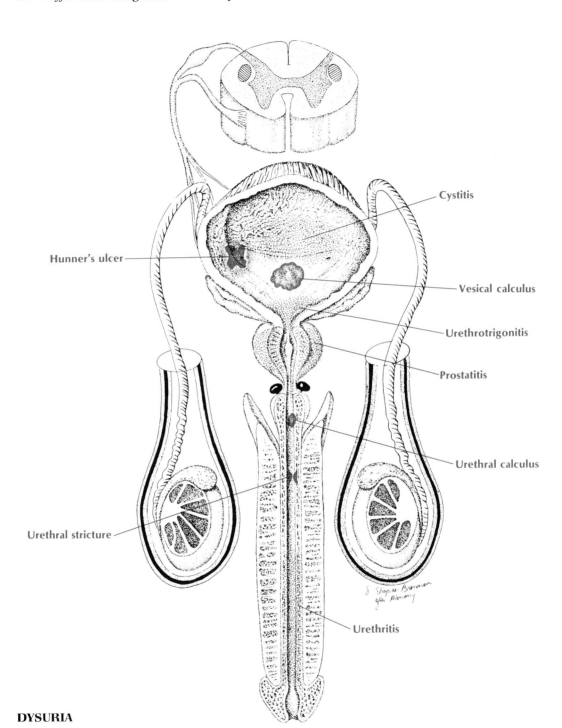

Cystitis

Hunner's ulcer

Vesical calculus

Urethrotrigonitis

Prostatitis

Urethral calculus

Urethral stricture

Urethritis

DYSURIA

EARACHE

The analysis of earache is much like that of dysuria: that is, it is **anatomical** and **inflammation** accounts for the vast majority of causes. Thus, otitis externa would be like urethritis and otitis media like cystitis, and so forth.

Like cystitis, otitis media is often initiated by obstruction (*e.g.*, swollen adenoids). Foreign bodies in the ear, like foreign bodies in the bladder, must always be looked for. Unlike dysuria, earache is often caused by referred pain. Thus parotitis (*e.g.*, mumps) temporomandibular joint syndrome, pharyngitis, and dental caries or abscesses may cause earache.

Inflammation further up includes petrositis and mastoiditis. Neoplasms and degenerative diseases do not usually cause earache.

Approach to the Diagnosis

The approach to the diagnosis requires ear, nose, and throat examination, culture of any discharge, x-ray film of the mastoids, petrous bone, temporomandibular joints, and, in some cases, the sinuses and teeth. A careful neurological examination is necessary in unexplained otalgia. Referral to an otolaryngologist or neurologist is probably best for the busy physician who is unable to find the cause on a routine examination.

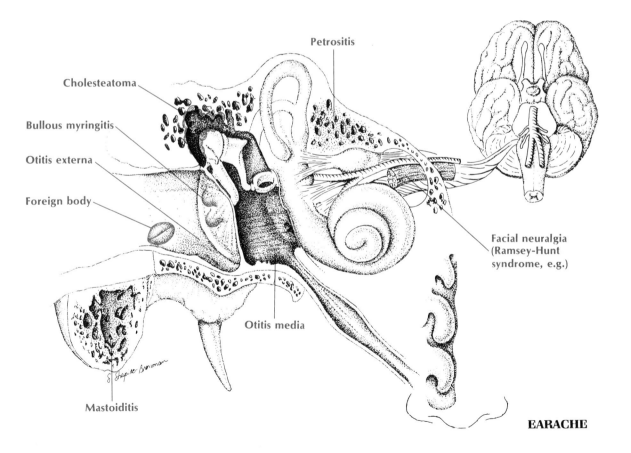

Cholesteatoma

Bullous myringitis

Otitis externa

Foreign body

Mastoiditis

Petrositis

Otitis media

Facial neuralgia (Ramsey-Hunt syndrome, e.g.)

EARACHE

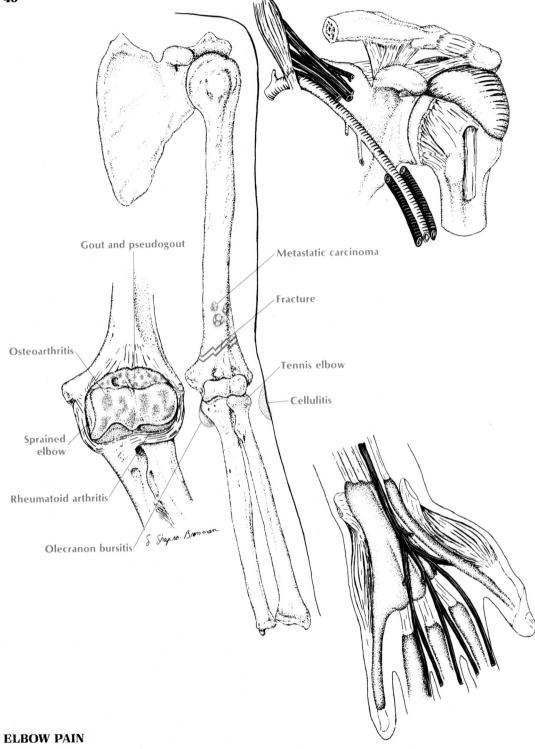

Gout and pseudogout

Metastatic carcinoma

Fracture

Osteoarthritis

Tennis elbow

Cellulitis

Sprained elbow

Rheumatoid arthritis

Olecranon bursitis

S. Shapiro-Bronman

ELBOW PAIN

ELBOW PAIN ■

A painful elbow really does not require a detailed analysis of the anatomy to discover the various causes, almost all of which are bursal or bone and joint disorders. Of course, the skin may be involved by trauma and infection, just like the skin of the hands (see p. 52). The arteries, veins, muscles, and nerves are rarely the cause of pain here.

The simplest and most expedient approach is to use the mnemonic **MINT** and apply it to the bones, joints, and bursae.

M—Malformations are usually acquired, such as the Charcot's joints of syphilis and syringomyelia. Bleeding into the joint in a hemophiliac is also classified here.

I—Inflammation should signal **bursitis,** particularly radiohumeral (popularly called tennis elbow), and olecranon bursitis. One should also recall arthritis of the elbow joint, particularly rheumatoid arthritis, gout, and osteoarthritis; surprisingly enough, rheumatic fever frequently affects the joint, and tuberculosis should be considered along with other forms of septic arthritis.

N—Neoplasms are unusual but osteosarcomas and metastatic carcinomas nevertheless occur.

T—Trauma suggests fractures, dislocations, and elbow sprains.

Approach to the Diagnosis

In the approach to the diagnosis the traumatic conditions and arthritic disorders will probably stand out. A real diagnostic dilemma is at hand when the elbow looks normal and has good movement. But most of these cases are caused by tennis elbow or myositis and fasciitis. Thus a simple injection at the trigger point will assist the diagnosis and give the patient immediate and sometimes lasting re-

lief. Appendix I may be consulted for a workup of the more difficult diagnostic problems.

EYE PAIN ■

Applying the mnemonic **MINT** to the various anatomical parts of the eye will aid in systematically developing a list of diagnostic possibilities for eye pain.

M—Malformations most certainly suggest glaucoma and all the refractive disorders (*e.g.,* astigmatism, myopia, hypermetropia).

I—Inflammation accounts for most cases. One anatomically recalls conjuctivitis, keratitis, scleritis, corneal ulcers, iridocyclitis, and optic neuritis. Do not forget inflammation of the orbit. Vasculitis from temporal arteritis must be considered with obstruction of the retinal veins or arteries.

N—Neoplasms are unlikely causes but must be considered.

T—Trauma should suggest abrasions and foreign bodies, particularly those of the cornea.

Eye pain, like earache, may be referred. Cerebral neoplasms, migraine, and sinusitis may all present with orbital or retro-orbital pain.

An additional category of etiologies that is not common in earache is systemic disease. Any febrile disease may cause bilateral eye pain, particularly viral influenza.

Approach to the Diagnosis

The approach to the diagnosis of eye pain involves a careful search for inflammation of the various anatomical structures; then a drop or two of fluorescent dye is inserted and the cornea inspected for lacerations, herpes ulcers, and foreign bodies. Finally, tenometry may be done. Referral to an ophthalmologist is often necessary, but the astute clinician will want to x-ray the sinuses, ask about a history of migraine, do a visual field, and rule out systemic diseases beforehand.

FACIAL PAIN

Visualize the structures of the face in a systematic fashion to develop a differential diagnosis of facial pain. With the **skin,** herpes

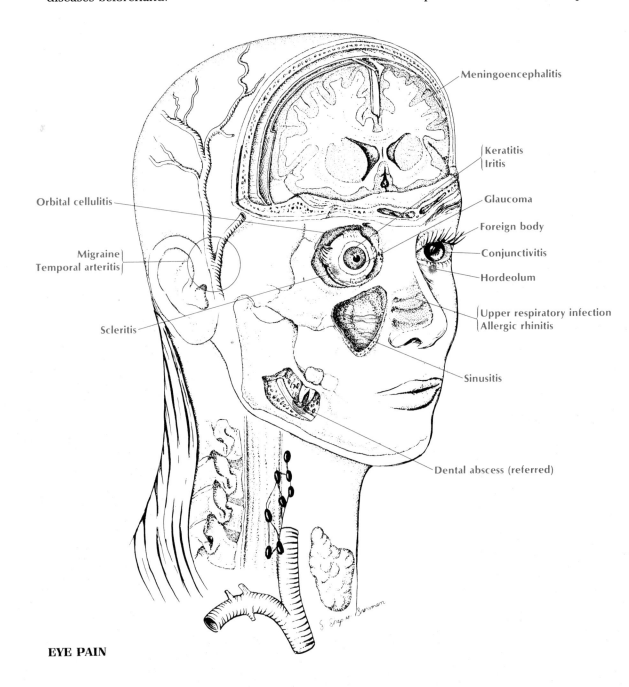

- Meningoencephalitis
- Keratitis
- Iritis
- Glaucoma
- Foreign body
- Conjunctivitis
- Hordeolum
- Upper respiratory infection
- Allergic rhinitis
- Sinusitis
- Dental abscess (referred)
- Orbital cellulitis
- Migraine
- Temporal arteritis
- Scleritis

EYE PAIN

zoster and carbuncles come to mind. Next, the **internal maxillary artery** suggests histamine cephalalgia and arteritis, just as the **nerves** suggest trigeminal neuralgia, herpes zoster, and the atypical facial neuralgias encountered in multiple sclerosis, Wallenberg's syndrome, and other central nervous system conditions. These will almost invariably be associated with other neurological findings. With reference to the **bones,** one should recall temporomandibular joint syndrome, sinusitis, and dental caries or abscesses. Disor-

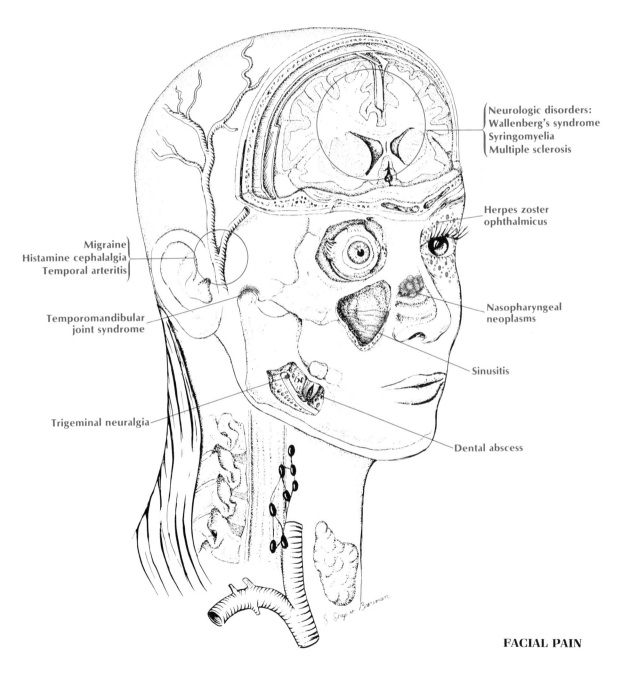

Neurologic disorders:
Wallenberg's syndrome
Syringomyelia
Multiple sclerosis

Herpes zoster
ophthalmicus

Migraine
Histamine cephalalgia
Temporal arteritis

Nasopharyngeal
neoplasms

Temporomandibular
joint syndrome

Sinusitis

Trigeminal neuralgia

Dental abscess

FACIAL PAIN

44

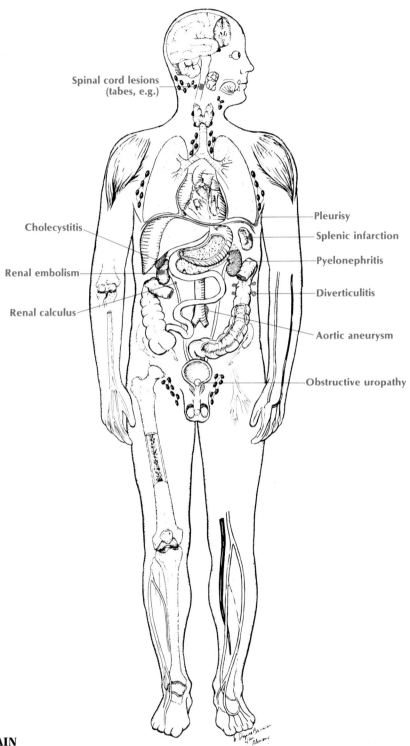

Spinal cord lesions
(tabes, e.g.)

Cholecystitis

Renal embolism

Renal calculus

Pleurisy

Splenic infarction

Pyelonephritis

Diverticulitis

Aortic aneurysm

Obstructive uropathy

FLANK PAIN

ders of the eye that cause face pain are included in the section on Eye Pain.

Of course, one could apply the mnemonic **VINDICATE** to the differential diagnosis and come up with an extensive list. Thus, **V—Vascular** conditions suggest histamine cephalalgia, **I—Inflammatory** conditions suggest herpes zoster, sinusitis, and dental abscesses, and, **N—Neoplasms** suggest Schmincke tumors and carcinoma of the tongue, and so forth. This procedure, however, is more involved than is necessary.

Approach to the Diagnosis

The approach to the diagnosis of face pain includes a careful history and physical with a good neurological examination. The sinuses are transilluminated and may be x-ray films taken. The teeth and occlusion are examined carefully and possibly roentgenographed. A histamine test may be indicated. The busy physician may want to refer the patient to a neurologist immediately but this will obviously take away the challenge.

FLANK PAIN

Most cases of flank pain are associated with inflammation of the kidney. As is shown in Table 1-7, however, jumping to that conclusion in any given case may be hazardous.

Inflammation of the **skin** (herpes zoster), the **colon** (diverticulitis and colitis), the **gallbladder** (cholecystitis), and the **spine** (epidural abscess and Pott's disease) may also cause flank pain, in addition to the kidney (pyelonephritis and perinephric abscess). The mnemonic **VINDICATE** also suggests several vascular disorders that are significant causes of flank pain. These include aortic aneurysms, embolic nephritis, and mesenteric thrombosis. Neoplasms of the kidney and colon are

less likely to produce pain unless they are complicated by infection. However, trauma of the kidney and spine and renal calculi—whether due to hyperparathyroidism, idiopathic etiologies, or hyperuricemia—are important causes. Neoplasms of the spinal cord and tabes dorsalis must also be considered.

Approach to the Diagnosis

The diagnosis of flank pain usually involves careful examination of the urine and a urine culture, an IVP, and plain films of the abdomen and spine. If these are negative, bone scans, arteriography, and other tests may be required (Appendix I). Computerized axial tomography has eliminated the need for exploratory laparotomy in many cases.

FOOT, HEEL, AND TOE PAIN

Many patients presenting with pain in the foot or toes have joint disease (see pp. 64 and 146 for a discussion of these differentials). Other anatomical components of the foot and toes may cause pain as well, so a consideration of the differential diagnosis of foot and toe pain must include diseases of these structures.

Let us develop our list by moving from the skin inward. Many of these conditions are illustrated on page 48 (Table 1-8). Painful conditions of the **skin** include warts, calluses, bunions, and corns, conditions often caused by bad posture and poor-fitting shoes. Ingrown toenails may be found. Herpes zoster in this location is unusual. Moving to the **subcutaneous tissue** and **fascia,** cellulitis and plantar fasciitis are suggested. In plantar fasciitis, a spur of the calcaneus will be found on the roentgenogram. Achilles bursitis and tendonitis are suggested in this layer. The **veins** may be involved by phlebitis and hemorrhage.

The **arteries** may be inflamed in Buerger's disease and periarteritis nodosa; they are painfully obstructed in the arteriolar sclerosis of diabetes mellitus and arteriosclerosis. Emboli may be a cause of pain in the foot. Raynaud's disease may also affect the foot. The **nerves** of the foot may be involved by the many causes of peripheral neuropathy, as well as herniated lumbosacral discs and cauda equina tumors; the radiation of the pain should suggest the latter two conditions. Trapping of the plantar tibial nerve may cause

TABLE 1-7.   FLANK PAIN

	V Vascular	I Inflammatory	N Neoplasm	D Degenerative
Skin		Cellulitis Herpes zoster		
Muscle and Fascia		Trichinosis		
Colon	Mesenteric thrombosis	Colitis	Carcinoma	
Gallbladder		Cholecystitis Cholangitis	Carcinoma	
Adrenal Gland				
Kidney	Embolism Thrombosis	Pyelonephritis Perinephric abscess	Wilms' tumor Hypernephroma	
Aorta	Aneurysm			Atheromas Dissecting aneurysm
Vena Cava	Thrombosis			
Spine		Osteomyelitis Tuberculosis	Metastatic carcinoma	Osteoarthritis
Spinal Cord and Nerves	Anterior spinal artery occlusion	Tabes dorsalis Myelitis Epidural abscess	Spinal cord tumor	

pain just like the carpal tunnel syndrome in the hand. Metatarsalgia may be caused by a plantar digital neuroma. Tracing the arteries centrally will suggest Leriche's syndrome, while tracing the nerves centrally will suggest a thalamic syndrome.

Finally, the **bones** may be involved by fractures, by deformities such as pes planus, pes cavus, talipes equinovarus and hallux valgus, and by many postural defects. Kohler's disease is aseptic bone necrosis in the calcaneus (considered under Joint Pain, p. 64.)

I Intoxication Idiopathic	C Congenital Acquired Malformation	A Autoimmune	T Trauma	E Endocrine
			Contusion Laceration	
	Hernia	Dermatomyositis	Contusion	
	Diverticulitis Appendix	Ulcerative colitis Granulomatous colitis	Contusion Laceration	
				Hemorrhage Infarction Tumors
Gout Toxic nephritis Crush syndrome	Obstruction Infection due to malformation	Periarteritis nodosa Vasculitis of other causes	Contusion Laceration	Calculi in hyperparathy- roidism
			Rupture	
		Marie–Strümpell's disease	Fracture Herniated disc	
Arsenic poisoning Porphyria	Syringomyelia	Guillain–Barré syndrome	Hematoma	

TABLE 1-8. FOOT, HEEL, AND TOE PAIN

	M Malformation	I Inflammation
Skin	Ingrown toenail	Herpes zoster Cellulitis
Subcutaneous Tissue and Fascia		Cellulitis Plantar fascitis
Arteries		Vasculitis
Veins	Varicose veins	Thrombophlebitis
Nerves	Hypertrophic polyneuritis Peroneal muscular atrophy Plantar entrapment syndrome	Tuberculosis of spine
Bones	Pes planus Pes cavus Talipes equinovarus	Osteomyelitis Kohler's disease
Joints		Rheumatoid arthritis Gout Osteoarthritis Pseudogout

Approach to the Diagnosis

Special considerations in the approach to the diagnosis of foot pain include examining the shoes for abnormal areas of wear and tear, measuring the arches, palpating the joints for maximal tenderness, and ordering laboratory tests for joint disease (Appendix I). Nerve blocks and lidocaine injections in the plantar fascia and other areas of maximum tenderness will assist in diagnosis. A therapeutic trial of proper-fitting shoes and arches may be indicated. Weight control is essential in the obese. Referral to a podiatrist or orthopedic surgeon is often necessary.

GROIN PAIN

The anatomical components of the groin consist of the skin, subcutaneous tissue, fascia, lymph nodes, the femoral nerve, arteries and veins, and underneath, the hip bones. With these components in mind, it should be easy to develop a differential diagnosis of groin pain because most of the lesions are inflammatory or traumatic.

The **skin** is affected by intertrigo, scabies, furuncles, and herpes zoster, among other things. The **subcutaneous tissue** may be in-

N Neoplasm	T Trauma	S Systemic Disease
	Calluses Bunions	
	Hemorrhage Contusion Aneurysm	Diabetes Periarteritis nodosa Buerger's disease
	Hemorrhage	Buerger's disease
Neuroma Cauda equina tumor	Contusion Compression Laceration	Diabetic neuropathy
Primary and metastatic neoplasms	Fractures	Hyperparathyroidism Sickle cell anemia
	Traumatic synovitis	Gout Rheumatic fever Reiter's syndrome

volved by cellulitis and a tuberculous abscess. When the **fascia** is weak or torn, femoral or inguinal hernias develop. More likely causes of groin pain are inflamed **lymph nodes** that may be from any venereal disease (such as gonorrhea or chancroid) or infections of other portions of the genitalia. The **femoral nerve** may be affected by viral neuritis, diabetic neuropathy, and disease of the spine (fracture, disc, or tumors). The **femoral artery** may be involved by a thrombosis, embolism, or dissecting aneurysm, whereas the **vein** may be thrombosed. Finally, the underlying **hip bones** can be involved by any form of arthri-

tis, and infections or metastatic tumors of the bone. Fractures and other traumatic disorders affect the bones of the hip also.

It would be a gross omission if referred pain to the groin were not considered. Pain may be referred to the groin in pyelonephritis, renal colic, regional ileitis, appendicitis, salpingitis, and many other abdominal disorders.

Approach to the Diagnosis

In the approach to the diagnosis of groin pain, a mass or tender structure is usually present in the groin. If the mass is a lymph node, care-

(*Text continues on p. 52*)

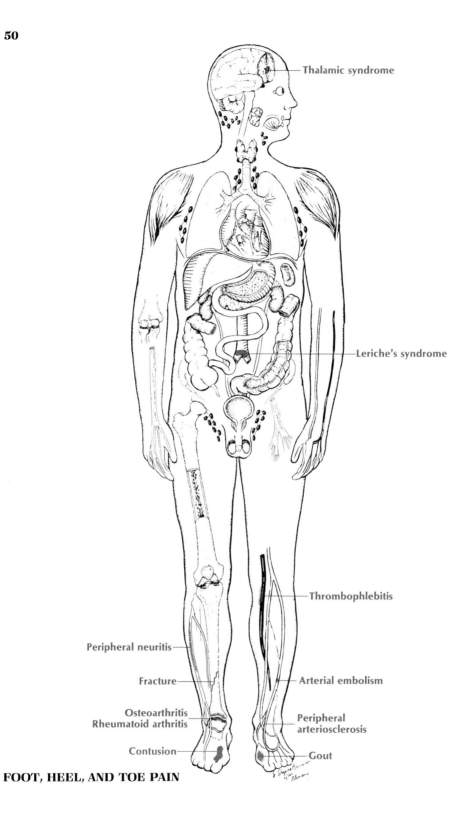

Thalamic syndrome

Leriche's syndrome

Thrombophlebitis

Peripheral neuritis

Fracture

Osteoarthritis
Rheumatoid arthritis

Contusion

Arterial embolism

Peripheral
arteriosclerosis

Gout

FOOT, HEEL, AND TOE PAIN

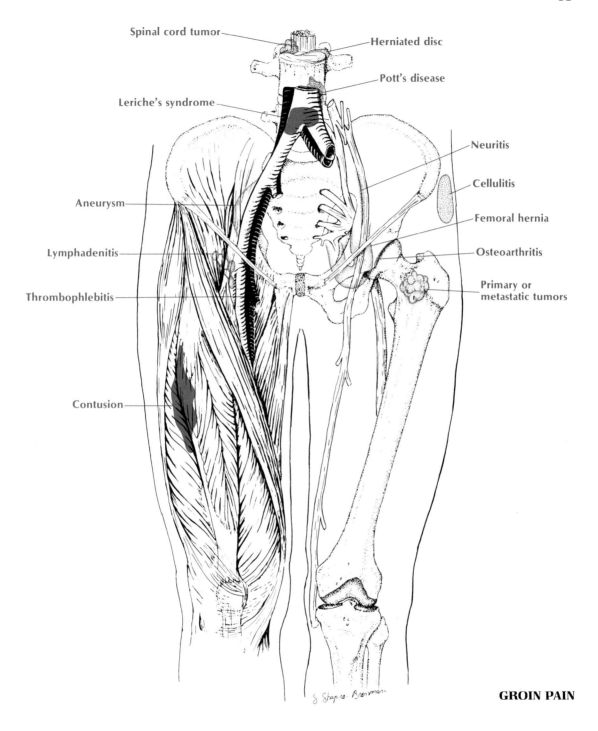

Spinal cord tumor

Herniated disc

Pott's disease

Leriche's syndrome

Neuritis

Cellulitis

Aneurysm

Femoral hernia

Lymphadenitis

Osteoarthritis

Thrombophlebitis

Primary or
metastatic tumors

Contusion

GROIN PAIN

ful examination of the genitalia and lower extremities will often show the cause, but a urethral or vaginal smear may be necessary to show gonorrhea. Investigation of the GU tract and GI tract for causes of referred pain is then undertaken. If the mass is reducible a hernia is likely and referral to a surgeon is in order. Incarcerated hernias, of course, demand immediate referral. Consult Appendix I in difficult diagnostic problems.

HAND AND FINGER PAIN ■

Visualize the anatomy when a patient presents with pain in the hand or fingers (Table 1-9). The **skin** may show a contact dermatitis, fungal infection, furuncle or cellulitis, or a traumatic lesion. An insignificant wound may be infected; if there are streaks going up the arm, lymphangitis has complicated the picture. Herpes zoster rarely occurs in this area. Underneath the skin, the many **tendon sheaths** and **fascial pockets** are inviting sites for infection following a minor wound, but the swelling is obvious. One space particularly well known, the pulp space at the tip of the finger (usually the index finger), may develop a felon. A paronychia infection that involves the nail is very painful. A hematoma under the nail is perhaps even more painful.

The **arteries** of the hand may go into intermittent painful spasms in Raynaud's phenomena, which occurs for example in macroglobulinemia, menopause, and rheumatoid arthritis. It also occurs in a primary form called Raynaud's disease. This is an extremely painful condition associated with cold, blue hands intermittently and gangrene ultimately. The collagen diseases and Buerger's disease may cause a vasculitis of the arteries and Raynaud's phenonema. Finally, peripheral arterial emboli may occur here but they are more frequent in the lower extremities.

Surprisingly enough, the **veins** of the hand do not frequently develop thrombophlebitis, except in the hospitalized patient on frequent intravenous therapy. This may not be so unusual when one realizes that varicose veins are uncommon in the upper extremities. Buerger's disease also may involve the veins of the hand. The **tendons** are sometimes trapped in their sheaths and cause pain. De Quervain's stenosing tenosynovitis of the extensor pollucis tendon is a common form. The **muscles** of the hands are not commonly involved in myositis but are frequently traumatized and contused, particularly in contact sports.

Trapping of the **median nerve** in the carpal tunnel is a well-known cause of pain in the hand and fingers, particularly in the thumb, index, and middle fingers. Sensory changes involve these and the medial half of the ring finger; there may be significant atrophy of the thenar eminence with Tinel's sign. Remember that the **ulnar nerve** may be trapped also, causing pain in the little finger and associated sensory changes. The carpal tunnel syndrome may be caused by multiple myeloma, amyloidosis, acromegaly, rheumatoid arthritis, menopause, and a host of other conditions.

Symptoms similar to those of the carpal tunnel may come from high up the peripheral nerve tract. Compression of the **brachial plexus** by a cervical rib, a scalenus anticus muscle, or the clavicle (so-called costoclavicular syndrome) may be the culprit. Chronic bursitis or arthritis of the shoulder may ultimately lead to a causalgia syndrome, as will a peripheral nerve injury, and create pain in the hand and fingers. The frozen shoulder following pneumonia, myocardial infarctions, and other chest conditions can do the same. The brachial plexus may also be involved by Pancoast's tumors.

At a third site, compression of the **cervical nerve roots** by a herniated disc, cervical

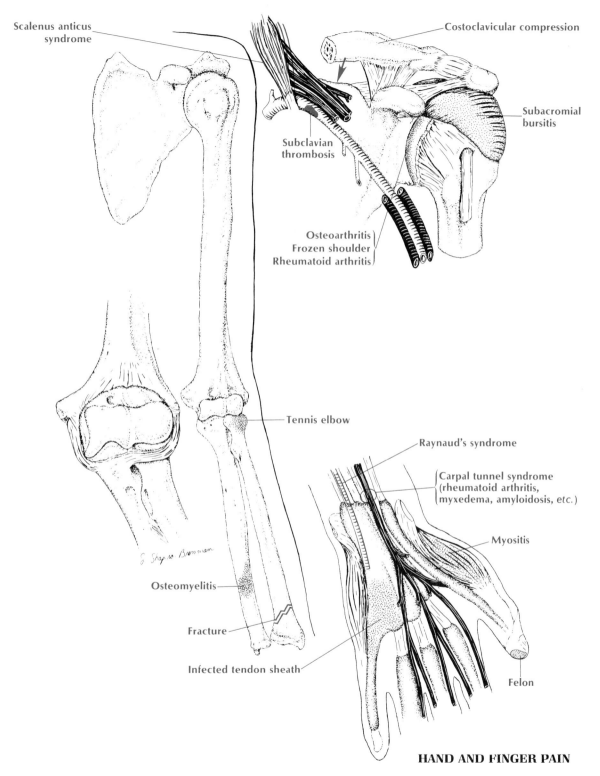

Scalenus anticus syndrome

Costoclavicular compression

Subclavian thrombosis

Subacromial bursitis

Osteoarthritis
Frozen shoulder
Rheumatoid arthritis

Tennis elbow

Raynaud's syndrome

Carpal tunnel syndrome
(rheumatoid arthritis,
myxedema, amyloidosis, *etc.*)

Myositis

Osteomyelitis

Fracture

Infected tendon sheath

Felon

HAND AND FINGER PAIN

53

spondylosis, tuberculosis, and primary and metastatic tumors may be the cause of hand and/or finger pain. Cord conditions like syringomyelia and brain stem involvement of the thalamus by embolism or thrombosis may occasionally cause pain in the hand, but in the latter condition there is usually an accompanying leg pain.

In the deepest penetration of our dissection of the hand we encounter the most

TABLE 1-9. HAND AND FINGER PAIN

	V Vascular	I Inflammatory	N Neoplasm	D Degenerative and Deficiency
Skin	Periarteritis nodosa Gangrene	Carbuncle Ulcers Folliculitis Herpes zoster	Carcinoma	
Fascia, Ligaments, Tendon Sheaths, Subcutaneous Tissue		Felon Abscess Cellulitis Tendon sheath infection	Sarcoma	
Arteries	Arteriosclerosis	Subacute bacterial endocarditis	Macroglobulinemia	
Veins		Thrombophlebitis		
Muscles		Myositis		
Peripheral Nerves (Carpal Tunnel)		Multiple myeloma		
Brachial Plexus	Ischemic neuritis Myocardial infarction	Bursitis Arthritis Pneumonia	Pancoast's tumor	
Spinal Cord and Cer- vical Roots		Tuberculosis	Primary, metastatic tumors of cord	Cervical spondylosis Syringomyelia
Bone		Gonococcal arthritis		Osteoarthritis

common structures that cause hand pain, the **bones** and **joints.** The bones may be fractured, dislocated, or contused or the joints may be sprained, but if the joints are painful, arthritis is the most likely cause. This may be rheumatoid arthritis, osteoarthritis, gout, or gonococcal arthritis. More rarely it is associated with psoriatic arthritis, lupus erythematosus, and other systemic diseases.

I Intoxication	C Congenital	A Autoimmune Allergic	T Trauma	E Endocrine
		Contact dermatitis Erythema multiforme	Contusion	
De Quervain stenosing tenosynovitis	Ganglion	Scleroderma	Hematoma Contusion Ruptured tendon	
	Buerger's disease	Vasculitis Rheumatoid arthritis	Laceration Contusion	Menopause
	Buerger's disease			
	Amyloidosis Rheumatoid arthritis		Laceration Contusion	Myxedema Acromegaly Diabetes
Scalenus anticus syndrome	Cervical rib		Costoclavicular compression	
		Rheumatoid spondylitis	Herniated disc Fracture	
Gout		Rheumatoid arthritis Lupus erythematosus	Fracture Sprain Contusion	

Approach to the Diagnosis

In diagnosis, most of these conditions will be obvious on inspection. The difficulty arises when the hand looks normal. Then one must check for:

1. Carpal tunnel syndrome by tapping the volar aspect of the wrist (Tinel's sign).
2. Brachial plexus neuralgia and scalenus anticus syndrome by Adson's tests.
3. Causalgia by stellate ganglion block to see if pain is relieved.
4. Cervical spine disease by a roentgenogram, possibly a myelogram or magnetic nuclear imaging (MRI), and nerve blocks of the various roots. Referral to a neurologist is often necessary. In early rheumatoid arthritis, the joints may be normal on inspection but pain and stiffness of the hands and fingers in the morning is an excellent clue.

Other useful tests for the workup of hand and finger pain are listed in Appendix I.

HEADACHE

This symptom is best analyzed by utilizing **anatomy,** Tables 1-10 and 1-11, but differentiation by pathophysiology is interesting, particularly in muscle traction headaches, and migraines.

Moving by layers from the **skin** to the center of the brain is the local application of the anatomical process. Thus, sunstroke is a cause of headache originating in the sunburnt skin, as is herpes zoster. Abscesses of the scalp are uncommon but significant causes of head pain. Moving to the **muscles** one encounters the most common cause of headache, muscle traction headache, which may be secondary to other conditions (*e.g.,* mi-graine or eyestrain), or primarily due to nervous tension or constantly holding the head in one position. Fibromyositis (usually of rheumatic etiology) may also cause a headache.

The next most common type of headache, migraine, originates from the **superficial arteries.** It usually involves the superficial temporal arteries, but it can involve the internal carotid arteries (Horton's cephalalgia or cluster headaches), the occipital artery, and the intracranial arteries (*e.g.,* hemiplegic migraine). Temporal arteritis and hypertension are two other important causes of headache originating from the **extracranial arteries.** The adjacent superficial **nerves** are a less common but important cause of headache. Occipital neuralgia may result from inflammation or compression of either the minor or major occipital nerve and is often involved secondarily in muscle contraction headache. This etiology is established by blocking these two nerves (medially and laterally). Trigeminal neuralgia is no less important.

Moving to deeper layers, one encounters the **skull,** where osteomyelitis (*e.g.,* tuberculous or syphilitic), primary and metastatic carcinomas, cranial stenosis, Paget's disease, and skull fractures are important etiologies of headache. The **temporomandibular joint** is the origin of headache in the temporomandibular joint syndrome (usually caused by malocclusion) and rheumatoid arthritis. Important causes of headache affect the **cervical spine.** Cervical spondylosis is a major cause in the elderly, but rheumatoid arthritis, spondylitis, spinal cord tumors, and metastatic disease of the vertebrae are also etiologies to consider.

Several common causes of headache come to mind when considering the organs of the head. Thus the **eyes** are affected by refractive errors, astigmatism, and glaucoma, all etiologies of headache. The **ear** is affected by otitis media, mastoiditis, acoustic neuromas, and

(*Text continues on p. 60*)

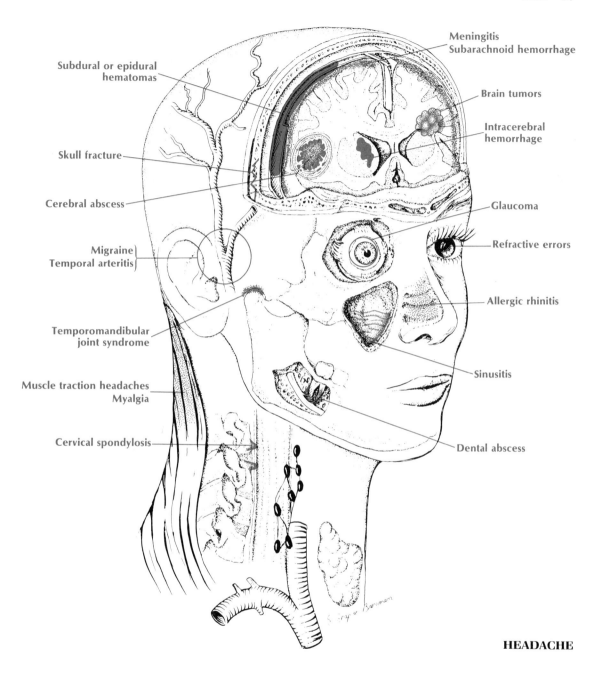

Subdural or epidural hematomas

Meningitis
Subarachnoid hemorrhage

Brain tumors

Intracerebral hemorrhage

Skull fracture

Cerebral abscess

Glaucoma

Refractive errors

Migraine
Temporal arteritis

Allergic rhinitis

Temporomandibular joint syndrome

Sinusitis

Muscle traction headaches
Myalgia

Cervical spondylosis

Dental abscess

HEADACHE

TABLE 1-10. HEADACHE—EXTRACRANIAL AND CRANIAL

	V Vascular	I Inflammatory	N Neoplasm	D Degenerative and Deficiency
Skin		Herpes zoster Abscess (scalp)		
Muscle and Fascia				
Superficial Arteries	Migraine			
Superficial Nerves		Occipital neuralgia		
Skull		Tuberculosis Osteomyelitis	Osteomas Metastatic carcinoma Multiple myeloma	
T-M Joint				
Cervical Spine		Tuberculosis	Cord tumors Metastasis	Osteoarthritis
Sinuses		Sinusitis	Sinus tumor or polyps	
Eyes	Retinal artery or vein occlusion	Uveitis Retinitis Scleritis	Orbital tumor	
Ears		Otitis media Mastoiditis Petrositis	Acoustic neuroma Cholesteatoma	
Teeth		Abscess		Dental caries
Nose	Wegener's granuloma- tosis	Rhinitis Mucormycosis	Schmincke tumor	

I Intoxication Idiopathic	C Congenital	A Autoimmune Allergic	T Trauma	E Endocrine
Sunstroke				
Muscle traction head- ache Fibromyositis				
Migraine Histamine cephalalagia		Temporal arteritis		
Trigeminal neuralgia Sphenopalatine gan- glion neuralgia				
Paget's Disease Cranial stenosis Hyperostosis frontalis			Skull fracture	Hyperparathyroidism
Temporomandibular joint syndrome	Malocclusion	Rheumatoid arthritis		
Cervical spondylosis		Rheumatoid arthritis		
Vacuum sinus head- ache Caffeine withdrawal		Allergic sinusitis	Fracture	
Glaucoma Refraction error	Glaucoma Astigmatism	Uveitis Scleritis	Orbital trauma Corneal erosion	
			Basilar fracture	
			Irritation of nerve root by filling	
Toxic rhinitis (*e.g.,* nicotine)	Deviated septum	Allergic rhinitis	Broken nose	

cholesteatomas. The **nose** is involved by infectious rhinitis, allergic rhinitis, Wegener's granulomatosis, nicotine toxicity, fractures and deviated septum, all causes of headache. Sinusitis (both the purulent and the vacuum type), sinus polyps, and tumors make checking the nasal sinuses important in analyzing the cause of headaches. Finally, the **teeth** should be investigated for caries, abscesses,

and fillings that may be too close to the nerve root.

Intracranially there are very important but less common causes of headache. The **meninges** are the site of subarachnoid hemorrhages, subdural and epidural hematomas, meningitis, and hydrocephalus. Missing one of these is a grave error. The **cerebral arteries** are the site of cerebral hemorrhages,

TABLE 1-11.   HEADACHE—INTRACRANIAL

	V Vascular	I Inflammatory	N Neoplasm	D Degenerative and Deficiency
Meninges	Subarachnoid hemorrhage	Meningitis Cystic hygroma Epidural abscess Rocky Mountain spotted fever	Meningioma Hodgkin's disease	
Cerebral Arteries	Hemorrhage Thrombosis Embolism			
Cerebral Veins		Venous sinus thrombosis		
Cranial Nerves				
Brain	See above Hypertensive encephalopathy	Lues Encephalitis Parasites Tuberculoma Cerebral abscess	Primary and metastatic tumors	
Systemic Disease	Hypertension CHF	Fever of any cause	Leukemia Hodgkin's disease Metastasis	

thrombosis, and emboli, as well as aneurysms and arteriovenous anomalies. The **cerebral veins,** especially the venous sinuses, may become inflamed and thrombosed, producing a headache. The **cranial nerves** are the site of trigeminal neuralgia mentioned above and glossopharyngeal neuralgia.

Although the **brain** itself is not tender, lesions of the brain cause increased intracranial pressure or traction on other painful structures, such as the intracranial arteries, venous sinuses, or nerves. A third of the cases of brain tumors present with a headache. Encephalitis produces a headache by the associated fever or meningeal irritation. Concussions, pituitary tumors, toxic encephalopathy from alcohol, bromides, and other substances are important causes, in addition to the cerebral

I Intoxication Idiopathic	**C** Congenital	**A** Autoimmune Allergic	**T** Trauma	**E** Endocrine
Hydrocephalus Meningocele	Hydrocephalus Others		Subdural and epidural hematoma Lumbar puncture headache	
	Aneurysm A-V anomaly	Arteritis		
			Subdural hematoma	
Trigeminal and glossopha- ryngeal neuralgia		Optic neuritis		
Benign intracranial hyper- tension Bromism Alcoholism Other drugs Gout			Concussion Contusion Postconcussion syn- drome	Pituitary tumors Acromegaly
Lead poisoning Drugs Uremia Jaundice Iodide toxicity		Collagen diseases		Diabetic acidosis Goiter Menstrual tension Menopause Hypothyroidism

hemorrhage, thrombosis, and emboli already mentioned. The various systemic diseases shown in Table 1-11 are too numerous to mention here, but fever of any etiology is an important cause and must not be forgotten, although it is usually obvious.

Approach to the Diagnosis

The approach to the diagnosis of a headache is primarily by history, but a thorough neurological examination is done to rule out brain tumors or other space-occupying lesions. Migraine is easily diagnosed when one considers the faimly history, the unilateral and throbbing nature of the pain, the associated aura, photophobia, and the nausea and vomiting. An arteriogram may be indicated when the "migraine" is consistently located on one particular side of the head to exclude an aneurysm. Muscle traction headache is usually associated with nervous tension or an occupational hazard such as typing. A lidocaine block of the occipital nerves will give temporary relief and will help in the diagnosis. Nerve blocks can also be useful in headaches originating from cervical spine disease, dental abscess or caries, and sphenopalatine ganglion neuralgia. A thorough spraying of the nasal turbinates with phenylephrine will often relieve the headache of rhinitis and help establish that diagnosis. A sedimentation rate to exclude temporal arteritis should be ordered in the elderly.

It should become obvious from the above that **seeing the patient during an attack** of headache is valuable in diagnosis. Compression of the temporal arteries will usually relieve a migraine attack temporarily.

Relief from ergotamine tartrate by injection is also helpful in diagnosis. Checking the eyeball for tension may diagnose glaucoma. Compression of the jugular veins will often relieve postspinal headache.

Ancillary diagnostic procedures such as skull, sinus, and cervical spine x-ray films and blood tests are usually negative, but if there is any doubt at all about a brain tumor or other cerebral pathology, a computerized axial tomography (CT) scan should be done even if the neurological exam is negative. Frequent follow-up visits and repeat neurological exams will also be helpful in ruling out serious pathology.

HEARTBURN

True heartburn (see also Indigestion, p. 338 and Anorexia, p. 228) may be defined as a burning pain in the substernal area or midepigastrium which is usually increased by swallowing and which is almost invariably due to esophagitis from gastric reflux. There are other causes, however, and the problem for the diagnostician is how best to recall these in the clinical situation. From an etiological standpoint **inflammation** is almost invariably the culprit, although myocardial infarction or angina pectoris are two frequent causes which are not inflammatory.

Anatomically, the best approach is to move in a target-like fashion from the intrinsic portion of the esophagus and stomach peripherally. Thus, in the **first zone** one encounters esophagitis, gastritis, and gastric ulcers. In the **second zone** one encounters hiatal hernia (which, of course, predisposes to esophagitis), pericarditis, mediastinitis, and gastrojejunostomy complications. In the **third zone** one visualizes cholecystitis (which probably induces a bile esophagitis), pancreatitis, myocardial infarction or coronary insufficiency, pleurisy, and intestinal obstruction. In the **fourth zone,** one recalls systemic diseases such as uremia, severe emphysema, cirrhosis, and congestive heart failure (which probably causes gastritis or gastric ulcers).

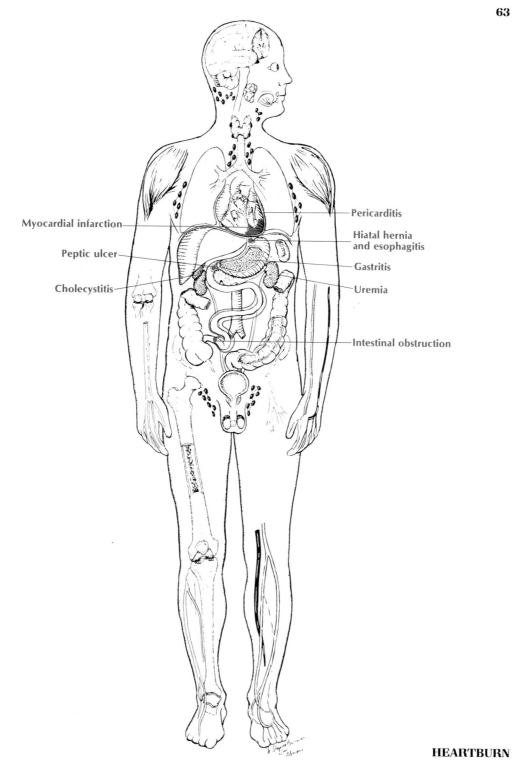

Myocardial infarction

Peptic ulcer

Cholecystitis

Pericarditis

Hiatal hernia
and esophagitis

Gastritis

Uremia

Intestinal obstruction

HEARTBURN

Approach to the Diagnosis

The approach to the diagnosis of heartburn is similar to that for any gastrointestinal complaint, but a few clinical tricks will help decide whether it is intrinsic or extrinsic, especially if the upper GI series is negative. Always order an esophagram. If the patient has the pain when he is in the office, administer a tablespoon or two of lidocaine (Xylocaine viscus). If he gets relief in 5 to 10 minutes, the heartburn is probably caused by esophagitis. Further confirmation can be obtained by a Bernstein test. In this test, solutions of normal saline and 0.10 normal hydrochloric acid are administered by intravenous tubing into the lower esophagus, alternating one with the other. If the patient invariably experiences pain when the 0.10 normal HCl is administered, esophagitis is confirmed. Esophagoscopy and gastroscopy will diagnose most intrinsic lesions with certainty but occasionally they are normal in esophagitis. Manometric studies of the esophagus are the best way to diagnose esophageal reflux. If the episodes are frequent but relatively brief, a trial of nitroglycerin may diagnose angina pectoris. Coronary insufficiency may also be confirmed by an exercise tolerance test. A cholecystogram and liver and pancreatic function studies may also be indicated.

JOINT PAIN

Because most joints may be affected by the same etiological processes, a general discussion of the differential diagnosis of joint pain will be undertaken, followed by a discussion of exceptions which apply to certain joints.

Anatomical and histological breakdown of the joint is not of much value in the differential diagnosis. It is sufficient to say that extrinsic lesions about the joint, such as cellulitis, bursitis, and tendonitis must be considered in the differential diagnosis. Nonarticular rheumatism or fibromyositis comes to mind here also.

To develop a differential list of intrinsic conditions of the joints the mnemonic **VINDICATE** is useful.

V—Vascular suggests hemophilia and scurvy as well as aseptic bone necrosis (Osgood–Schlatter disease, and so forth).

I—Inflammatory suggests several infectious lesions, but gonorrhea, streptococcus, tuberculosis, and syphilis are most likely.

N—Neoplastic disorders to be ruled out are osteogenic sarcoma and giant cell tumors.

D—Degenerative disorders bring to mind degenerative joint disease or osteoarthritis, which is so common that it is often the first condition to be considered in joint pain.

I—Intoxication suggests gout (uric acid) and pseudogout (calcium pyrophosphate). Drugs infrequently initiate joint disease but the lupus syndrome of hydralazine (Apresoline) and procainamide and the "gout syndrome" of diuretics should be kept in mind.

C—Congenital and acquired malformations would bring to mind the joint deformities of tabes dorsalis and syringomyelia and congenital dislocation of the hip. Alkaptonuria–ochronosis is also considered here.

A—Autoimmune indicates another commonly encountered group of diseases. Rheumatoid arthritis is the most prevalent of these, but serum sickness, lupus erythematosus, rheumatic fever, Reiter's syndrome, ulcerative colitis, regional ileitis, and psoriatic arthritis must be also considered.

T—Trauma suggests numerous disorders. In addition to traumatic synovitis, one must consider tear or rupture of the collateral or cruciate ligaments, subluxation or lacera-

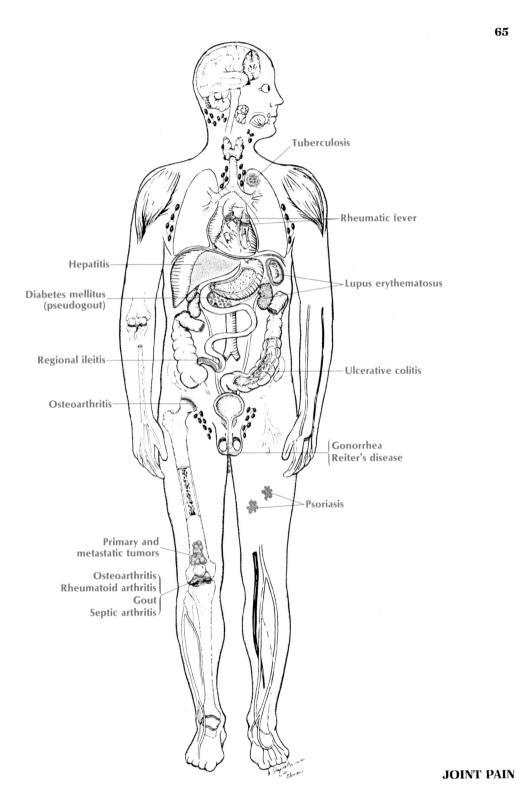

Tuberculosis

Rheumatic fever

Hepatitis

Lupus erythematosus

Diabetes mellitus
(pseudogout)

Regional ileitis

Ulcerative colitis

Osteoarthritis

Gonorrhea
Reiter's disease

Psoriasis

Primary and
metastatic tumors

Osteoarthritis
Rheumatoid arthritis
Gout
Septic arthritis

JOINT PAIN

tion of the meniscus (semilunar cartilage), dislocation of the joints or patella, a sprain of the joint, and fracture of the bones of the joint.

E—Endocrine disorders that affect the joints include acromegaly, menopause, and diabetes mellitus (pseudogout).

Now it is useful to consider individual joints where special etiologies apply. The **temporomandibular joint** is often affected by malocclusion. The **cervical spine** is affected by cervical spondylosis, a condition where hypertrophic lipping of the vertebrae occurs in response to degeneration of the discs. Inflammation of the **sacroiliac joint** occurs most commonly in Marie–Strümpell's disease, psoriatic arthritis, Reiter's disease, and regional ileitis.

Approach to the Diagnosis

The approach to the diagnosis of joint pain includes a careful history and examination for other signs such as swelling, redness, and hyperthermia of the joints. If multiple joints are involved, look for rheumatoid arthritis, lupus, and osteoarthritis. Single joint involvement suggests gonorrhea, septic arthritis, tuberculosis, or gout, among other things. Small joints are involved more frequently in rheumatoid arthritis, Reiter's syndrome, and lupus, although the large joints are more frequently involved in osteoarthritis, gonorrhea, tuberculosis, and other infections. Remember, however, that both osteoarthritis and gonorrhea may involve the small joints of the hands and feet. Rheumatic fever presents a migratory arthritis and this is a helpful differential point. When the knee joint is involved, the astute clinician will always examine for a torn or subluxated meniscus and loose cruciate or collateral ligaments. For the laboratory, Appendix I gives the most valuable diagnostic tests. Synovialysis for uric acid and calcium

pyrophosphate, the character of the mucin clot, a white cell count, and culture can be done in the office and may make the diagnosis almost immediately the eliminate the need for hospitalization.

A therapeutic trial of aspirin or colchicine is useful in diagnosing rheumatic fever and gout, respectively. If the joint fluid examination is nonspecific and no systemic signs of infection are evident, the injection of steroids into the joint is not unreasonable while the physician waits for the results of more sophisticated diagnostic tests.

LEG PAIN

Again, anatomical breakdown of the leg into its various anatomical components is the basis of a sound differential diagnosis (Table 1-12). Before that, however, one should determine if the pain is actually originating from the hip or if it is the result of knee joint disease. If so, the differential diagnosis of these must be considered (see pp. 64 and 146).

Beginning with the **skin,** consider herpes zoster and various dermatological conditions. In the **subcutaneous tissue,** one encounters cellulitis and occasionally filariasis, which may produce a similar picture. Beneath this layer the **muscle** and **fascia** suggest numerous causes of leg pain. There may be hematomas of the muscle, trichinosis or cysticercosis, nonarticular rheumatism, or fibromyositis. Muscle cramping from low sodium or other electrolyte disturbances must be considered.

The superficial and deep **veins** are the site of thrombophlebitis, a prominent cause of leg pain. The **arteries** may be involved by emboli (from auricular fibrillation, acute myocardial infarction, and subacute bacterial endocarditis), thrombosis (especially in Buerger's dis-

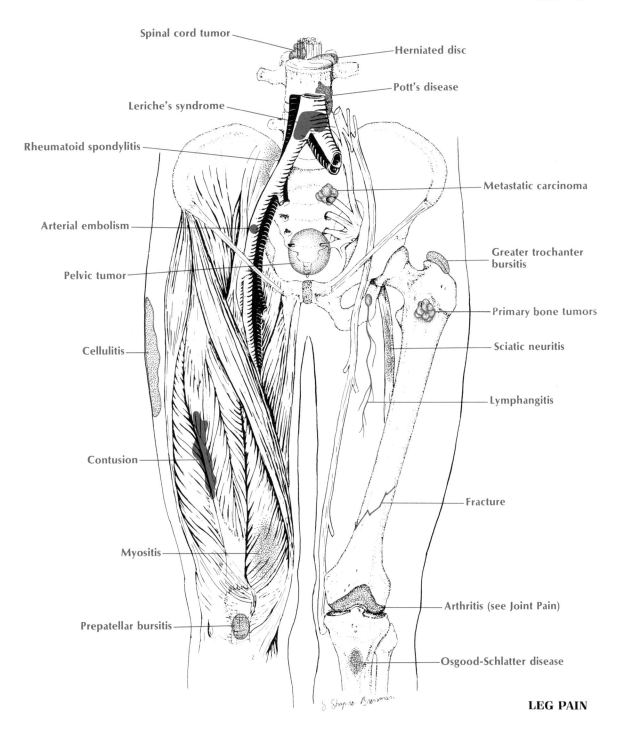

Spinal cord tumor

Herniated disc

Pott's disease

Leriche's syndrome

Rheumatoid spondylitis

Metastatic carcinoma

Arterial embolism

Greater trochanter bursitis

Pelvic tumor

Primary bone tumors

Sciatic neuritis

Cellulitis

Lymphangitis

Contusion

Fracture

Myositis

Arthritis (see Joint Pain)

Prepatellar bursitis

Osgood-Schlatter disease

LEG PAIN

ease and blood dyscrasias), and vasculitis (from arteriosclerosis and collagen diseases). Acute trauma to the artery or veins may cause pain. As usual, when one moves centrally along the arterial pathways additional causes of pain come to mind. A Leriche's syndrome and dissecting aneurysm must be considered.

When superficial or deep infections of the leg spread to the lymphatics, lymphangitis is important in the differential.

The **nerves** may be involved locally, centrally, or systemically. Buerger's disease, cellulitis, and osteomyelitis may involve the nerve locally. Neuromas may occasionally cause fo-

TABLE 1-12. LEG PAIN

	V Vascular	I Inflammatory	N Neoplasm	D Degenerative
Skin	Embolism	Herpes zoster Carbuncle	Kaposi's sarcoma	
Subcutaneous Tissue		Cellulitis Filariasis		
Muscle, Fascia, and Bursa		Tetanus Trichinosis Cysticercosis Epidemic myalgia		
Veins and Capillaries		Thrombophlebitis Subacute bacterial endocarditis	Hemangioma	Scurvy
Arteries	Leriche's syndrome Dissecting aneurysm Embolism	Subacute bacterial endocarditis		Arteriosclerosis
Lymphatics		Lymphangitis Filariasis	Hodgkin's disease Lymphangioma	
Nerves	Ischemic neuropathy Buerger's disease	Viral neuritis Tabes dorsalis	Pelvic tumor Neuroma Cord tumor Metastatic tumor	
Bone	Aseptic necrosis	Osteomyelitis Relapsing polychon- dritis	Osteogenic sarcomas Metastatic carcinoma Multiple myeloma	Scurvy Paget's disease

cal pain in the distribution of the nerve involved. More important are the central causes of nerve pain in the limbs. Probably herniated discs of the lumbar spine account for most of these cases, but Pott's disease, lumbar spondylosis (osteoarthritis?), metastatic and primary tumors, multiple myeloma, fractures, spondylolisthesis, and osteomyelitis of the spine all may compress the cauda equina and cause pain in the lower limbs.

Pelvic tumors, endometriosis, and sciatic neuritis are in a sense "central" causes of leg pain and all patients deserve a rectal and pelvic examination when the diagnosis is ob-

I Intoxication	C Congenital	A Autoimmune Allergic	T Trauma	E Endocrine
		Pyoderma gangren- osum Periarteritis nodosa	Contusion Laceration	
		Weber–Christian disease	Hematoma	
Low sodium from di- uretic Black widow spider bite	McArdle syndrome Myositis ossificans	Dermatomyositis Fibrositis	Hematoma Laceration Rupture	Tetany
	Varicose veins Buerger's disease		Hemorrhage	
		Periarteritis nodosa	Hemorrhage	
	Milroy's disease			
	Obturator hernia Porphyria Blood dyscrasias		Fracture Hematoma Ruptured disc	Diabetic neur- opathy
Radiation osteitis	Sickle cell anemia Osteogenesis imper- fecta		Fracture Hematoma	Osteomalacia Polyosteotic fi- brosa cystica Osteoporosis

scure. Pelvic inflammatory disease and obturator hernias may rarely involve the obturator nerve. Meralgia paresthetica from diabetes mellitus and other causes must be considered in thigh pain, and also in causalgia. Finally, the thalamic syndrome and diseases of the cervical spine must be considered. Dissecting the limb layer by layer, we have finally reached the **bone,** which suggests osteomyelitis, bone tumors, Osgood–Schlatter disease, tuberculous osteomyelitis, and Paget's disease.

Systemic diseases that may involve the nerves causing pain in the legs include tabes dorsalis, periarteritis nodosa, diabetes mellitus, metabolic and nutritional neuropathies, and blood dyscrasias.

Approach to the Diagnosis

The approach to the diagnosis of leg pain involves numerous ancillary examinations that one may not routinely do. Thus, arterial pulses must be checked all the way up. One should look for a positive Moses or Homans' sign. Straight leg raising (SLR) and meticulous mapping of sensory changes are valuable. The SLR sign may be negative and the patient could still have a herniated disc higher up. Thus, a femoral stretch test is done* and when positive suggests a herniated disc at L2–L3, or L3–L4. Edema associated with phlebitis or atrophy associated with a herniated disc can be detected only with careful measurement of the calf and thigh. Arterial circulation is best evaluated with an ultrasound flow study and thermography. Venography and arteriography may be necessary if plain x-ray films are unremarkable. One should almost always x-ray the spine, hips, knee joints, and, in difficult cases, the entire legs.

---

* Wiles P, Sweetnam R: Essentials of Orthopedics. Boston, Little, Brown, 1965.

LOW BACK PAIN ▪

Nothing is more challenging to diagnose than a case of low back pain. That is why it is so important to have an extensive list of causes in mind before approaching the patient. **Anatomy** forms the basis for developing such a list (Table 1-13).

Moving posteriorly from the skin inwards, one encounters the muscle and fascial planes, the lumbosacral spine and its ligaments, the spinal cord and cauda equina, the abdominal aorta and its branches, the rectum, and prostate in the male, the uterus and pelvic organs in the female, and finally the bladder.

The **skin** may be involved by a pilonidal cyst, contusions and lacerations, or herpes zoster. The **muscle** and **fascia** are involved by fibromyositis, trichinosis, contusions and lacerations, strains or sprains, and herniation of fat through the subfascial plain. (The latter has been espoused as a common cause of lumbago.) A more important cause of muscle spasms and irritation is faulty posture. Slumping over a typewriter, wearing the wrong shoes (*e.g.,* very high heels), and having one leg shorter than the other may cause this.

The next "layer" is the **lumbosacral spine.** Vascular lesions are infrequent here, but inflammation caused by osteomyelitis and tuberculosis (Pott's disease) is still seen in some countries. More common lesions of the spine inducing low back pain are metastatic carcinoma, herniated discs, rheumatoid spondylitis, or lumbar spondylosis (often erroneously labeled osteoarthritis). Osteoarthritis and other arthritides may involve the facets of the zygapophyseal joints and produce back pain ("facet syndrome"). Multiple myeloma is not an uncommon cause and should be looked for in each case. Fractures are particularly frequent in association with this disease. Fractures are also seen with osteoporosis, osteitis fibrosa cystica, and osteomalacia. Paget's disease, gout, and sprung back (in which the interspinous ligament is torn) are less common causes of low back pain originating in the spine. Congenital anomalies such as spondylolisthesis and scoliosis are important causes. In the **spinal cord** arteriovenous anomalies, myelitis, epidural abscesses, and primary tumors are important causes.

Moving deeper, one encounters the aorta, and arteriosclerotic and dissecting aneurysms come to mind. Disease of the **rectum** may refer pain to the low back, particularly hemorrhoids, fissures, perirectal abscesses,

and carcinomas. In the **prostate,** prostatitis and prostatic carcinoma are frequent causes. Prostatic carcinoma, however, produces low back pain most frequently by metastasis. The **bladder** and **urethra** are infrequent causes of low back pain, but a urinalysis and culture may be necessary to rule out infections.

To diagnose low back pain in women the **uterus** and other **pelvic organs** must be examined. Dysmenorrhea (functional) is often the cause but tubo-ovarian abscess, ovarian cysts, endometriosis, fibroids, retroversion or flexion, and uterine carcinomas must be looked for.

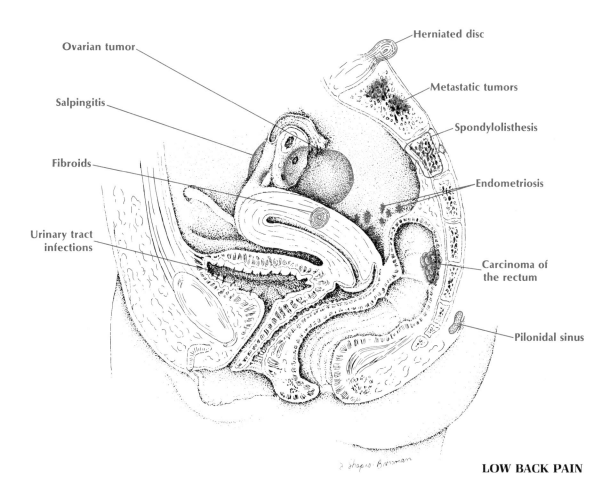

LOW BACK PAIN

Approach to the Diagnosis

The approach to the diagnosis of back pain involves a careful history and a physical examination, including a rectal and pelvic. During the physical examination, a search for a herniated disc is particularly important. A positive SLR suggests an L4–L5 or L5–S1 disc. A positive femoral stretch test suggests an L3– L4 disc. Achilles and knee reflexes and sensory dermatomes for these nerve roots are examined. Sacrospinalis muscle spasms should be looked for; they are particularly important when they are unilateral. The best way to find muscle spasm is to examine the patient standing in the "at ease" position.

A simple measurement of leg length may reveal the cause of low back pain, but watch-

TABLE 1-13. LOW BACK PAIN

	V Vascular	I Inflammatory	N Neoplasm	D Degenerative and Deficiency
Skin		Herpes zoster		
Muscle and Fascia, Ligaments		Fibromyositis Trichinosis		
Lumbosacral Spine		Tuberculosis Osteomyelitis	Hodgkin's disease Metastatic carcinoma Multiple myeloma	Osteomalacia Osteoporosis Osteoarthritis Lumbar spondylosis
Spinal Cord and Cauda Equina	A-V anomaly	Epidural abscess Myelitis	Primary and meta- static tumors	
Aorta	Aortic aneurysm			Dissecting aneurysm
Rectum	Hemorrhoid	Anal fissures Perirectal abscess	Carcinomas	
Uterus, Tubes, and Ovaries		Endometritis Tubo-ovarian abscess	Fibroids Carcinoma Endometriosis Ovarian cyst	
Bladder and Prostate		Cystitis Urethritis Prostatitis	Prostatic carcinoma	

ing the patient walk may identify faulty posture as the cause. Blocking the various nerve roots with lidocaine is also useful in diagnosis, but this procedure is usually done by a neurologist.

X-ray films of the lumbosacral spine often reveal degenerated discs, osteoarthritis, metastatic carcinoma, and other conditions, but when the roentgenograms are negative a myelogram, CT scan, EMG, and thermography must be done if a herniated disc is to be excluded. Even then a few discs will be missed and discography, selective lumbar angiography and venography, or surgery must be performed.

A sedimentation rate will be useful in diagnosing rheumatoid spondylitis or multiple myeloma. Bone scans may diagnose early

I Intoxication Idiopathic	C Congenital and Acquired Anomaly	A Autoimmune Allergic	T Trauma	E Endocrine
	Pilonidal cyst		Contusion Laceration	
	Herniation of subfascial fat Faulty posture		Contusion Tears Lumbosacral sprain	
Paget's disease Alkaptonuria Gout	Herniated disc Spina bifida Spondylolisthesis Coccydynia Scoliosis	Rheumatoid spondylitis	Herniated disc Fracture Sprung back Coccydynia	Osteitis fibrosa cystica
	A-V anomaly			
	Fistula			
	Retroversion or retroflexion			Dysmenorrhea
			Ruptured urethra or bladder	

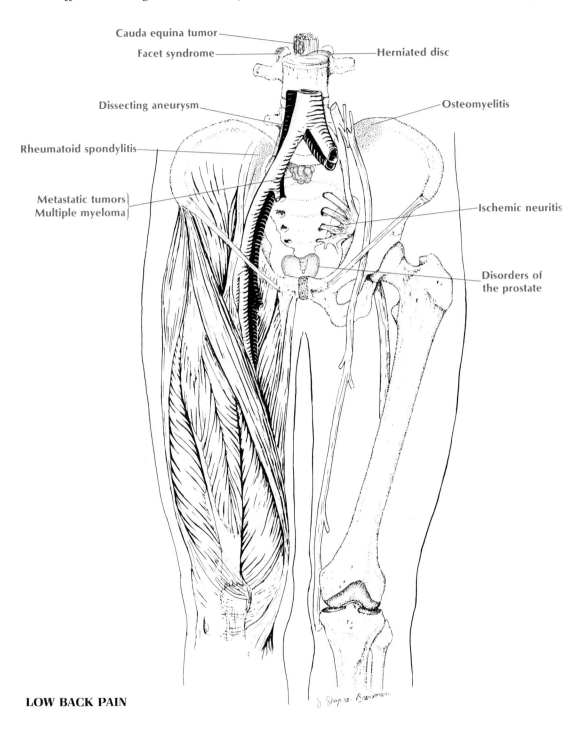

Cauda equina tumor

Facet syndrome

Herniated disc

Dissecting aneurysm

Osteomyelitis

Rheumatoid spondylitis

Metastatic tumors
Multiple myeloma

Ischemic neuritis

Disorders of
the prostate

LOW BACK PAIN

rheumatoid spondylitis. Other useful laboratory procedures are noted in Appendix I.

NECK PAIN ■

The analysis of the cause of neck pain is similar to that of headache. First, the anatomical
components are distinguished, then the various etiologies are applied to each (Table 1-
14). Moving from the skin to the spinal cord
layer by layer, we encounter the fascia, muscles, arteries, veins, brachial and cervical
plexus, and lymph nodes. Next are the esophagus, trachea, and thyroid gland. Finally,
there is the cervical spine encircling the spinal cord and meninges and designed to allow
uninfringed exit of the cervical nerve roots.

Taking each of these structures and applying the etiologic categories of **MINT,** we can
arrive at a respectable differential diagnosis of
neck pain. Inflammation and trauma are the
principal causes. The **skin** may be involved by
herpes zoster, cellulitis, contusions, and lacerations. An infected bronchial cleft cyst may
occasionally be the offender. In the **muscle
and fascia,** one encounters not only fibromyositis, dermatomyositis, and trichinosis
but also traumatic contusions and pulled or
torn ligaments (strains). The muscles may be
involved by tension headache, poor posture,
and occasionally by epidemic myalgia.
Meningitis causes nuchal rigidity and neck
pain. Torticollis causes painful spasms, but
the jerking of the neck makes the condition
obvious.

The **arteries** of the neck are infrequently
tender or painful as are most aneurysms
(aside from dissecting aneurysms) unless they
compress adjacent structures. Arteritis is unusual here, but a common carotid thrombosis
may be tender and painful. Referred pain
from angina pectoris is not uncommon.

Like the arteries it is rare for the **jugular
veins** and smaller veins of the neck to cause
pain by thrombosis or rupture, but it occasionally happens in superior vena caval obstruction. The **lymph nodes,** on the other
hand, are a frequent site of neck pain. They
are usually enlarged and tender in association
with pharyngitis, otitis media, sinusitis, dental
abscesses, and mediastinitis.

The **brachial plexus** may be involved by a
primary neuritis or by compression from a
scalenus anticus syndrome, a Pancoast's tumor, the clavical (costoclavicular syndrome),
or a cervical rib. More often the roots are compressed by diseases of the **spine,** such as a
herniated disc, fracture, cervical spondylosis,
tuberculous or nontuberculous osteomyelitis,
and primary or metastatic tumors of the spine
and spinal cord. In the case of the **spinal
cord** one should also remember the meninges as a cause of neck pain in meningitis,
arachnoiditis, and subarachnoid hemorrhage.
Rheumatoid arthritis of the spine will cause
neck pain without compression.

The esophagus is not usually a cause of
neck pain, but pain may be referred to the
neck from a hiatal hernia or subdiaphragmatic abscess. Pulsion diverticuli of the
esophagus may also compress adjacent structures and cause painful symptoms. Like the
esophagus, the **trachea** is an infrequent
source of neck pain but occasionally acute laryngotracheitis will be the source of severe
pain. Finally, **subacute thyroiditis** and inflammatory or obstructive lesions of the salivary glands may be the offenders in neck pain,
even though the patient complains of a sore
throat.

Approach to the Diagnosis

When diagnosing neck pain look for an associated mass or enlargement of the lymph
nodes or thyroid. If there are no specifically
tender areas in the muscles, check the mobil-

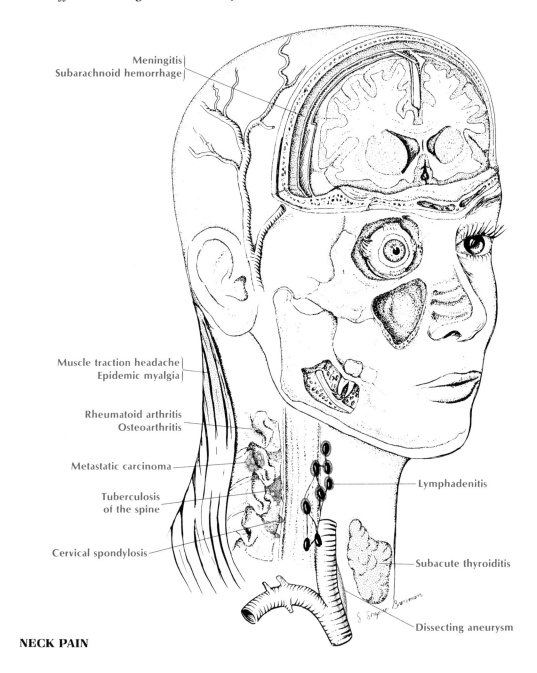

Meningitis
Subarachnoid hemorrhage

Muscle traction headache
Epidemic myalgia

Rheumatoid arthritis
Osteoarthritis

Metastatic carcinoma

Tuberculosis
of the spine

Cervical spondylosis

Lymphadenitis

Subacute thyroiditis

Dissecting aneurysm

NECK PAIN

ity of the neck and each cervical nerve root for tenderness. In numerous cases, an x-ray of the cervical spine will confirm the diagnosis of a herniated disc or cervical spondylosis. Sometimes a cervical myelogram, thermography or MRI will be necessary to exclude a herniated disc. However, a dermatomal hypal- gesia or hyperalgesia will usually be demonstrated in these cases. EMG will help diagnose these root syndromes in doubtful cases. Keep in mind referred pain from the heart or diaphragm, and, in the acute case, look for nuchal rigidity to rule out meningitis or subarachnoid hemorrhage, as well as infections

TABLE 1-14. NECK PAIN

	M **Malformations**	**I** **Inflammation**	**N** **Neoplasm**	**T** **Trauma**
Skin		Herpes zoster Cellulitis Carbuncles		Contusion Laceration
Muscle and Fascia		Epidemic myalgia Trichinosis		

Arteries	Dissecting aneurysms
	Subarachnoid hemor-
	  rhage from cerebral
	  aneurysm
		Temporal arteritis		Hemorrhage

Veins		Thrombophlebitis		Hemorrhage
Lymph Nodes		Lymphadenitis Tuberculosis	Hodgkin's disease Metastatic car- cinoma	

Nerves	Cervical rib
	Scalenus anticus syn-
	  drome
		Brachial plexus neuri-
		  tis
			Pancoast's tumors	Contusion
				Lacerations
				Compression

Thyroid		Subacute thyroiditis Riedel's struma	Metastatic thyroid carcinoma	Ruptured colloid cyst
Esophagus	Congenital diverticu- lum	Esophagitis	Carcinoma	Pulsion diverticulum

Cervical Spine	Platybasia	Rheumatoid arthritis
		Tuberculosis
		Osteoarthritis
			Metastatic car-
			  cinoma
			Spinal cord
			  tumors
				Fracture
				Herniated disc

in the upper respiratory tract. Appendix I summarizes many useful tests that may be indicated in the workup.

PENILE PAIN

Perhaps no other pain will bring a patient to the doctor more quickly in this age of sexual candor. Most cases will be caused by **inflammation,** so a mnemonic of etiologies is, for the most part, superfluous. Utilization of **anatomy** is valuable, however. Let us begin, then, with the **head of the penis** and proceed upward to the prostate, the bladder, and the kidney.

The **head of the penis** may be inflamed by a painful chancroid ulcer or lymphogranuloma venereum, but one must remember that a chancre (syphylitic ulcer) is not painful. Herpes progenitalis, on the other hand, is extremely painful. Balanitis is usually caused by a nonspecific infection, but one should caution the uncircumcised patient about proper cleaning of the area and rule out Reiter's disease. (Look for conjunctivitis and joint symptoms.) Trauma to the head of the penis should be obvious, but some patients may be too shy to mention its origin without careful questioning. Carcinoma of the penis rarely causes pain, but like all carcinomas it will often be painful when it is secondarily infected.

Next, let us consider the **urethra.** Inflammation here is probably the most common cause of penile pain. It is almost invariably associated with a discharge, and the smear will usually disclose the typical gram-negative intracellular diplococci of gonorrhea. The clinician is reminded that nonspecific urethritis is more frequently encountered each year and that chlamydia and mimae polymorphia are common etiologies. Reiter's disease must also

be considered. Passage of a stone through the urethra causes pain in the penis.

The **shaft** of the penis is one of the few areas in which a vascular lesion may account for penile pain. Thrombosis of the corpus cavernosis is not infrequently encountered in blood dyscrasias (particularly leukemia), and the resulting permanent erection may be enviable and even humorous to the observer but not to the patient. Peyronie's disease will cause a painful erection.

Moving to the **prostate,** one hardly needs to be reminded that both acute and chronic prostatitis are frequent causes of penile pain. On the other hand, carcinoma and hypertrophy of the prostate are rarely associated with pain unless there is associated infection.

The **bladder** is another common source of penile pain, but because there is often an associated urethritis it is uncertain whether pure cystitis causes penile pain by itself except on urination. Bladder stones cause pain in the penis, especially on urination. Carcinoma of the bladder will not usually cause penile pain unless it is complicated by infection. Hunner's ulcer, on the other hand, causes great pain in the penis at times. Occasionally, ureteral and renal stones will cause penile pain but pyelonephritis is very unlikely to do so. Referred pain from the rectum caused by hemorrhoids and fissures is not uncommon.

Approach to the Diagnosis

Examination of the penis, prostate, and urine will usually determine the cause of penile pain, but certain other diagnostic procedures should be used if the diagnosis is obscure. An IVP and voiding cystogram, examination of the urethral discharge after prostatic massage, and cystoscopy may sometimes be necessary. Other useful tests are listed in Appendix I.

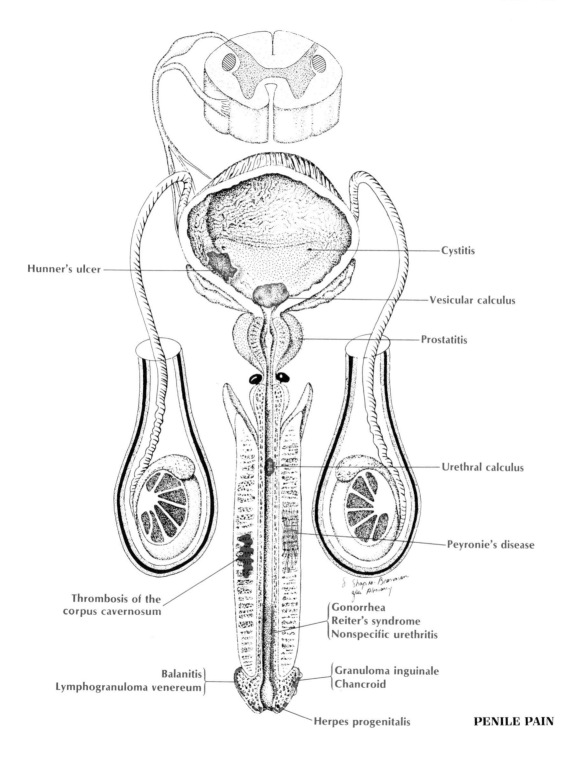

Cystitis

Vesicular calculus

Prostatitis

Hunner's ulcer

Urethral calculus

Peyronie's disease

Thrombosis of the
corpus cavernosum

Gonorrhea
Reiter's syndrome
Nonspecific urethritis

Balanitis
Lymphogranuloma venereum

Granuloma inguinale
Chancroid

Herpes progenitalis

PENILE PAIN

RECTAL PAIN

Practically the whole specialty of proctology is devoted to taking care of patients with rectal pain. To develop the differential diagnosis it is useful first to divide the conditions into **extrinsic** and **intrinsic.** To recall the **extrinsic** causes one simply visualizes the structures around the rectum. Noting the tubes and ovaries, one considers salpingitis, ovarian cysts, and ectopic pregnancy. Visualize the coccyx, and the coccydynia is brought to mind. Just as important a cause of rectal pain is prostatitis or prostatic abscess. A pelvic appendix or ruptured diverticulum may inflame the rectum extrinsically.

Intrinsic causes are developed by the mnemonic **VINDICATE.**

V—Vascular suggests hemorrhoids.

I— Inflammation suggests proctitis, anal ulcers, and perirectal abscess.

N—Neoplasms are not usually painful until late.

D—Degenerative is suggested but there are no degenerative diseases causing rectal pain.

C—Congenital and **acquired malforma-**

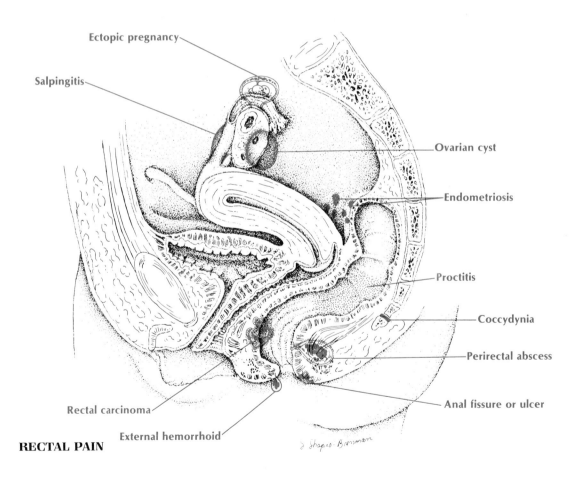

RECTAL PAIN

tions suggest fistula in ano, diverticulum, and intussusception.

A—Autoimmune diseases suggest ulcerative proctitis and granulomatous colitis.

T—Trauma should bring to mind fecal impactions and foreign bodies or introduction of the male organ into the rectum.

E—Endocrine disorders suggest nothing other than the ovarian cysts and ectopic pregnancy already mentioned.

Approach to the Diagnosis

The cause of rectal pain is usually obvious on examination with an anoscope or proctoscope. Careful palpation may be necessary to discover a perirectal abscess, coccydynia, or an ectopic pregnancy. Anal fissures may be missed unless all quadrants of the anus are examined with the slit-anoscope.

SHOULDER PAIN ■

The differential diagnosis of shoulder pain, like other forms of pain, is best established by **anatomy,** working from the outside in (Table 1-15). Beginning with the **skin,** one immediately thinks of cellulitis and herpes zoster. The **muscles** and **tendons** come next, and epidemic myalgia and the myalgias secondary to many infectious diseases lead the list. However, **trichinosis, dermatomyositis, fibromyositis,** and **trauma** must always be considered. Proceeding to the **blood vessels,** keep in mind thrombophlebitis, Buerger's disease, vascular occlusion from periarteritis nodosa, and other forms of vasculitis.

Inflammation of the **bursae** is probably the most common cause of shoulder pain. This should be considered traumatic because in most cases the torn ligamentum teres rubs

the bursa and causes the inflammation. Interestingly enough, aside from gout, the bursae are rarely involved in other conditions. The **shoulder joint** itself is also a frequent site of pain. Osteoarthritis, rheumatoid arthritis, gout, lupus, and various bacteria all may involve this joint, but dislocation of the shoulder, fractures, and frozen shoulder should also be considered. If the **bone** is the site of pain, there is usually a fracture involved. Osteomyelitis and metastatic tumors, however, ought to be ruled out.

Neurological causes are not the last to be considered just because anatomically they come last. The **brachial plexus** may be compressed by a cervical rib, a large scalenus anticus or pectoralis muscle, or the clavical (costoclavicular syndrome). When the **cervical sympathetics** are irritated or disrupted, a shoulder—hand syndrome develops. The **cervical spine** is the site or origin of shoulder pain in cervical spondylosis, spinal cord tumors, tuberculosis and syphilitic osteomyelitis, ruptured discs, or fractured vertebrae.

It would be a grave error to omit the **systemic causes** of shoulder pain. Thus, coronary insufficiency, cholecystitis, Pancoast's tumors, pleurisy, and subdiaphragmatic abscesses should be ruled out.

Approach to the Diagnosis

The approach to ruling out various causes is most often clinical, provided x-ray films of the shoulder and cervical spine are negative. In the classical case of subacromion bursitis, in which passive movement is much less restricted than active movement and a point of maximum tenderness can easily be located, lidocaine and steroid injections into the bursa (at the point of maximum tenderness) may be done without roentgenograms. Cervical root blocks, stellate ganglion blocks for shoulder—hand syndrome, and aspiration and injection of the shoulder joint with lido-

(Text continues on p. 84)

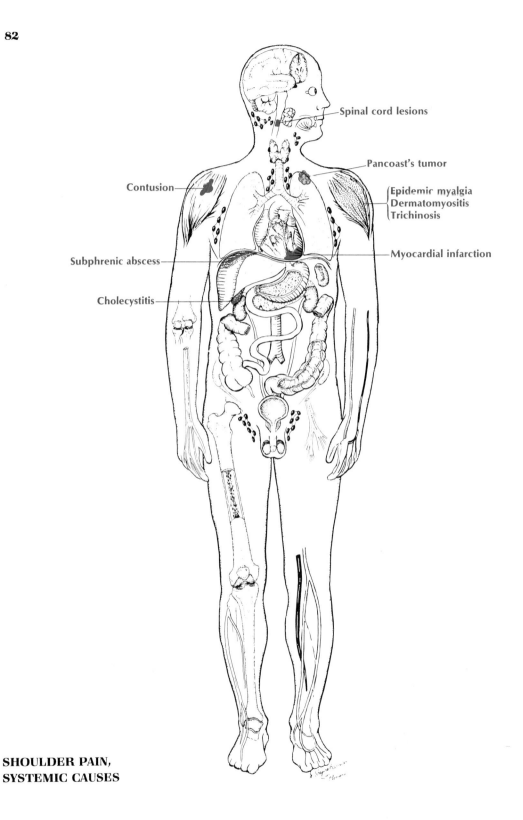

Spinal cord lesions

Pancoast's tumor

Contusion

Epidemic myalgia
Dermatomyositis
Trichinosis

Subphrenic abscess

Myocardial infarction

Cholecystitis

**SHOULDER PAIN,
SYSTEMIC CAUSES**

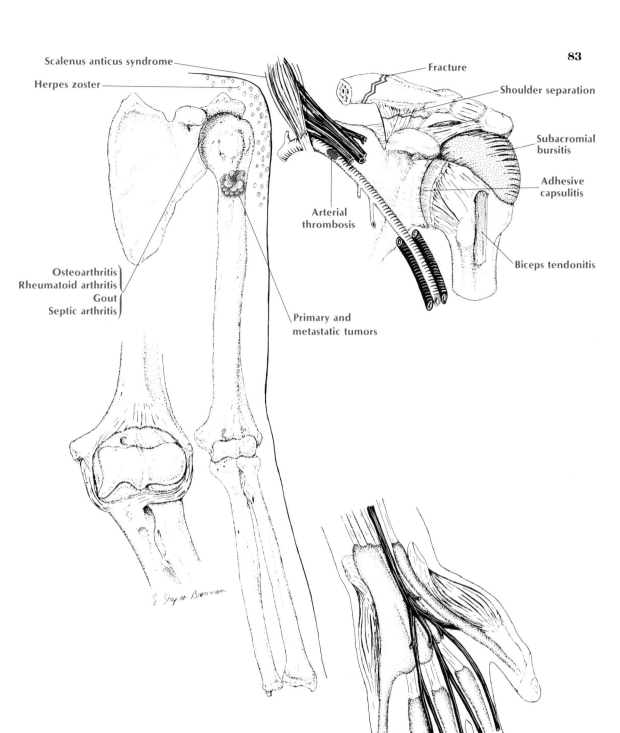

Scalenus anticus syndrome

Herpes zoster

Fracture

Shoulder separation

Subacromial bursitis

Adhesive capsulitis

Arterial thrombosis

Biceps tendonitis

Osteoarthritis
Rheumatoid arthritis
Gout
Septic arthritis

Primary and metastatic tumors

**SHOULDER PAIN,
LOCAL CAUSES**

caine and steroids may also be useful in establishing the cause. Adson maneuvers will help establish the diagnosis of scalenus anticus syndrome, but the clinician must bear in mind that there are many false positives for this test and the job is not finished until tests for pectoralis minor and costoclavicular compression are also done. The history will help

TABLE 1-15. SHOULDER PAIN

	V Vascular	I Inflammatory	N Neoplasm	D Degenerative and Deficiency
Skin		Herpes zoster		
Muscle and Tendons		Epidemic myalgia Trichinosis Tendonitis biceps		
Blood Vessels	Arterial thrombosis Buerger's disease Dissecting aneurysm	Phlebitis		
Bursae		Bursitis		
Shoulder Joint		Purulent arthritis		Osteoarthritis
Bone	Aseptic bone necrosis	Osteomyelitis	Primary and metastatic tumors	
Brachial Plexus and Sympathetics		Neuritis	Lymphoma	
Cervical Spine		Osteomyelitis Tuberculosis Syphilis	Cord tumor (primary and metastatic)	Osteoarthritis
Systemic Causes	Coronary insufficiency Aortic aneurysm	Cholecystitis Pleurisy Subdiaphragmatic abscess	Pancoast's tumor	

diagnose systemic causes, but checking for dermatomal hyperalgesia or hypalgesia and other sensory changes will be most helpful in diagnosing disease of the cervical spine. Remember that a negative cervical spine x-ray film does not rule out a herniated disc. If the pain is increased by pressure on the top of the head or by coughing and sneezing,

I Intoxication Idiopathic	C Congenital	A Autoimmune Allergic	T Trauma	E Endocrine
Fibromyositis		Dermatomyositis	Contusion Ruptured tendon	
	Hemophilia	Vasculitis		
Gout				Pseudogout
Gouty arthritis Frozen shoulder		Rheumatoid arthritis Rheumatic fever Lupus	Shoulder dislocation Shoulder separation Torn ligaments	
			Fracture	
Shoulder–hand syndrome	Cervical ribs Scalenus anticus syndrome		Traumatic neuromas	
Cervical spondylosis	Klippel–Feil syndrome		Ruptured disc Fracture	

then a disc must be ruled out by myelography.

SORE THROAT

Breaking down the orophraynx, nasopharynx, and larynx into anatomical components is not very valuable in developing a differential diagnosis of sore throat. What is useful is to use the word **VINDICATE** to establish the etiologies. Further analyzing the differential (because so many causes of sore throat are infectious), one may recall the inflammatory etiologies in a systematic fashion by starting with the smallest organism and working to the largest.

Let us begin with **VINDICATE.**

V—Vascular reminds one of blood dyscrasias like leukemia, agranulocytosis of numerous causes, and Hodgkin's disease.

I—Inflammatory diseases include the most common causes of sore throat, streptococcal or viral pharyngitis, but one must also consider the less frequent infectious diseases here. Beginning with the smallest organism and moving to the largest, one thinks of viral pharyngitis, particularly herpangina (due to Coxsackie virus), pharyngoconjunctival fever (due to eight or more viruses), and infectious mononucleosis. Viral influenza may begin with a sore throat. Moving to a larger organism, one should remember that Eaton agent (mycoplasma) pneumonia may be associated with pharyngitis.

Next, **bacterial causes** such as group A hemolytic streptococcus (with or without scarlet fever), diphtheria, listeria monocytogenes, and meningococcemia should be considered. Gonorrhea is increasingly a cause of sore throat. Tuberculosis should also be mentioned, although it is rare in contemporary affluent societies. Consider among bacterial causes sinusitis, tonsillar or peritonsillar abscesses (quinsy), and retropharyngeal abscess. Staphylococcus may cause these but it rarely causes the common sore throat.

Moving to the next largest organisms, the spirochetes, think of syphilis and Vincent's angina. Remember finally, the fungi, including thrush (moniliasis) and actinomycosis.

N—Neoplasm and carcinomas may include Hodgkin's disease and leukemia. The Schmincke tumor is of particular interest here.

D—Degenerative diseases are an unlikely cause of sore throat, just as they are unlikely to cause pain anywhere.

I—Intoxication brings to mind chronic alcoholism and smoker's throat. Agranulocytosis may also be included in this category, since it is so often drug-induced.

C—Congenital diseases are also an infrequent cause of sore throat, but a hiatal hernia with reflux esophagitis may cause recurrent sore throat, because there may be reflux of gastric juice all the way to the posterior pharynx in the recumbent position. An elongated uvula may also be responsible.

A—Allergic diseases include angioneurotic edema of the pharynx or uvula and allergic rhinitis. Otherwise, this category is a rare etiology of sore throat.

T—Trauma brings to mind foreign bodies such as chicken bones and tonsillolithes.

E—Endocrine causes of sore throat should remind one of subacute thyroiditis; even though the pain is really in the neck, the patient will often say he has a "sore throat."

Approach to the Diagnosis

In diagnosing the cause of sore throat, it has been traditional to do a throat culture and possibly a cbc and differential and start the patient on penicillin until the culture comes

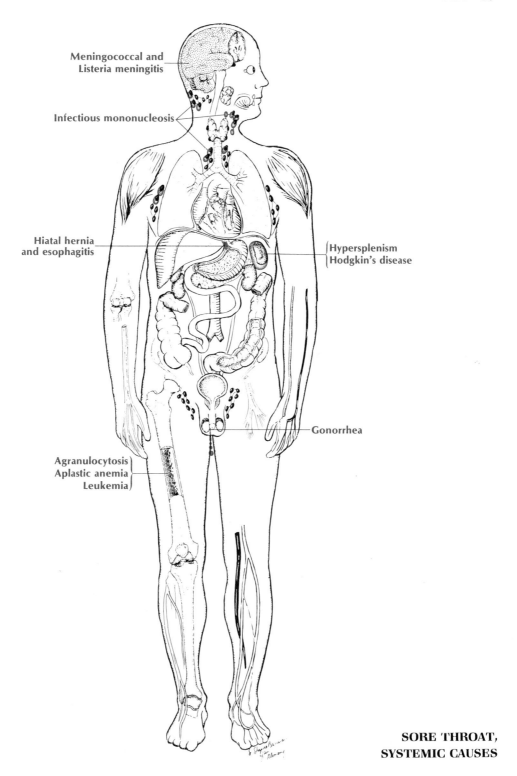

Meningococcal and
Listeria meningitis

Infectious mononucleosis

Hiatal hernia
and esophagitis

Hypersplenism
Hodgkin's disease

Gonorrhea

Agranulocytosis
Aplastic anemia
Leukemia

**SORE THROAT,
SYSTEMIC CAUSES**

back. Now Abbott Laboratories has developed a rapid strept agglutination test on a throat swab. In resistant cases, repeated cultures (especially for diphtheria, gonorrhea, and listeria) and a Mono spot test will be useful. Since the titer for infectious mononucleosis may not be high initially, the differential test (Paul–Bunnell) or a repeat Mono spot test 1 to 3 weeks later may be necessary.

TESTICULAR PAIN

It is helpful but unnecessary to do an anatomical breakdown in developing this differential diagnosis. The mnemonic **MINT** brings the most important causes to mind instantly.

M—Malformation suggests hernias, varicocele, and torsion of the testicle.

I—Inflammation recalls epididymitis and epididymo-orchitis.

N—Neoplasms of the testicles may be virtually painless, but the mass will give them away. Tuberculosis is also unlikely to cause significant pain.

T—Traumatic lesions are common in contact sports, but occasionally a boy will deny a history of trauma.

Referred pain from renal calculi is a significant cause of testicular pain. Any condition that irritates the T_{12} nerve root (*e.g.*, osteoarthritis and herniated disc) and the course of the peripheral portion of this nerve (appendicitis) may cause testicular pain, but these are uncommon causes.

Approach to the Diagnosis

The approach to the diagnosis of testicular pain involves searching for a mass; if it is present, certain questions must be answered.

Does it transilluminate (hydrocele)? Can one get above the swelling (testicular mass)? Is it reducible (hernia)? Does supporting the testicle relieve the pain (torsion)? A search for prostatic hypertrophy or prostatitis should be made, particularly in older men. Smears of urethral discharge, urinalysis and urine culture, cystoscopy, and an intravenous pyelogram may be indicated in selected cases. An exploration for torsion or hernia may be the only way to establish these diagnoses.

TONGUE PAIN

Examination of the tongue is a time-honored important diagnostic aid, but in my experience it is unusual for patients to present with pain in the tongue. Nevertheless, there is a plethora of causes. The mnemonic **VINDICATE** lends itself best to prompting the recall of these causes.

V—Vascular suggests pernicious and iron deficiency anemia.

I—Inflammation recalls Vincent's stomatitis, herpes simplex, tuberculosis, and syphilis. The referred pain from gingivitis and abscessed teeth should also be considered here.

N—Neoplasms remind one that carcinoma of the tongue often presents with pain.

D—Degenerative and **deficiency** diseases remind one of pellagra and other avitaminosis.

I—Intoxication and **idiopathic** call to mind tobacco, plumbism, mercurialism, and glossopharyngeal or trigeminal neuralgia.

C—Congenital anomalies of the tongue are rare.

A—Allergic and **autoimmune** diseases, on the other hand, suggest dermatomyositis and angioneurotic edema.

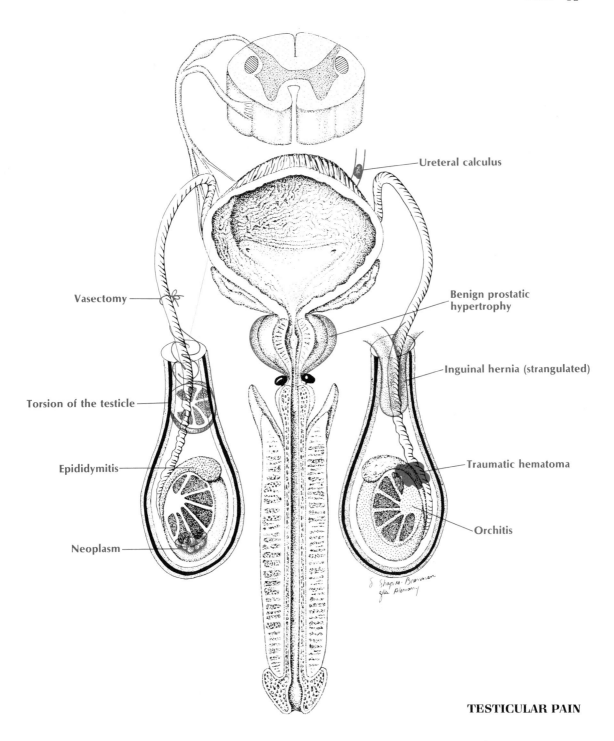

Ureteral calculus

Vasectomy

Benign prostatic hypertrophy

Torsion of the testicle

Inguinal hernia (strangulated)

Epididymitis

Traumatic hematoma

Neoplasm

Orchitis

TESTICULAR PAIN

T—Trauma suggests the numerous times we bite our tongues and may prompt a search for epilepsy when a patient presents with syncope.

E—Endocrine reminds one of hypothyroidism.

Approach to the Diagnosis

The approach to the diagnosis includes a cbc, sedimentation rate, serology, tuberculin test, and perhaps biopsy of the lesion. A trial of vitamin therapy may be indicated.

TOOTHACHE

Toothache is included here not only because dentists might read this book but also because physicians are occasionally called on to manage toothache until a dentist can be reached. A **histological analysis** of the tooth and surrounding structures will supply the differential diagnosis. Most commonly, the **pulp** may be exposed by dental caries, but then the pain is intermittent. When the pulp is infected (pulpitis) the pain is continuous, and the pulp may subsequently become abscessed. The **periapical tissue** may be inflamed, and an alveolar abscesss may ensue. Finally an **osteomyelitis** of the **jaw** or **maxillary bones** may occur. The **gingiva** may be inflamed and pyorrhea will result. What is often not appreciated by physicians is that the tooth can be sore and inflamed without objective evidence on examination. A common cause of this situation is a filling which is close to or in apposition with the pulp.

Referred pain is as important here as it is in other structures of the head. Thus, sinusitis, otitis media, and temporomandibular joint disease may cause pain in the tooth. Trigeminal neuralgia and other neurological disorders must occasionally be considered.

Approach to the Diagnosis

This is simple. Refer the patient to a dentist. If infection is suspected, an antibiotic may be started if there is a delay in getting an appointment. If the dentist cannot find the cause, referral to a neurologist would be appropriate.

MASS OR SWELLING
Chapter 2

GENERAL DISCUSSION

With few exceptions, **anatomy** and **histology** are the basic sciences that are most useful in developing a differential diagnosis of a mass or swelling. Visualizing the anatomical structures in any given part of the body and then breaking down each structure into its histological components is the key.

When the physician is examining a mass anywhere in the body, he should ask himself what it could be composed of. It could be composed of one or more of the following:

1. An increased amount of extracellular fluid (*e.g.*, edema or ascites) from inflammatory or noninflammatory causes.
2. Hemorrhage into the organ or space.
3. Increased amount of air in the tissues (subcutaneous emphysema).
4. Hypertrophy or hyperplasia of one or more of the cellular components of the organ or tissues in the area caused by neoplasia or a reaction to infection (granuloma).
5. The presence of an organ that normally is found elsewhere (*e.g.*, pelvic kidney).
6. The invasion of the area by a tissue that is normally found elsewhere (*e.g.*, metastatic carcinoma).
7. Obstruction of a duct leading from the area, causing an increase in the amount of a fluid normally present (*e.g.*, hydrops of the gallbladder).
8. Obstruction of the veins or lymphatics leading from the area or dilatation of the artery or vein.
9. Remnant of a congenital tissue (*e.g.*, dermoid cyst or thyroglossal duct cyst) that gradually hypertrophies.
10. The presence of an abnormal solid in the

area (*e.g.*, cystine or urate deposits) or an increase in the amount of a solid normally present (*e.g.*, feces). The physician's diagnostic acumen in dealing with mass lesions will be enhanced if he keeps these principles in mind.

The etiologies of most masses are either malformations, inflammation, neoplasm, or trauma. The mnemonic **MINT** allows quick recall of these.

M—Malformations might lead one to consider congenital cysts (*e.g.*, polycystic kidneys).

I—Inflammation should suggest abscesses, swellings of an organ caused by inflammation and granulomas.

N—Neoplasms can include hyperplasia (benign or malignant) of any type of tissue in the body. Thus proliferation of liver parenchyma would suggest a hepatoma, proliferation of epidermis would suggest a squamous cell carcinoma, and proliferation of connective tissue would indicate a sarcoma.

T—Trauma suggests fracture-dislocations, herniated discs, hematomas, and rupture of muscle, ligaments, or fascia. These concepts will be expanded as each symptom is developed.

Once a group of possibilities is recalled, the next step is to eliminate as many as possible by a thorough history and physical examination. The presence or absence of other symptoms and signs is important in establishing the exact diagnosis. An acute onset of the mass would suggest trauma or infection, whereas a gradual onset suggests neoplasm. Painful masses are likely to be inflammatory, traumatic, or vascular lesions, painless lesions are often congenital malformations or neoplasms.

The laboratory workup of each mass is listed in Appendix I. Certain procedures may apply in the workup of all masses. These are x-ray films, computerized axial tomography (CT scans), ultrasonography, angiography, phlebography, needle biopsy or exploration, and open biopsy. The workup of specific mass lesions such as carcinoma of the pancreas or hypernephroma can be found in Appendix II.

These, then, are the steps to be taken in diagnosing a mass.

1. Develop a list of causes to be considered.
2. Take a thorough history and physical examination with these causes in mind.
3. Group the signs and symptoms together in order to include or exclude certain causes in the list.
4. Order appropriate laboratory tests to exclude unlikely causes or pinpoint the most likely diagnosis.

ABDOMINAL MASS

Abdominal Mass, Generalized

As the physician examines the abdomen, how can he recall all of the causes of a mass or swelling? He should ask himself what a mass may be composed of. It may be **air,** in which case he would think of air in the peritoneum with rupture of a viscus, particularly a peptic ulcer; or it may be air in the intestinal tract from focal or generalized distention, in which case he would recall gastric dilatation, intestinal obstruction related to numerous causes (p. 3), or paralytic ileus. The mass may be **fluid,** in which case he would recall fluid in the abdominal wall (anasarca), the peritoneum (ascites, p. 94) and its various causes, and fluid (urine) accumulation in the bladder or intestine or cysts of other abdominal organs. The

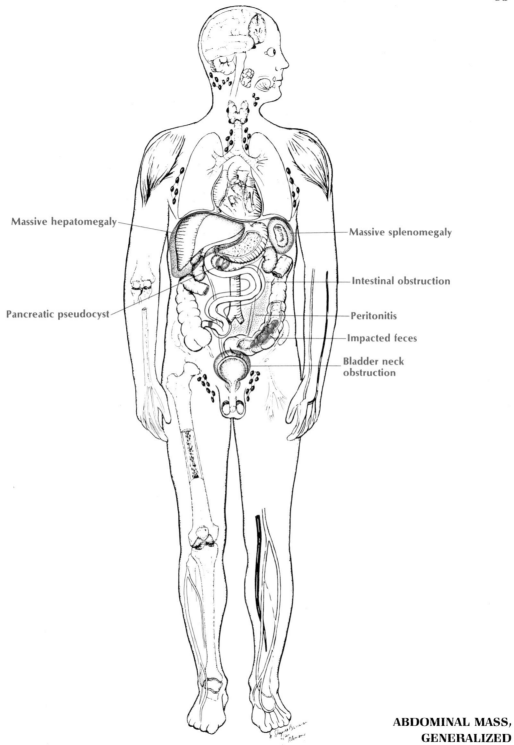

Massive hepatomegaly

Massive splenomegaly

Intestinal obstruction

Pancreatic pseudocyst

Peritonitis

Impacted feces

Bladder neck
obstruction

**ABDOMINAL MASS,
GENERALIZED**

latter brings to mind ovarian cysts, pancreatic cysts, and omental cysts. The mass may be **blood** in the peritoneal wall, the peritoneum, or any of the organ systems of the abdomen. The mass may be a solid **inorganic substance,** such as the fecal accumulation in celiac disease and Hirschsprung's disease. Finally, the mass may be a **hypertrophy, swelling,** or **neoplasm** of any one of the organs or tissues in the abdomen.

This is where **anatomy** comes in. In the abdominal wall there may be an accumulation of fat (obesity). The **liver** may be enlarged by neoplasm or obstruction of its vascular supply (*e.g.,* Budd-Chiari syndrome or cardiac cirrhosis), or by obstruction of the biliary tree with neoplasms or biliary cirrhosis. The **spleen** may become massively enlarged by hypertrophy, hyperplasia in Gaucher's disease, infiltration of cells in chronic myelogenous leukemia and myeloid metaplasia, and by inflammation in kala-azar. The **kidney** rarely enlarges to the point where it causes a generalized abdominal swelling in hydronephrosis, but a Wilm's tumor or carcinoma may occasionally become extremely large.

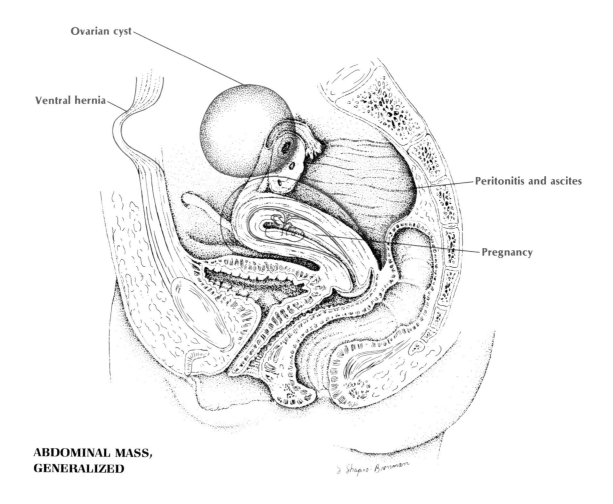

Ovarian cyst

Ventral hernia

Peritonitis and ascites

Pregnancy

ABDOMINAL MASS, GENERALIZED

J. Shapiro-Brennan

The **bladder,** as mentioned above, may be enlarged sufficiently to present a generalized abdominal swelling when it becomes obstructed, but neoplasms of the bladder will not present as a huge mass by themselves. The **uterus** presents as a generalized abdominal mass in late stages of pregnancy, but ovarian cysts should be first considered in huge masses arising from the female genital tract. Pancreatic cysts and pseudocysts are another possible cause of a generalized abdominal swelling, although they are usually localized to the right upper quadrant or epigastrium. It would be unusual for an aortic aneurysm to grow to a size sufficient to cause a generalized abdominal mass, but it is frequently mentioned in differential diagnosis texts.

The above method is one method of developing a differential diagnosis of generalized abdominal swelling or mass. Sticking solely to anatomy and cross-indexing the various structures with the mnemonic **MINT** is another. This is suggested as an exercise for the reader. Take each organ system as a tract. Thus, the **gastrointestinal tract** presents most commonly with a diffuse swelling in intestinal obstruction and paralytic ileus; the **biliary tract** and pancreas with hepatitis, neoplasms, and pancreatic pseudocysts. The **urinary tract** presents with a diffuse "mass" in bladder neck obstruction. The female genital tract may be the cause of a huge abdominal mass in ovarian cysts, neoplasms, and pregnancy. Apply the same technique to the spleen and abdominal wall to complete the picture.

There are, in addition, certain conditions that cause abdominal swelling that is more apparent than real. Lumbar lordosis causes abdominal protuberance, as does visceroptosis. A huge ventral hernia or diastasis recti may mimic an abdominal swelling. Psychogenic protrusion of the belly by straining is another cause.

Approach to the Diagnosis

What can be done to work up a diffuse abdominal swelling? It is important to catheterize the bladder if there is any question at all that this may be the cause. A flat plate of the abdomen and lateral decubiti and upright films will help in diagnosing intestinal obstruction, a ruptured viscus, or peritoneal fluid. If pregnancy or ovarian cysts can be definitely excluded by CT scans and/or ultrasonography, then a diagnostic peritoneal tap may be helpful in the diagnosis. Other useful tests for the differential diagnosis are listed in Appendix I.

Right Upper Quadrant Mass

When the clinician lays his hand on the right upper quadrant (RUQ) and feels a mass, he should visualize the anatomy and the differential diagnosis should become clear to him. Proceeding from the skin, he encounters the subcutaneous tissue, fascia, muscle, peritoneum, liver, hepatic flexure of the colon, gallbladder, duodenum, pancreas, kidney, and adrenal gland. The blood vessels and lymphatics to these organs should be considered and also the bile and pancreatic ducts. Then, because masses are caused by a more limited number of etiologies, apply the mnemonic **MINT** to each organ. The differential using these methods is developed in Table 2-1.

Skin malformations do not usually cause a mass, but inflammation of the skin is manifested by cellulitis and carbuncles and neoplasms are manifested as carcinomas, both primary and metastatic. Trauma of the skin is usually manifested by the obvious contusions or laceration. A mass of the **subcutaneous tissue** may be a lipoma, fibroma, metastatic carcinoma, cellulitis, or contusion. A mass disease of the **fascia** is usually the result of a hernia. The causes of hepatomegaly are reviewed on page 139, but if the mass is in the **liver** it is usually hepatitis, amebic or septic abscess, carcinoma (primary or metastatic), contusions, or laceration. A Riedel's lobe should not be mistaken for a large gallbladder. The **hepatic flexure of the colon** may be enlarged by a diverticulitis, carcinoma, patch of granulomatous colitis, contusion, or volvulus. Malrotation may cause a mass in infants. Retrocaecal appendix should not be forgotten here either.

An enlarged gallbladder accounts for the mass in the RUQ in many cases; it may be caused by cholecystitis, obstruction of the neck of the cystic duct by a stone causing gallbladder hydrops, or a Courvoisier gallbladder caused by obstruction of the bile duct by a carcinoma of the head of the pancreas. Cholangiocarcinoma may cause an enlarged gallbladder.

The **pancreas** may be enlarged in **M—Malformations** by congenital or acquired pancreatic cysts, **I—Inflammation** of an acute or chronic pancreatitis, **N—Neoplasm,** and **T—Traumatic** pseudocysts.

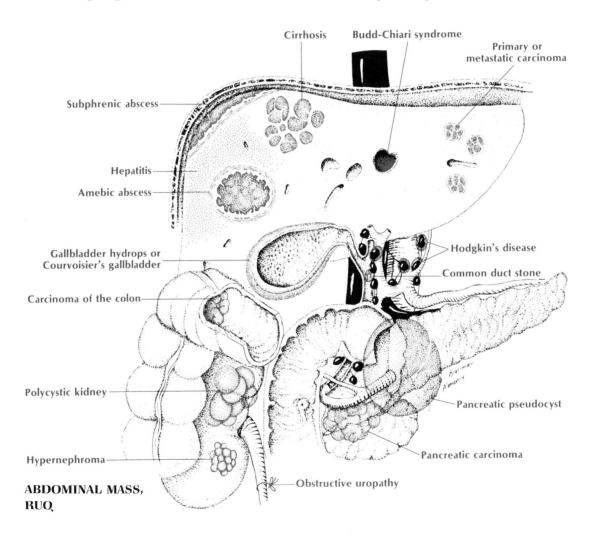

ABDOMINAL MASS, RUQ

TABLE 2-1. RIGHT UPPER QUADRANT MASS

	M Malformation	I Inflammation	N Neoplasm	T Trauma
Skin	Sebaceous cyst	Abscess	Carcinomas (primary or metastatic)	Contusion
Subcutaneous Tissue and Fascia	Hernia	Cellulitis	Metastatic carcinoma Lipoma	Contusion
Muscle		Myositis		Contusion
Liver	Cysts Riedel's lobe	Abscess Hepatitis	Carcinoma (primary and metastatic)	Contusion Laceration
Hepatic Flexure of Colon	Diverticulum Malrotation	Diverticulitis Retrocaecal appendix	Carcinoma of the colon	Contusion Perforation
Gallbladder and Ducts	Hydrops	Cholecystitis Cholelithiasis	Pancreatic carcinoma Cholangioma Choledochal carcinoma	Contusion
Duodenum		Perforation of ulcer with subphrenic abscess		
Pancreas	Pancreatic cysts	Acute and chronic pancreatitis	Carcinoma of the head of the pancreas	Traumatic pseudocyst
Kidney	Renal cyst Hydronephrosis Polycystic kidney	Hydronephrosis Pyonephrosis Perinephric abscess	Wilm's tumor Hypernephroma	Contusion Laceration
Adrenal Gland			Neuroblastoma Pheochromocytoma Adrenal carcinoma	
Lymph Nodes			Hodgkin's disease Metastatic carcinoma	

A **duodenal** diverticulum is not usually felt as a mass, but a perforated duodenal ulcer may manifest itself by a palpable subphrenic abscess in the right anterior intraperitoneal pouch. Malformations of the **kidney** often cause hydronephrosis, whereas inflammation may cause a perinephric abscess and thus an RUQ mass. Carcinoma or Wilm's tumor of the kidney is frequently responsible for a large kidney.

Carcinomas of the **adrenal gland** are not usually palpable until late in the disease process but a neuroblastoma is palpable early. Other lesions of the adrenal gland are not usually associated with a mass.

Aneurysms, emboli, and thrombosis of the vessels supplying these organs usually do not produce a mass, but a thrombosis of the hepatic vein (the well-known Budd–Chiari syndrome) causes hepatomegaly, and emboli and thrombi of the mesenteric vessels of the colon may cause focal enlargement from obstruction and infarction. Visualizing the lymphatics should remind one of Hodgkin's disease in the portal area.

Approach to the Diagnosis

To diagnose a right upper quadrant mass, first look for associated signs and symptoms. If jaundice is present, is it obstructive or parenchymal? Is there associated pain or blood in the stool? The answers to these questions and the laboratory workup in Appendix I will usually pin down the diagnosis. If a certain disease is immediately suspected by the history and physical examination, the specific tests to confirm it will be found in Appendix II. A surgical consultation is wise from the outset.

Left Upper Quadrant Mass

The differential diagnosis for left upper quadrant (LUQ) masses is not a great deal different from that of the right upper quadrant. The anatomy is similar: just replace the liver with the spleen and the gallbladder with the stomach. The presence of the aorta on the side of the abdomen should not be forgotten. Again, **anatomy** is the key, as shown in Table 2-2. Cross-index the various organs and tissues with the etiologies using **MINT** as the mnemonic.

M—Malformations of the skin, subcutaneous tissue, fascia, and muscle are primarily hernias; for the spleen they are **aneurysms;** for the splenic flexure of the colon, they are mainly volvulus, intussusceptions, and diverticuli. Gastric dilatation of the stomach is secondary to obstruction or pneumonia. Cysts are common for the pancreas, just as polycystic disease, single cysts, and hydronephrosis are for the kidney. There is no common malformation for the adrenal gland.

I—Inflammatory conditions of the skin, subcutaneous tissue, muscle, and fascia are primarily abscesses and cellulitis. In the spleen a host of systemic inflammatory lesions can cause enlargement (see p. 169) but actual primary infections of the spleen are unusual. The colon may be inflamed by diverticulitis, granulomatous colitis, and occasionally by tuberculosis. Inflammatory disease of the stomach does not usually produce a mass, but if an ulcer perforates or if a diverticulum ruptures, a subphrenic abscess may form in the left hypochondrium. Inflammatory pseudocysts may form in the tail of the pancreas. A palpable perinephric abscess and an enlarged kidney from acute pyelonephritis or tuberculosis may be felt, but inflammatory lesions of the adrenal gland are rarely palpable.

N—Neoplasms of the organs mentioned above account for most of the masses in the LUQ. A carcinoma of the stomach or colon, Hodgkin's disease and chronic leukemias involving the spleen, Wilm's tumor, or carcinoma of the kidney and neuroblastoma must be considered. A retroperitoneal sarcoma is occasionally responsible for an LUQ mass.

T—Trauma to the spleen or kidney will produce a tender mass in the LUQ. Less common traumatic lesions here include contusion of the muscle and perforation of the stomach or colon. It should be noted that the left lobe of the liver may project into the LUQ so that tumors and abscess of the liver must be considered.

Approach to the Diagnosis

The approach to the diagnosis involves a search for associated symptoms and the use of Appendix I for the laboratory workup. A surgical consultation is wise at the outset.

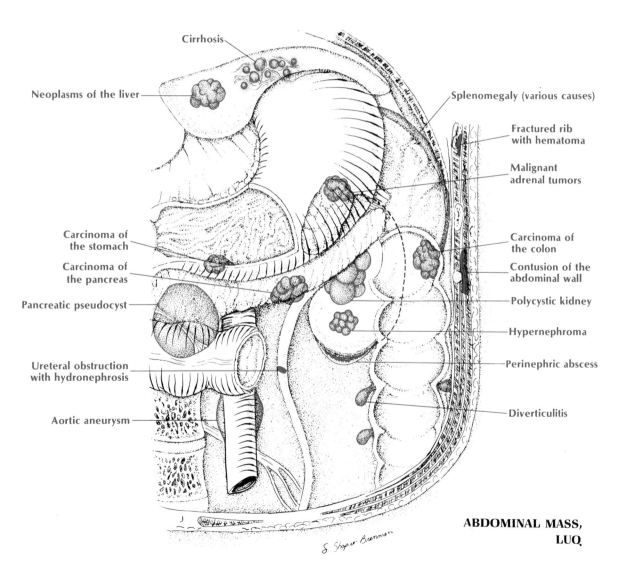

ABDOMINAL MASS, LUQ

TABLE 2-2. LEFT UPPER QUADRANT MASS

	M Malformation	I Inflammation	N Neoplasm	T Trauma
Skin	Sebaceous cyst	Abscess	Carcinoma (primary or metastatic)	Contusion
Subcutaneous Tissue and Fascia	Hernia	Cellulitis	Metastatic tumors Lipoma	Contusion
Muscle		Myositis		Contusion
Spleen	Aneurysms Accessory spleens	Tuberculosis Systemic disease Malaria	Hodgkin's disease Chronic leukemia	Contusion Laceration
Stomach	Gastric dilatation	Perforated ulcer with subphrenic abscess	Carcinoma of the stomach	Perforation
Splenic Flexure of the Colon	Diverticulum Volvulus Intussusception	Diverticulitis	Carcinoma of the colon	Contusion Perforation
Pancreas	Pancreatic cysts	Pseudocyst from pancreatitis	Carcinoma of the pancreas	Traumatic pseudocyst
Kidney	Hydronephrosis Polycystic kidney Renal cyst	Hydronephrosis Pyonephrosis Perinephric abscess	Wilm's tumor Hypernephroma	Contusion Laceration
Adrenal Gland			Neuroblastoma Pheochromocytoma Adrenal carcinoma	
Lymph Nodes			Hodgkin's disease Retroperitoneal lymphosarcoma	
Blood Vessels	Aortic aneurysm			

Right Lower Quadrant Mass

Anatomy is once again the key to developing a differential diagnosis of a right lower quadrant (RLQ) mass. Underneath the skin, subcutaneous tissue, fascia, and muscle, lie the caecum, appendix, terminal ileum, iliac artery and vein, and the ilium. In the female, the tube and ovary should be included. Occasion-

ally a ptosed kidney will be felt here also. Now apply the etiological mnemonic **MINT** to each organ and you should have a reliable differential diagnosis, like that in Table 2-3. The important lesions to remember here are the following:

M—Malformations like inguinal and femoral hernias may be present.

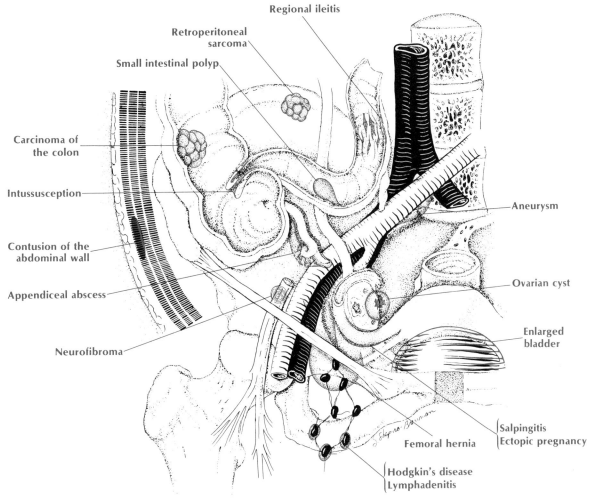

Regional ileitis

Retroperitoneal sarcoma

Small intestinal polyp

Carcinoma of the colon

Intussusception

Contusion of the abdominal wall

Appendiceal abscess

Neurofibroma

Aneurysm

Ovarian cyst

Enlarged bladder

Salpingitis
Ectopic pregnancy

Femoral hernia

Hodgkin's disease
Lymphadenitis

ABDOMINAL MASS, RLQ

I—Inflammations include acute appendicitis with abscess, tubo-ovarian abscesses, and regional ileitis,

N—Neoplasms to be considered in this area are carcinoma of the caecum and tumors of the ovary.

T—Traumatic lesions include fracture or contusion of the ileum and perforation of the bowel from a stab wound.

The lymph nodes may be involved with tuberculosis or actinomycosis. The caecum may also be enlarged by accumulation of ascaris or other parasites. The omentum can contribute to adhesions of the bowel to form a mass or it may develop cysts in its substance.

Approach to the Diagnosis

A complete history, a careful rectal and vaginal examination, and a check for the presence or absence of other signs like metorrhagia, bloody stools, fever and chills will do much to pin down the diagnosis, but with a differen-

TABLE 2-3.   RIGHT LOWER QUADRANT MASS

	M Malformation	I Inflammation	N Neoplasm	T Trauma
Skin	Sebaceous cysts	Abscess	Primary or metastatic carcinomas	Contusions
Subcutaneous Tissue and Fascia	Hernias	Cellulitis	Metastatic carcinomas Lipoma	Contusions
Caecum	Intussusception Diverticulum Intestinal obstruction	Diverticulitis Granulomatous colitis Parasites Amebiasis Ulcerative colitis	Carcinoma of the caecum	Perforation Contusion
Muscle		Psoas abscess Myositis		Contusion
Appendix	Fecalith	Appendicitis Appendiceal abscess	Carcinoid	Perforation
Terminal Ileum	Intussusception Meckel's diverticulum Intestinal obstruction	Regional ileitis Typhoid Tuberculosis	Polyps Carcinoid Sarcomas	Perforation Contusion
Iliac Blood Vessels	Aneurysms	Thrombophlebitis		
Lymph Nodes		Tuberculous adenitis	Metastatic tumors	
Ilium		Osteomyelitis	Sarcoma	Fracture or contusion

tial diagnosis in mind before beginning, one is in a better position to ask the right questions and perform the right examinations. Appendix I provides a list of diagnostic tests to utilize the workup. If a certain disease is strongly suspected, Appendix II provides a list of more specific tests that should be ordered.

Left Lower Quadrant Mass

To quickly develop a list of etiologies of a left lower quadrant (LLQ) mass, visualize the **anatomy** of the area. Compared to the RUQ, the number of organs there is few. Beneath the skin, subcutaneous tissue, fascia, and

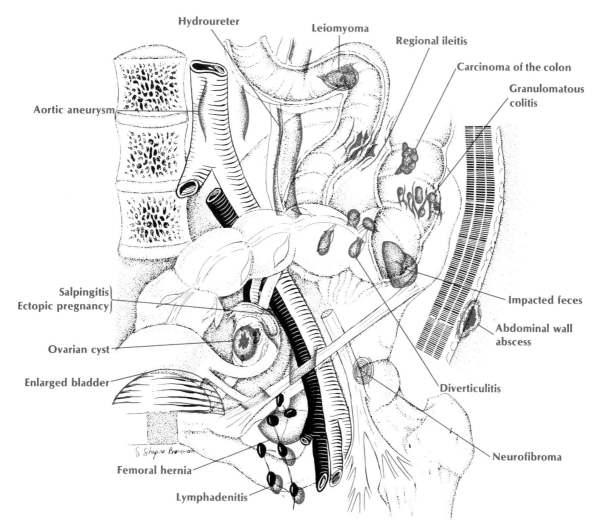

ABDOMINAL MASS, LLQ

muscle, are the sigmoid colon, the iliac artery and veins, the aorta, and the ileum. In the female, one must remember the tube and ovary. Occasionally, the kidney drops into this region (nephroptosis) and the omentum may cause adhesion. Now apply the mnemonic **MINT** to each organ and the list of possibilities in Table 2-4 is completed without any difficulty.

Lesions of the **skin** and **fascia** are similar to those in upper quadrants with one exception: because of the inguinal and femoral canals, hernias (especially indirect inguinal hernias) are much more frequent. In the **sigmoid colon** the following conditions should be considered:

M—Malformations include diverticuli and volvulus.

TABLE 2-4. **LEFT LOWER QUADRANT MASS**

	M Malformation	I Inflammation	N Neoplasm	T Trauma
Skin	Sebaceous cysts	Abscess	Primary and metastatic carcinoma	Contusion
Subcutaneous Tissue and Fascia	Hernia	Cellulitis	Metastatic carcinomas Lipomas	Contusion
Muscle		Myositis		Contusion
Sigmoid Colon	Diverticuli Volvulus Intestinal obstruction	Diverticulitis and abscess Tuberculosis Granulomatous and ulcerative colitis	Carcinomas and polyps	Perforation Contusion Foreign body
Tube and Ovary	Hydatid cyst of Morgagni Ectopic pregnancy	Tubo-ovarian abscess	Ovarian cysts and carcinomas	
Iliac Artery and Veins and Aorta	Aneurysms	Thrombophlebitis		
Lymph Nodes		Tuberculous and acute infectious adenitis	Metastatic tumors	
Ilium		Osteomyelitis	Sarcoma	Fracture or contusion

I—**Inflammatory** conditions to be considered are diverticulitis, abscesses, and granulomatous and ulcerative colitis.

N—**Neoplasms** such as polyps and carcinomas may be present.

T—**Trauma** to this area may involve perforations and contusions.

This list excludes an important consideration, that of fecal impaction. If the patient is given an enema the mass will often disappear. Less common causes of masses in the sigmoid colon are tuberculosis, amebiasis, and other parasites.

There may be aneurysms of the **iliac artery** or **aorta** and thrombosis of the **iliac vein,** although the latter is not usually palpable. The **iliac lymph nodes** may enlarge from Hodgkin's disease, metastatic carcinoma, or tuberculosis. **Tubal** and **ovarian** lesions that should come to mind are malignant and benign ovarian cysts, tubo-ovarian abscesses, ectopic pregnancy, and endometriosis. A sarcoma or other tumors of the **ilium** may be palpable but abscesses of the sacroiliac joint rarely are.

Approach to the Diagnosis

The approach to this diagnosis includes a careful pelvic and rectal examination, a search for the presence of blood in the stool, weight loss, tenderness of the mass, fever and other symptoms, and a laboratory workup. As mentioned above, an enema may diagnose and treat a fecal impaction. Stool examination (for blood, ova, and parasites), sigmoidoscopy, and barium enemas are the most useful diagnostic procedures other than a colonoscopy. Arteriography and gallium scans (for diverticular and other abscesses) and the CT scan have become useful additions to the diagnostic armamentarium. Peritoneoscopy and exploratory laparotomy are still necessary in many cases.

Epigastric Mass

In developing the differential diagnosis of an epigastric mass, one merely needs to visualize the anatomy of the epigastrium from skin to spine. The conditions are presented in outline form in Table 2-5, but the important conditions are emphasized in the following discussion.

1. **Abdominal wall.** Here the physician must consider ventral hernias, contusions in the wall, the xiphoid cartilage (that occasionally fools the novice), and lipomas or sebaceous cysts.
2. **Diaphragm.** A subphrenic abscess may be felt here.
3. **Liver.** The liver extends over into the epigastrium and even occasionally into LUQ, thus any cause of hepatomegaly (p. 139) may present as an epigastric mass.
4. **Omentum.** This may be enlarged by a cyst, a mass of adhesions, tuberculomas, or metastatic carcinoma.
5. **Stomach.** The acute dilatation in pneumonia or pyloric stenosis needs to be recalled. One usually thinks of carcinoma of the stomach or a perforated ulcer, however, when this organ is visualized.
6. **Colon.** Carcinoma, toxic megacolon, or diverticulitis may cause a mass in this organ but a hard chunk of feces may do so too.
7. **Pancreas.** Important conditions that must be considered here are carcinoma of the pancreas and pancreatic cysts. Chronic pancreatitis may present as a mass occasionally.
8. **Retroperitoneal lymph nodes.** Lymphoma, retroperitoneal sarcoma, and metastatic tumors may make these nodes palpable.
9. **Aorta.** An aortic aneurysm may be felt but more often the examiner is fooled by a normal or slightly enlarged aorta.

10. **Spine.** Deformities of the spine (e.g., lordosis) may make it especially prominent, but a fracture, metastatic neoplasm, myeloma, or arthritis may do the same.

Approach to the Diagnosis

This is similar to the approach for all abdominal masses. The association of other symptoms and signs is important in pinpointing the diagnosis. For example, a mass with anorexia and vomiting suggests gastric or pancreatic carcinoma. A painful mass suggests a perforated, walled-off ulcer or pancreatitis. Diagnostic procedures include examining stools for occult blood, ordering an upper GI series and a barium enema, and performing gastroscopy and duodenoscopy and liver function tests. Total body computerized axial tomography has allowed a definitive diagno-

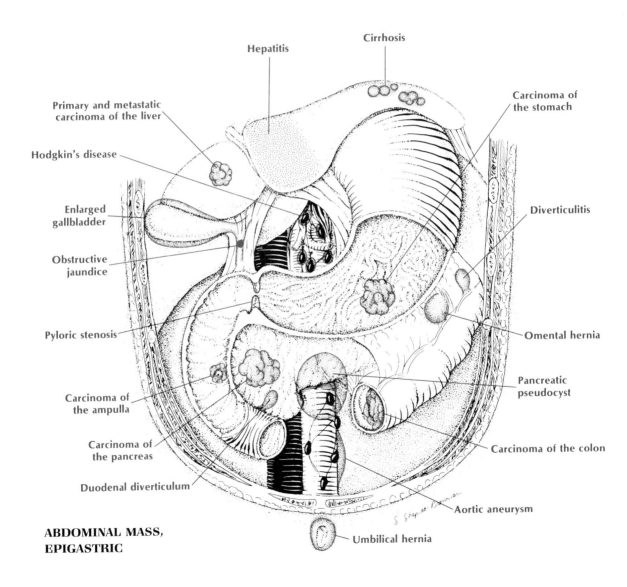

Hepatitis

Cirrhosis

Primary and metastatic
carcinoma of the liver

Carcinoma of
the stomach

Hodgkin's disease

Enlarged
gallbladder

Diverticulitis

Obstructive
jaundice

Pyloric stenosis

Omental hernia

Pancreatic
pseudocyst

Carcinoma of
the ampulla

Carcinoma of
the pancreas

Carcinoma of the colon

Duodenal diverticulum

Aortic aneurysm

**ABDOMINAL MASS,
EPIGASTRIC**

Umbilical hernia

TABLE 2-5. EPIGASTRIC MASS

	M Malformation	I Inflammation	N Neoplasm	T Trauma
Abdominal Wall	Hernia	Cellulitis Carbuncles	Lipoma Sebaceous cysts	Contusions
Diaphragm	Hiatal hernia	Subphrenic abscess		
Liver	Cysts Hemangiomas	Abscess Hepatitis	Hepatoma Metastatic carcinoma	Contusion Laceration
Omentum	Adhesions Cysts	Peritonitis Tuberculoma	Metastatic carcinoma	Traumatic fat necrosis Hemorrhage
Stomach	Hypertrophic pyloric stenosis	Gastric ulcer Gastric dilatation Gastric syphilis	Gastric carcinomas	Hemorrhage Stab wounds
Colon	Hirschsprung's disease Intussusception Volvulus	Diverticulitis Toxic megacolon	Colon carcinoma Polyps	Contusion Laceration
Pancreas	Cyst Pseudocyst	Pancreatitis	Carcinoma of pancreas	Contusion
Retroperitoneal Lymph Nodes		Tuberculosis	Lymphoma Sarcoma Metastatic carcinoma	
Aorta	Aneurysm			
Spine	Lordosis Scoliosis	Tuberculosis Arthritis Osteomyelitis	Metastatic carcinoma Myeloma Hodgkin's disease	Fracture Herniated disc Hematoma

sis in many cases prior to exploratory laparotomy. Other tests are listed in Appendix I.

Hypogastric Mass

More physicians have been fooled by a hypogastric mass than by a mass in any other area. How many times can you recall the mass disappearing on the operating table after catheterization of the bladder? More often than not the mass is more apparent than real because of a lumbar lordosis or a diastasis recti.

Anatomy is the key to the differential diagnosis. There really are not many organs here normally. Under the skin, subcutaneous tissue, fascia, and rectus abdominus muscles, the bladder, terminal aorta, and lumbosacral spine may be palpated in a thin male. In the female, the uterus may be palpated on bimanual pelvic examination. When there is visceroptosis the transverse colon will be palpated.

Under pathological conditions, however, the lymph nodes, sigmoid colon, tube and ovary, and small intestines may be palpated as well as a pelvic kidney. Applying the mnemonic **MINT** to these organs results in the extensive differential diagnosis in Table 2-6. The discussion that follows mentions only the most significant causes of a hypogastric mass.

Lipomas of the skin, ventral hernias, and

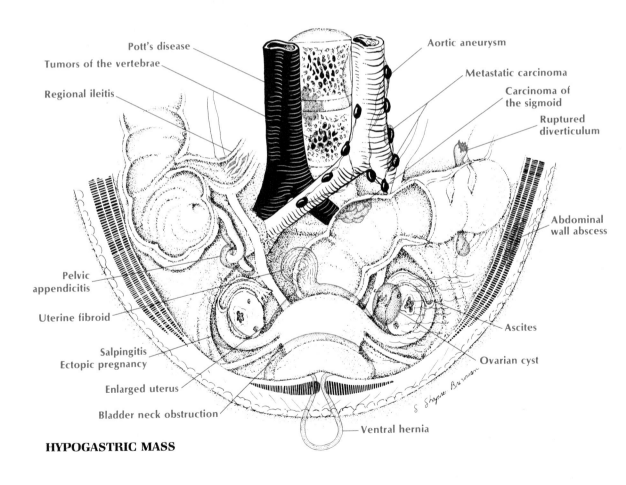

Pott's disease
Tumors of the vertebrae
Regional ileitis
Pelvic appendicitis
Uterine fibroid
Salpingitis Ectopic pregnancy
Enlarged uterus
Bladder neck obstruction

Aortic aneurysm
Metastatic carcinoma
Carcinoma of the sigmoid
Ruptured diverticulum
Abdominal wall abscess
Ascites
Ovarian cyst
Ventral hernia

HYPOGASTRIC MASS

TABLE 2-6. MASS IN THE HYPOGASTRIUM

	M Acquired or Congenital Malformation	I Inflammation	N Neoplasm	T Trauma
Skin	Sebaceous cyst	Abscess	Primary and metastatic tumors Lipomas	Contusion
Subcutaneous Tissue and Fascia	Ventral hernia	Cellulitis	Primary and metastatic tumors Lipomas Neurofibromas	Contusion
Muscle	Diastasis recti	Myositis		Contusion
Bladder	Diverticulum Obstruction Stone		Carcinoma of bladder or prostate Prostatic hypertrophy	Ruptured bladder
Transverse Colon	Diverticulum Volvulus Intussusception	Diverticular abscess Granulomatous colitis Toxic megacolon	Carcinoma of colon	Contusion or perforation
Uterus	Pregnancy Endometriosis	Endometritis and parametritis	Fibroids Endometrial carcinoma Cervical carcinoma Choriocarcinoma	Perforation Contusion
Tube and Ovary	Ectopic pregnancy	Tubo-ovarian abscess	Ovarian cysts (benign and malignant)	Perforation Rupture
Aorta	Aneurysm Leriche's syndrome Arteriosclerosis			Perforation
Lumbosacral Spine	Spondylolisthesis Lordosis	Pott's disease Osteomyelitis	Metastatic tumors	Herniated disc
Pre-aortic Lymph Nodes		Tuberculous adenitis	Metastatic carcinoma or Hodgkin's disease	Herniated disc

Peritoneum	Obstruction of
	   portal vein with
	   ascites
		Ascites from tubercu-
		   losis or gonorrhea
			Metastatic carcinoma
			   with ascites
				Bloody ascites
				   from perfora-
				   tion of viscus

diastasis recti form the most frequently encountered disorders in the covering of the hypogastrium. The **bladder** may be obstructed by strictures and prostatism (p. 165) but bladder carcinoma and stones may also be palpable. Bladder rupture should be considered in trauma to the perineum. The **uterus** may be enlarged by pregnancy, endometritis, fibroids, choriocarcinomas, and endometrial carcinoma. An **ovarian** or **tubal** mass may come from a benign or malignant ovarian cyst, an ectopic pregnancy, or a tubo-ovarian abscess. The **aorta** may present a mass in aneurysms or thrombosis and severe arteriosclerosis of the terminal aorta. Finally, the **lumbosacral spine** may present as a hypogastric mass in severe lordosis of Pott's disease, spondylolithesis, metastatic carcinoma, and lumbar spondylosis. The **pre-aortic lymph nodes** may greatly enlarge in tuberculosis, Hodgkin's disease, and metastatic carcinoma. If the **transverse colon** drops to the hypogastrium, a carcinoma or inflamed and abscessed diverticulum may be felt. Volvulus may present a mass here.

Ascites from cirrhosis of the liver, ruptured abdominal viscus, or bacterial or tuberculous peritonitis is often encountered and is difficult to differentiate from an ovarian cyst and a distended bladder. Careful percussion and ultrasonic evaluation will be extremely helpful, but a peritoneoscopy or a peritoneal tap in the lateral quadrants may be necessary.

Approach to the Diagnosis

The approach to the diagnosis of a hypogastric mass is similar to that for any mass in the abdomen (p. 95). Obviously, catheterization of the bladder and an enema must be done after a thorough history and physical examination with both pelvic and rectal examinations. Next sigmoidoscopy, a barium enema, and an upper GI series with a small bowel follow-through are axiomatic if a gynecological cause

has been ruled out (*e.g.,* pregnancy). Colonoscopy and peritoneoscopy with CT scans and diagnostic ultrasound are the most recent additions to the diagnostic armamentarium and have eliminated the need for an exploratory laparotomy in many, but not all, cases.

ANAL MASS

Aside from the common external hemorrhoids (which will not be seen in many cases unless the patient is asked to bear down), anal masses may include any of the following:

1. **Skin tags** from previous ruptured or incised hemorrhoids
2. **Sentinel piles** from rectal fissures
3. **Perirectal abscesses**
4. **Condyloma latum** (syphilitic warts)
5. **Condyloma acuminatum** or **viral warts**
6. **Rectal prolapse**

It is important to keep all of them in mind when the anus is being examined because often you will not seem them unless you remember to look for them.

AXILLARY MASS

When the physician palpates a mass in the right axilla, his first thought is that it is a lymph node. Although in most cases this is probably right, it is a good idea to first think of the **anatomy.** There are the skin and its glands, the lymph nodes, the axillary artery, subcutaneous tissue, muscles, and ribs. Thus, in addition to an enlarged lymph node, one must consider skin conditions such as sebaceous cysts and hidradenitis suppurativa; lesions of the subcutaneous tissue such as cellulitis, lipomas, and accessory breast tissue; and axillary aneurysms and primary and metastatic tumors of the ribs.

The lymph nodes are involved primarily by infection or malignancy. If other groups of lymph nodes are involved (*e.g.*, anterior cervical or groin), then consider the differential under generalized lymphadenopathy (p. 148). For focal lymphoadenopathy look for infection in the areas that feed the gland. There may be a minor wound of the arm and hand that has become infected or there may be an infection in the lung, breast, or back. Tularemia often causes axillary adenopathy even though the wound in the hand is insignificant. The node may be involved with tuberculosis or a fungal infection such as actinomycosis, but there is also usually a site of infection in the lung.

If infection has been excluded then malignancy must be considered. Hodgkin's disease, carcinoma of the breast, and carcinoma of the lung are the chief offenders, but lymphosarcomas and metastasis from other sites must be considered.

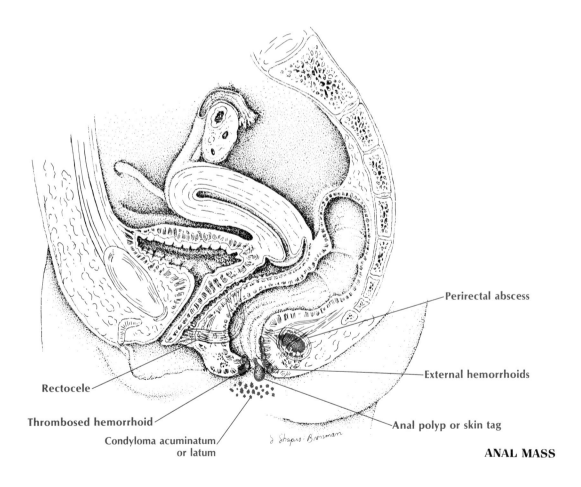

Perirectal abscess

External hemorrhoids

Rectocele

Thrombosed hemorrhoid

Condyloma acuminatum or latum

Anal polyp or skin tag

ANAL MASS

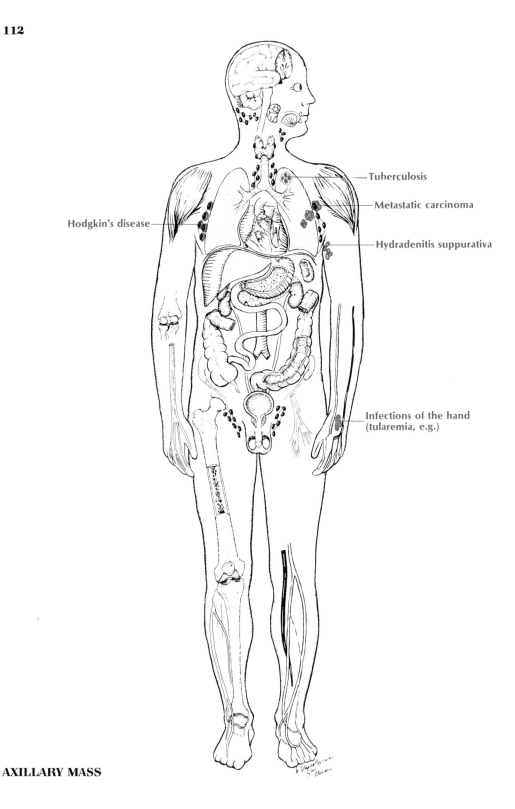

Tuberculosis

Metastatic carcinoma

Hydradenitis suppurativa

Hodgkin's disease

Infections of the hand
(tularemia, e.g.)

AXILLARY MASS

Approach to the Diagnosis

Lymph node biopsy is the most expedient method to apply in diagnosis once it is certain that the gland is a lymph node and no other primary site can be found. Nevertheless, mammography should always be done, even when palpation of the breast is negative. Lymphangiography may be considered before biopsy. Lesions of the skin are best treated by the dermatologist, whereas an axillary aneurysm can be handled by the vascular surgeon. Appendix I lists some other procedures that may be applied in individual cases.

BACK MASS ▪

It is not uncommon for a patient to complain of a lump on his back. Most of the time the lesion is a sebaceous cyst or lipoma. But there are other types of masses here and a simple method of recall is needed. **Anatomy** is the key. If the mnemonic **MINT** is applied to most of these structures, all of the important lesions can be recalled.

1. **Skin.**
   M—Malformations include pilonidal cysts and sebaceous cysts.
   I—Inflammation suggests carbuncles and furuncles.
   N—Neoplasms include hemangiomas, neurofibromas, lipomas, and metastatic tumors.
   T—Trauma, of course, suggests contusions.
2. **Subcutaneous tissue and fascia.**
   M—Malformations include hernias of Petit's triangle.
   I—Inflammatory suggests lesions such as rheumatoid nodules and abscesses.

   N—Neoplasms encompass those mentioned above.
   T—Trauma includes contusions and lacerations. Anasarca may produce edema of the back.
3. **Muscle.** Muscle is frequently nodular in fibromyositis and a bursa may occasionally swell significantly. Rupture of a muscle or ligament and contusions are traumatic lesions that may present a mass. Muscle spasm from back injuries is often significant enough to cause a "mass."
4. **Bone.** Lesions of the bone are usually responsible for the deeper masses in the back.
   M—Malformations include spina bifida, which may be occult or manifest as a swelling such as meningocele or meningomyelocele.
   I—Inflammation suggests the gibbus of Pott's disease (tuberculosis of the spine).
   N—Neoplasm suggests metastatic neoplasm and multiple myeloma of the spine which may protrude from beneath the skin.
   T—Trauma suggests the obvious mass of a fracture dislocation or hematoma of the periosteum of the spine.
5. **Retroperitoneal tumor.** Wilm's tumors of the kidney and perinephric abscesses may present as a mass in the back.

Approach to the Diagnosis

With skin lesions excision or biopsy is frequently the best approach. Masses of the deeper structures cannot be approached so aggressively until certain conditions have been ruled out by roentgenograms and bone scans. If a meningocele or similar congenital lesion is suspected a neurosurgeon must be consulted.

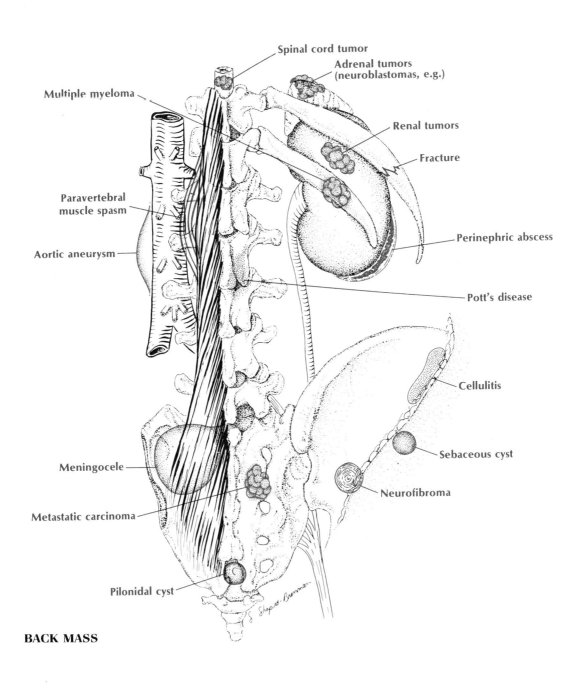

Spinal cord tumor

Adrenal tumors
(neuroblastomas, e.g.)

Multiple myeloma

Renal tumors

Fracture

Paravertebral
muscle spasm

Aortic aneurysm

Perinephric abscess

Pott's disease

Cellulitis

Sebaceous cyst

Meningocele

Neurofibroma

Metastatic carcinoma

Pilonidal cyst

BACK MASS

BREAST MASS
OR SWELLING ■

Developing a differential of this condition can be done either histologically or with the mnemonic **MINT.** After all, once each structure or tissue is identified the significant lesions are either inflammatory or neoplastic. Let us apply the histological method.

A **skin** or **subcutaneous mass** is most commonly an abscess, sebaceous cyst, lipoma, or neurofibroma. (For a more detailed discussion of masses of the skin see p. 166) The **supporting tissue** of the breast may be involved by cellulitis, fatty necrosis, fibromas, or sarcomas. The **breast tissue** itself can be inflamed by bacteria in **acute mastitis,** obstructed and inflamed on a chronic basis in cystic mastitis, diffusely and painfully swollen

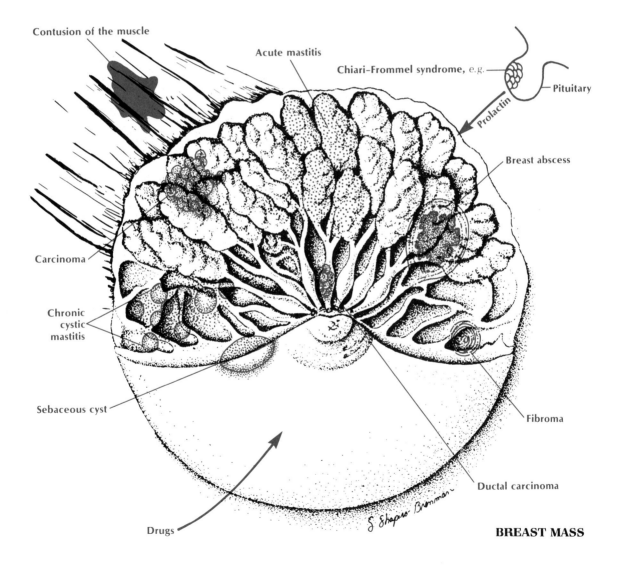

Contusion of the muscle

Acute mastitis

Chiari–Frommel syndrome, *e.g.*

Pituitary

Prolactin

Breast abscess

Carcinoma

Chronic cystic mastitis

Fibroma

Sebaceous cyst

Ductal carcinoma

Drugs

G. Shapiro-Brennan

BREAST MASS

bilaterally by drugs such as chlorpromazine and alpha-methyldopa or in endocrine disturbances (*e.g.*, pregnancy or Chiari–Frommel syndrome). Carcinoma of the breast usually forms a nontender, firm swelling in one breast. Ductal carcinoma presents with a mass and often with a bloody discharge.

Trauma may involve any of the histological components of the breast but the history and physical examination usually make the diagnosis clear.

Approach to the Diagnosis

When faced with a mass in the breast, the physician's first step should be a careful examination of the breasts and the surrounding area. If the mass is tender it is likely to be inflammatory or traumatic. If it is not tender one should suspect tumor. If it transilluminates it is probably a cyst. Obviously the concern of both physician and patient is primarily whether it is a neoplasm. A careful search for enlarged lymph nodes in the axilla and the neck or a mass in the other breast is important. Mammography and ultrasonography are the next most important steps, but a breast biopsy is still necessary in most cases. A truly cystic mass may be punctured for fluid analysis and Papanicolaou's smears.

CARDIOMEGALY ■

If an x-ray film demonstrates cardiomegaly, the physician must find out what is causing this condition (Table 2-7). You have already listened to the patient and he does not have a murmur. That seems to exclude the fairly common groups of causes—congenital and rheumatic heart disease. (It really doesn't). The patient does not have hypertension and

denies symptoms of heart failure. His ECG is normal. Now what do you do?

This situation is all too common and I hope this chapter will remedy that situation. The basic sciences, **histology** and **physiology** are, of course, the key to an immediate differential diagnosis. Remember that the heart is divided into three basic layers: endocardium, myocardium, and pericardium; each of these can be cross-indexed with the etiological classification using the mnemonic **VINDICATE.** The pathophysiological mechanism, **obstruction,** provides the remaining disorders in the differential diagnosis. This is applied to the pulmonary and systemic circulations and cross-indexed with the various etiological groups.

Beginning with the **endocardium,**

V—Vascular lesions include the ball—valve thrombosis.

I—Inflammatory lesions bring to mind acute and subacute bacterial endocarditis and syphilitic valvular disease.

N—Neoplasms suggest an atrial myxoma.

D—Degenerative disease signals atherosclerotic valvular disease.

I—Intoxication does not suggest any particular condition, as most toxins involve the myocardium.

C—Congenital suggests a host of valvular and septal defects and also transposition of the blood vessels of the heart.

A—Autoimmune suggests the important rheumatic carditis and also Libman-Sack's endocarditis of lupus erythematosus.

T—Trauma suggests all the valvular or septal defects that can occur from surgery.

E—Endocrine suggests the pulmonic and tricuspid valvular defects that result from carcinoid syndrome.

In the **myocardium,** one encounters a large number of diseases, thus only the most common ones will be mentioned here.

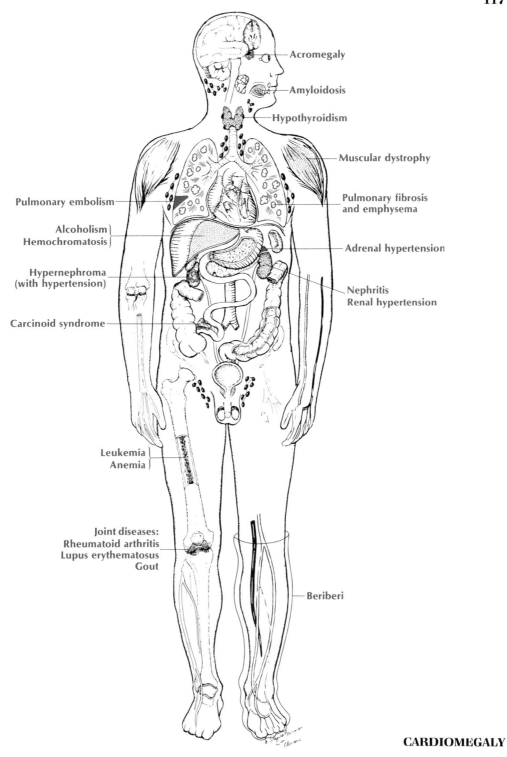

Acromegaly

Amyloidosis

Hypothyroidism

Muscular dystrophy

Pulmonary embolism

Pulmonary fibrosis
and emphysema

Alcoholism
Hemochromatosis

Adrenal hypertension

Hypernephroma
(with hypertension)

Nephritis
Renal hypertension

Carcinoid syndrome

Leukemia
Anemia

Joint diseases:
Rheumatoid arthritis
Lupus erythematosus
Gout

Beriberi

CARDIOMEGALY

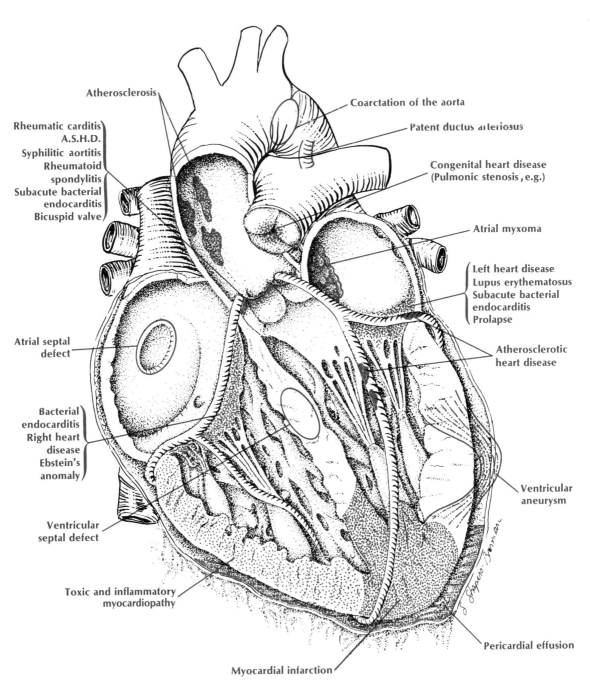

Atherosclerosis

Coarctation of the aorta

Patent ductus arteriosus

Rheumatic carditis
A.S.H.D.
Syphilitic aortitis
Rheumatoid
spondylitis
Subacute bacterial
endocarditis
Bicuspid valve

Congenital heart disease
(Pulmonic stenosis, e.g.)

Atrial myxoma

Left heart disease
Lupus erythematosus
Subacute bacterial
endocarditis
Prolapse

Atrial septal
defect

Atherosclerotic
heart disease

Bacterial
endocarditis
Right heart
disease
Ebstein's
anomaly

Ventricular
aneurysm

Ventricular
septal defect

Toxic and inflammatory
myocardiopathy

Pericardial effusion

Myocardial infarction

CARDIOMEGALY, LOCAL CAUSES

V—Vascular should immediately suggest coronary insufficiency and myocardial infarction.

I—Inflammation could indicate viral myocarditis, but it would hardly be expected to remind one of diphtheria and syphilitic myocarditis as these are now rarely seen.

N—Neoplasms of the myocardium are rare, thus the rhabdomyosarcoma needs only be mentioned here for completeness.

D—Degenerative and **Deficiency** disease should signal beriberi and muscular dystrophy, but these are also infrequently encountered.

I—Intoxicating and **Idiopathic** disorders of the myocardium are much more common, especially alcoholism. Others include hemochromatosis, alcoholism, amyloidosis, and gout.

C—Congenital disorders include von Gierke's disease and myocardial fibroelastosis.

A—Autoimmune again suggests rheumatic fever and the collagen diseases.

T—Trauma suggests the post-traumatic aneurysms.

E—Endocrine disorders include two treatable disorders, hyperthyroidism and hypothyroidism.

The **pericardium** is not frequently the cause of "cardiomegaly," but tuberculosis and idiopathic pericarditis should be considered as should hemopericardium, especially in the course of a myocardial infarction.

Obstruction in the pulmonary circulation from the following:

V—Vascular from pulmonary infarct

I—Inflammatory from chronic bronchitis and emphysema or from chronic infections such as tuberculosis and various fungi

N—Neoplastic from primary or metastatic carcinoma

D—Degenerative

I—Idiopathic or **Intoxication** in pulmonary fibrosis and primary pulmonary hypertension

C—Congenital disorders include pulmonic stenosis and hemangiomas.

A—Autoimmune diseases include collagen diseases.

T—Trauma may cause an arteriovenous aneurysm or pneumothorax obstructing the pulmonary circulation.

E—Endocrine disorders do not obstruct the pulmonary vasculature.

Under **systemic circulation** come essential or secondary hypertension caused by coarctation of the aorta, periarteritis nodosa, or the many renal and adrenal diseases. Dissecting aneurysms of the aorta may rupture into the pericardium causing cardiomegaly.

Approach to the Diagnosis

The approach to the diagnosis of cardiomegaly is much more sophisticated today than taking an ECG and chest roentgenogram with oblique views and a barium swallow. Echocardiography, phonocardiograms, vectorcardiology, radioactive isotopic scans of the myocardium, and angiography have allowed for almost 100% accurate diagnosis. Nevertheless, a careful history and physical examination are not replaced by these studies. For example, the family should be asked about alcohol intake before alcoholic myocardiopathy is ruled out. A snapping first heart sound at the apex should suggest mitral stenosis even without a murmur and a midsystolic click should suggest floppy mitral valve syndrome. A list of all the diagnostic tests that may be needed in the workup of cardiomegaly is given in Appendix I.

(Text continues on p. 122)

TABLE 2-7.   CARDIOMEGALY

	V Vascular	I Inflammatory	N Neoplasm	D Degenerative and Deficiency
Endocardium	Ball valve thrombus	Bacterial endocarditis Subacute bacterial en- docarditis Syphilis	Myxoma	Atherosclerotic val- vular disease
Myocardium	Coronary insuf- ficiency Myocardial infarc- tion Congestive heart failure	Diphtheria Trypanosomiasis Syphilis Viral myocarditis	Rhabdomyosarcoma	Beriberi Muscular dystrophy
Pericardium	Hemopericardium	Tuberculosis Viral pericarditis	Metastatic carcinoma	
Systemic Circu- **lation**	Renal artery steno- sis		Polycythemia vera Hypernephroma	Anemia Paget's disease
Pulmonary Circu- **lation**	Pulmonary embo- lism and infarc- tion	Chronic bronchitis and emphysema Tuberculosis Fungi	Carcinomatosis	

I Intoxication Idiopathic	C Congenital	A Autoimmune Allergic	T Trauma	E Endocrine
	Congenital valvular and septal defects	Lupus endocarditis Rheumatic fever	Valvular perforation or lacerating surgery	Carcinoid syndrome
Hemochromatosis Alcoholism Amyloidosis Gout	Hurler's disease von Gierke's disease Myocardial fibroelastosis Subaortic stenosis	Rheumatic fever Rheumatic arthritis scleroderma	Traumatic aneurysm Postmyocardotdotomy syndrome	Hyperthyroidism Diabetic arteriolar sclerosis Hypothyroidism
Idiopathic pericarditis		Rheumatic fever	Hemopericardium	
Essential hypertension Dissecting aneurysm	Coarctation of aorta Patent ductus	Periarteritis nodosa Glomerulonephritis	Arteriovenous fistula	Adrenal tumors
Pulmonary fibrosis Primary pulmonary hypertension				

CHEST WALL MASS ■

The differential diagnosis of this symptom and sign is similar to that of chest pain: **Anatomy** is the key to both. After visualizing all the organs of the chest and cross-indexing them with the mnemonic **MINT,** a convenient and extensive differential list can be constructed as in Table 2-8. The discussion that follows will also concentrate on the most significant of these.

The significant lesions of the **skin** and **subcutaneous tissues** include sebaceous cysts, cellulitis, neurofibromas, lipomas, and contusions. Unlike the abdomen, the chest seldom is the source of a hernia. In the **ribs,** look for fractures, contusions, multiple myeloma, and primary and metastatic tumors. In the **cartilage** there may be a protruding xiphoid process or a lump at the costochondral junctions in Tietze's syndrome. Years ago it was common for empyema, lung abscesses, pleural and pulmonary tuberculosis, and fungi (acti-

TABLE 2-8. MASS IN THE CHEST WALL

	M Malformations	I Inflammation
Skin and Subcutaneous Tissue	Neurofibroma Venous engorgement Sebaceous cysts	Cellulitis Abscess
Muscle		Myositis
Ribs	Pigeon breast Xiphoid prominence	Osteomyelitis Tuberculosis Tietze's syndrome
Lungs and Pleura		Tuberculosis Emphysema Lung abscess
Heart and Pericardium	Cardiomegaly Aneurysms	Tuberculous or idio- pathic pericarditis
Aorta	Aneurysms	
Mediastinum	Superior vena cava obstruc- tion	Mediastinitis

nomycosis especially) to work their way out to the skin and form a mass or fistula: This is now unusual. Carcinoma of the lung and mesentheliomas, however, may form a mass on the chest wall by direct extension. In the **mediastinal structures,** aortic aneurysms used to be a common cause of a pulsating chest wall mass, but they are now rarely seen. Cardiomegaly and pericardial effusions occasionally cause a noticeable protuberance of the precardium but not as frequently as in the past. Tumors of the mediastinum may also cause chest wall masses or protuberances.

Approach to the Diagnosis

The approach to this diagnosis is again a good clinical history and physical examination along with correlation of signs and symptoms. Chest x-ray films with special views and tomography will diagnose most cases, but a biopsy, arteriography, CT scans, and exploratory surgery may be necessary, especially if the lesion turns out to be noninfectious. It is important not to be fooled by a congenital anomaly (e.g., pigeon breast). Other tests for diagnosis will be found in Appendix I.

N Neoplasms	T Trauma
Lipomas	Contusion
(Rare)	Contusion
Osteoma Multiple myeloma Metastatic carcinoma	Fracture Contusion
Carcinoma or mesenthelioma with direct extension	Hemorrhage Pneumothorax Subcutaneous emphysema
Metastatic carcinoma to pericardium	Traumatic aneurysms
	Traumatic aneurysms
Hodgkin's disease Dermoid cyst	

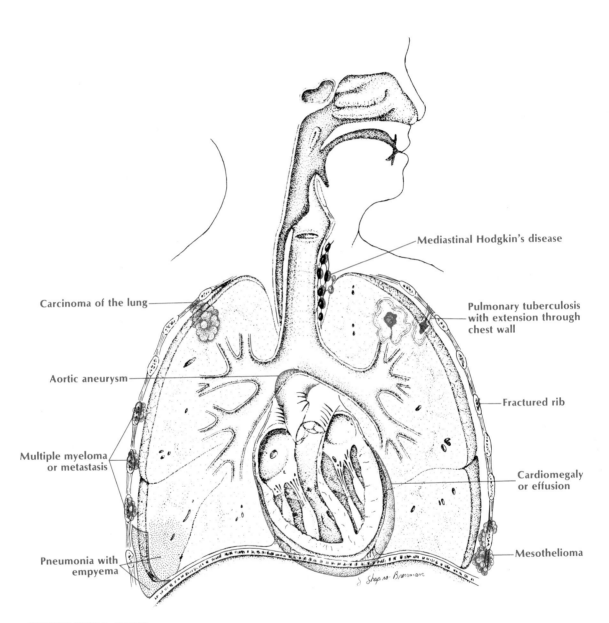

Mediastinal Hodgkin's disease

Carcinoma of the lung

Pulmonary tuberculosis with extension through chest wall

Aortic aneurysm

Fractured rib

Multiple myeloma or metastasis

Cardiomegaly or effusion

Mesothelioma

Pneumonia with empyema

CHEST WALL MASS

CLUBBING AND PULMONARY OSTEOARTHROPATHY

Although there has been argument in the past over whether clubbing and pulmonary osteoarthropathy are just two clinical manifestations of the same thing, I take the position that they are; their differential diagnosis, therefore, will be considered together.

When presented with a case of clubbing, one might simply use **anatomy** and think of all the major internal organs (except the kidney); one would then be closer to an accurate

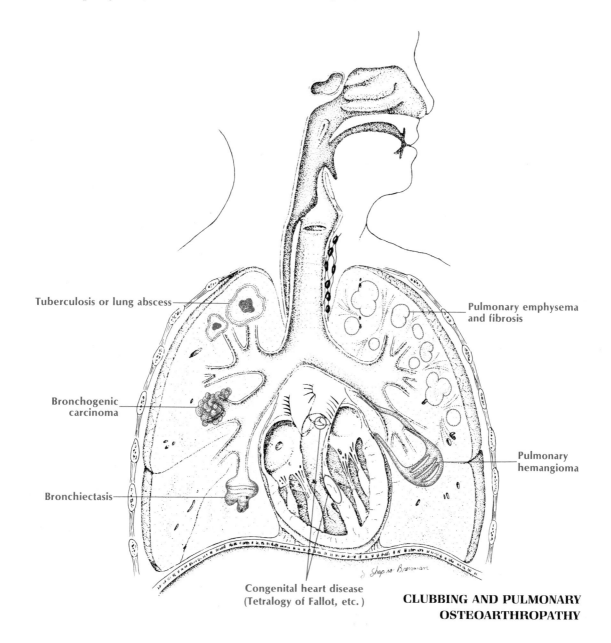

Tuberculosis or lung abscess

Pulmonary emphysema and fibrosis

Bronchogenic carcinoma

Pulmonary hemangioma

Bronchiectasis

Congenital heart disease (Tetralogy of Fallot, etc.)

CLUBBING AND PULMONARY OSTEOARTHROPATHY

TABLE 2-9. CLUBBING AND PULMONARY OSTEOARTHROPATHY

	V Vascular	I Inflammatory	N Neoplasm
Anoxic Anoxia (Pulmonary Disease)		Tuberculosis Lung abscess Emphysema Chronic bronchitis	Carcinoma of the lung
Shunt Anoxia (Cardiovascular Disease)	Pulmonary emboli		Pulmonary hemangioma
Anemic Anoxia		Amebiasis Ascaris Chronic osteomyelitis	Carcinoma of the GI tract Hodgkin's disease
Histotoxic Anoxia		Subacute bacterial endo- carditis	Carinoma of the GI tract
Miscellaneous	Aortic and brachial artery aneurysm		Polycythemia vera Nasopharyngeal tumors

and reliable differential diagnosis. To be more scientific apply basic physiology to provide an extensive and organized differential. The key basic science, then, is **physiology;** according to Mauer,* the principle common denominator is **anoxia.** Table 2-9 is developed on this basis. Anoxic anoxia or poor intake of oxygen would suggest the first category of disease, pulmonary; most significant among these are chronic diseases of the lung including chronic bronchitis and emphysema, empyema, pulmonary tuberculosis, carcinoma of the lung, pneumoconiosis, and pulmonary fibrosis. Acute pneumonia, pneumothorax, and bronchial asthma (where there may be many

short episodes of anoxia) do not usually lead to clubbing.

In the next group of disorders the lungs may be normal but a significant amount of blood never reaches the alveoli; I call this **shunt anoxia.** Here are classified the tetralogy of Fallot and other congenital anomalies of the heart, recurrent pulmonary emboli, cirrhosis of the liver (associated with small pulmonary arteriovenous shunts), and pulmonary hemangiomas. Many conditions associated with anemia may present with clubbing. Thus, anemic anoxia may be a factor in portal cirrhosis, biliary cirrhosis, Banti's disease, chronic malaria, and subacute bacterial endocarditis. It may also be a factor in disorders of the gastrointestinal tract, such as regional ileitis, ulcerative colitis, and carcinoma

*Mauer EF: Etiology of clubbed fingers. Am Heart J 34:852, 1947

D Degenerative and Deficiency	I Intoxication Idiopathic	C Congenital	A Autoimmune	T Trauma	E Endocrine
	Pulmonary fibrosis Emphysema	Cystic fibrosis Bronchiectasis	Sarcoidosis		
	Adhesive pericarditis	Congenital heart disease Tetralogy of Fallot Pulmonic stenosis			
	Cirrhosis of the liver		Regional ileitis Ulcerative colitis		
	Biliary cirrhosis				Myxedema
Syringomyelia	Idiopathic clubbing				

of the colon. Stagnant anoxia is not usually associated with clubbing, but this may be because severe anoxia in congestive heart failure and shock are usually transient.

Histotoxic anoxia is Mauer's other explanation for clubbing in patients without low arterial oxygen saturation. The theory is hindered by chronic inflammatory diseases. This group includes subacute bacterial endocarditis, myxedema, ulcerative colitis, intestinal tuberculosis, and amebic dysentery. Of course, this is a regular occurrence in chronic methemoglobinemia or sulfhemoglobinemia.

Approach to the Diagnosis

The clinical approach to clubbing involves being certain that clubbing is present. A curved fingernail is not good evidence, and the "drumstick" appearance (which makes the finger look like a true club) does not occur until late. Early clubbing is determined by the angle between the nail-covered portion of the dorsal surface of the terminal phalanx and the skin-covered portion. Normally this angle is 160°. When the angle becomes 180° and disappears, that is, when the terminal phalanx becomes flat, clubbing exists.

Careful examination for cyanosis and a thorough evaluation of the heart and lungs will determine the cause in most cases. Pulmonary function studies, and arterial blood gases before and after exercise and before and after 100% oxygen, will help confirm the diagnosis in many cases. Of course, lung scans and angiocardiography are frequently necessary. Blood cultures, stool culture and examination, and thorough roentgenographic studies of the GI tract will be necessary in obscure cases.

EDEMA OF THE EXTREMITIES ■

Edema of the extremities is a common symptom. Most physicians, therefore, have an immediate working diagnosis when the patient walks into the office: congestive heart failure if the edema is bilateral and deep vein phlebitis if it is unilateral. Many times this is right. But what if the heart and chest sound normal and there is a negative Homan's sign? Obviously, before he questions the patient the clinician needs a more complete list of diagnostic possibilities. **Physiology** is the key to that list.

Fluid is passing from the blood compartment into the subcutaneous tissues and back again all the time. Why does it stay in the subcutaneous tissues? There are four main physiological reasons and three minor ones.

1. **The pressure in the veins** may be so high that it overcomes the oncotic pressure of the albumin and other proteins in the blood. This is the explanation in phlebitis, venous thrombosis, pelvic tumors, and right-sided congestive heart failure (partially).

2. **The pressure in the arteries** may be so high that more fluid is pushed out than can be reabsorbed with a normal oncotic pressure. This may be the case in acute glomerulonephritis and malignant hypertension.

3. **The serum albumin** may be so low that the oncotic pressure drops to a point where it cannot reabsorb all the fluid being driven out by the forward pressure of the arteries or backward pressure of the veins. This is seen in conditions in which

either too little albumin is produced (cirrhosis of the liver) or too much albumin is lost in the urine (nephrotic syndrome of diabetes mellitus, lupus erythematosus, amyloidosis, and several other disorders of the kidney). It is also probably a component of the edema in beriberi and congestive heart failure.

4. **The lymphatic channels** that pick up any excess fluid that the veins cannot pick up may be blocked. This occurs notably in filariasis, Milroy's disease, and lymphedema following mastectomy, but other conditions may also block the lymphatics.

5. **An abnormal protein** (mucoprotein) may be deposited in the tissues and lead to edema. This results in the nonpitting edema of hypothyroidism (myxedema).

6. **A reduction in tissue turgor pressure** may be responsible for the edema of older people and beriberi (vitamin B_I deficiency).

7. **Retention of salt** as in primary and secondary aldosteronism is a minor factor because most cases of aldosterone secreting adenomas do not have significant edema.

It would be a serious omission not to mention local conditions such as cellulitis, burns (especially sunburn), contusions, and urticaria that may cause edema, but these are usually obvious.

Edema is classified according to the anatomical site of origin and the mechanisms that are responsible in Table 2-10.

Approach to the Diagnosis

The venous pressure and circulation time are useful in confirming congestive heart failure, as the ECG may be normal. Nephrosis and cirrhosis usually show characteristic patterns on an SMA-24. A urinalysis is helpful. Thyroid function studies need to be ordered. A pelvic examination is sometimes rewarding in fe-

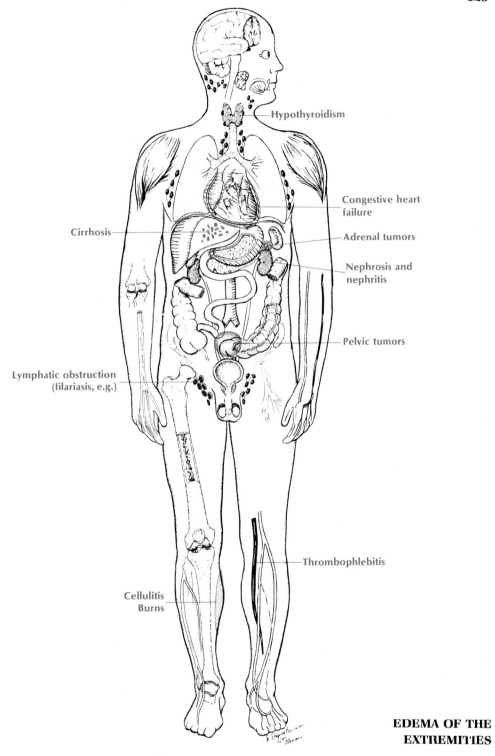

Hypothyroidism

Congestive heart failure

Cirrhosis

Adrenal tumors

Nephrosis and nephritis

Pelvic tumors

Lymphatic obstruction (filariasis, e.g.)

Thrombophlebitis

Cellulitis Burns

EDEMA OF THE EXTREMITIES

TABLE 2-10. PHYSIOLOGICAL MECHANISMS OF EDEMA

	Increased Venous Pressure	Increased Arterial Pressure	Decreased Serum Albumin
Congestive Heart Failure	√		√
Nephrosis			√
Cirrhosis	√		√
Pelvic Tumors	√		
Thrombophlebitis	√		
Filariasis			
Hypothyroidism			
Beriberi			√
Malignant Hypertension		√	
Acute Glomerulonephritis		√	
Toxemia of Pregnancy		√	√

males with bilateral pitting edema, because a large ovarian cyst may be found. Phlebography is valuable in diagnosing deep vein thrombosis, as are plethysomography and Doppler ultrasound studies.

EXOPHTHALMOS

The mnemonic **VINDICATE** is a useful and quick way to recall the causes of exophthalmos (for enophthalmos see Ptosis, p. 378).

V—Vascular disorders include a carotid-cavernous fistula and cavernous sinus thrombosis.

I—Inflammatory diseases recall orbital cellulitis, osteomyelitis, and sinusitis.

N—Neoplasms suggest hemangiomas, lymphangiomas, sarcomas, and metastatic carcinoma, and also nervous system tumors such as sphenoid ridge meningiomas.

D—Deficiency diseases suggest the retro-orbital hemorrhages of scurvy. **Degenerative** diseases suggest the apparent exophthalmos of facial palsy associated with progres-

Lymphatic Obstruction	Abnormal Protein in Subcutaneous Tissue	Loss of Tissue Turgor	Aldosteronism
			√
			√
			√
√			
	√		
		√	
			√
			√
			√

sive muscular atrophy and dystrophy in many forms.

I—Intoxication suggests the exophthalmos that develops or progresses on treatment in hyperthyroidism. **Idiopathic** diseases such as Paget's disease and fibrous dysplasia of the skull must also be considered.

C—Congenital brings to mind hydrocephalus, Hand–Schüller–Christian disease, meningoceles, and cleidocranial dystosis, all of which cause exophthalmos. In this category one should also include the genetic exophthalmos of the Blacks.

A—Autoimmune disorders suggest Wegener's granulomatosis.

T—Trauma suggests orbital fractures and hematomas, which will cause proptosis in many cases.

E—Endocrine disorders suggest that the most significant cause of exophthalmos is Grave's disease.

If exophthalmos can be classified as a result of a mass, then the causes can be recalled by the methods applied to any mass. The mass may be air (orbital emphysema), fluid (orbital

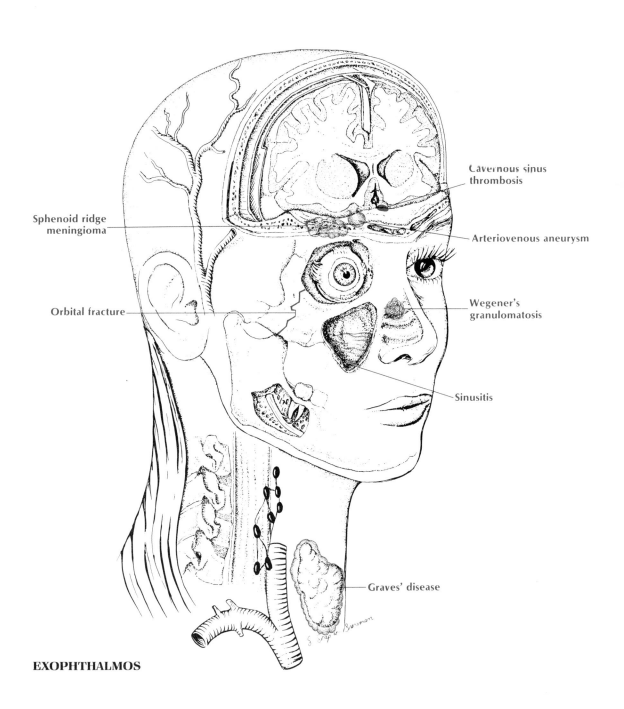

Cavernous sinus thrombosis

Arteriovenous aneurysm

Sphenoid ridge meningioma

Wegener's granulomatosis

Orbital fracture

Sinusitis

Graves' disease

EXOPHTHALMOS

abscess), blood (*e.g.,* hematomas from trauma, scurvy, hemophilia), a foreign substance (*e.g.,* echinococcal cyst), or hypertrophy of one of the tissues around the orbit. The latter can be developed by a histological analysis. Thus **fat** may hypertrophy or multiply in Hand–Schüller–Christian disease and in exophthalmic goiter. **Blood vessels** may become hypertrophied in cavernous sinus thrombosis, carotid-cavernous fistulae, and aneurysms and will undergo hyperplasia in hemangiomas. **Lymph tissue** and **connective tissue** may form sarcomas or granulomas. **Bone** may swell with a periosteitis and may undergo hyperplasia in Paget's disease, osteomas, metastatic carcinoma, and meningiomas. **Nerve tissue** may undergo hyperplasia in neurofibromatosis.

Approach to the Diagnosis

The approach to the diagnosis of exophthalmos involves a thyroid workup (see p. 398), roentgenograms of the skull and sinuses, special views of the orbit, and careful neurological and ENT examinations. CT scans and ultrasonography have proved to be very useful. One must listen for a bruit. If an orbital neoplasm or inflammatory lesion can be excluded and no bruit heard and the mass is not pulsatile, a thyroid disorder is likely and referral to an endocrinologist is wise even in the face of normal thyroid function studies.

EXTREMITY MASS ■

When the clinician tries to recall the causes of a mass in the extremities he should consider the **anatomy.** As he dissects downward from the skin, he encounters the subcutaneous tissue, veins, muscles and ligaments, bursae, arteries, lymph nodes, nerves, bones, and joints.

The common lesions causing a mass in each of these should easily come to mind.

1. **Skin.** Common lesions to consider here are sebaceous cysts, lipomas, and cellulitis. Other skin masses are considered on page 166.
2. **Subcutaneous tissue.** Rheumatic or rheumatoid nodules, tophi of gout, lipomas, and contusions are common.
3. **Veins.** Dilated veins (varicoceles) and thrombophlebitis present as mass lesions.
4. **Muscles and ligaments.** Contusions, nodules in myofascitis, ganglions, and partial or complete rupture of muscle (*e.g.,* rupture of the rectus femoris) are typical masses originating in the muscles and ligaments. Myositis ossificans may present with nodular masses.
5. **Bursae.** The bursae may be involved by gout, trauma, or rheumatic conditions and swell up with fluid.
6. **Arteries.** Aneurysms are the most likely cause of an extremity mass originating from the arteries. Severe arteriosclerosis may cause confusion occasionally.
7. **Lymph nodes.** Tuberculous adenitis, adenitis secondary to infections in the distal portion of the extremity, and metastatic tumors may cause enlargement of the lymph nodes.
8. **Nerves.** Traumatic neuromas, neurofibromas, and hypertrophy of the nerve in Dejerine–Sottas disease are typical "masses" arising from the peripheral nerve.
9. **Bone.** Trauma may lead to fractures and subperiosteal hematomas, callus formation following the fracture, or secondary osteomyelitis, all of which may cause a mass. Primary osteomyelitis, tuberculosis of the bone, syphilis of the bone, rickets, and acromegaly may cause bone masses. Typical tumors affecting the bone are chondromas, exostoses (osteomas), osteogenic sarcomas, fibrosarcomas, and meta-

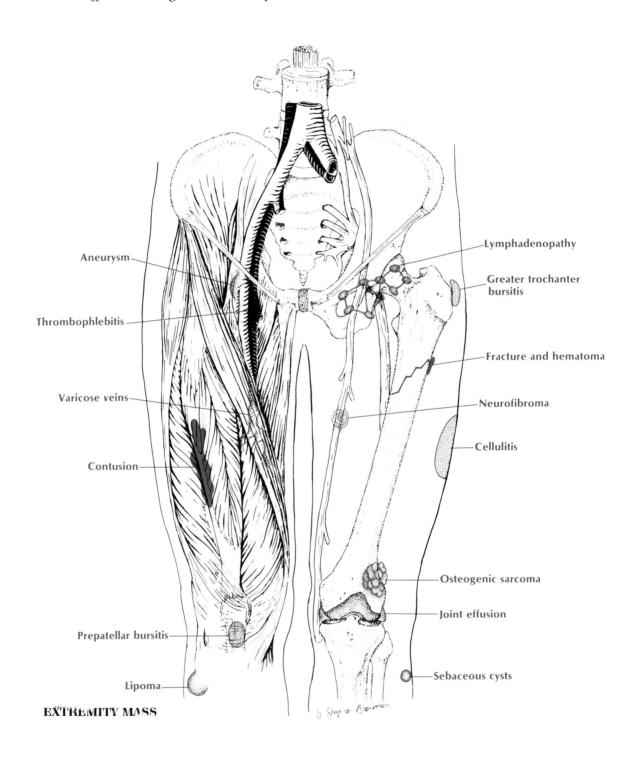

Aneurysm

Thrombophlebitis

Varicose veins

Contusion

Prepatellar bursitis

Lipoma

Lymphadenopathy

Greater trochanter bursitis

Fracture and hematoma

Neurofibroma

Cellulitis

Osteogenic sarcoma

Joint effusion

Sebaceous cysts

EXTREMITY MASS

static carcinomas, but there are several others. Paget's disease may present as an enlargement of the bone.

Approach to the Diagnosis

If the lesion is suspected to arise in the skin, simply biopsy or excision is the best approach. Deeper masses require careful examination, roentgenogram of the bones and soft tissue, bone scans, ultrasonic studies and phlebography, arteriography, or lymphangiography. Surgical exploration of the area may be the only means to accomplish a specific diagnosis.

GROIN MASS ■

A mass found on routine examination of the groin is most likely an enlarged lymph node. On the other hand, when the patient presents with a groin mass for diagnosis it is probably a hernia. But why diagnose by probability? A systemic approach will avoid misdiagnoses and should make medicine more fun.

Visualize the anatomy of the groin. There is skin, subcutaneous tissue, and the inguinal and femoral canal; underneath these are the saphenous and femoral veins, the femoral artery and nerve, and lymph nodes. In the next layer are the psoas and iliac muscles and the bones and ligaments of the hip joints. Apply the mnemonic **MINT** to these structures and the following list of possibilities may be arrived at.

M—Malformations suggest inguinal and femoral hernias in the fascia and hydroceles and undescended testicles in the inguinal canal. A saphenous varicocele and iliac aneurysm are also malformations to consider.

I—Inflammatory lesions include cellulitis, acute adenitis (usually secondary to venereal disease or skin disease) and chronic adenitis secondary to tuberculosis or a systemic disease (see p. 149). In addition, tuberculosis may cause a psoas abscess, there may be thrombophlebitis of the saphenous or femoral vein (especially postpartum), or there may be arthritis (rheumatoid, gouty, or osteoarthritis) of the joint. Finally, osteomyelitis of the hip bones must be considered.

N—Neoplasms suggest skin tumors (p. 166), lipomas, tumors of the lymph node such as Hodgkin's disease and metastatic tumors, and sarcomas of the bone.

T—Trauma would include a perforation of the femoral vein or artery, contusions and fractures, or dislocation of the hip.

Approach to the Diagnosis

Obviously, the approach to diagnosis involves differentiating enlarged lymph nodes from other conditions. Hernias are usually reducible; if they are not they are extremely tender and the patient often experiences GI complaints. They do not transilluminate and bowel sounds can often be heard over them. The location of inguinal hernias above the inguinal ligament should help differentiate them from lymph nodes and femoral hernias which are below the inguinal ligament. Lymphadenitis will usually be associated with a lesion on the genitalia (*e.g.*, chancre) or the lower extremity. Exploratory surgery and lymph node biopsy may be necessary to make a definitive diagnosis, but Appendix I suggests other tests that may be indicated in individual cases. Phlebography may be necessary to rule out venous thrombosis and angiography to rule out aneurysm.

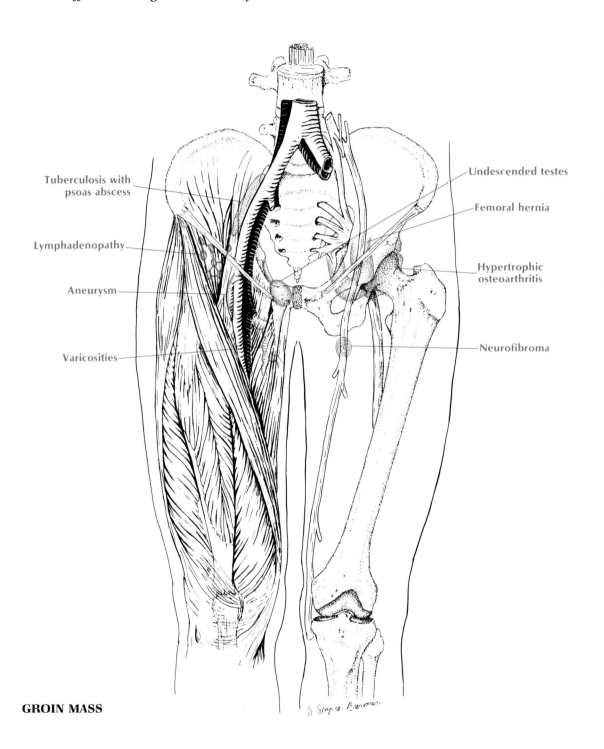

Tuberculosis with
psoas abscess

Lymphadenopathy

Aneurysm

Varicosities

Undescended testes

Femoral hernia

Hypertrophic
osteoarthritis

Neurofibroma

GROIN MASS

HEAD MASS ■

A localized mass on the head is usually a skin lesion, a lesion of the bone, or a protrusion of intracranial tissue through the bone. An extensive discussion of skin masses may be found on page 166, but most head masses originating from the skin are sebaceous cysts, caruncles, or lipomas. Lesions of the skull that may present as focal lesions are metastatic tumors, multiple myeloma, osteitis fibrosa cystica (hyperparathyroidism), and osteomas. Brain tumors, subdural hematomas, and epidural abscesses may cause proliferation of the bone over the lesion and produce a mass. Congenital meningoceles and meningoencephaloceles may protrude through defects in the skull, producing large focal lesions in the midline.

Approach to the Diagnosis

The approach to the diagnosis includes excision or biopsy of skin lesions, skull roentgenograms, bone scans, and, if need be, a bone biopsy.

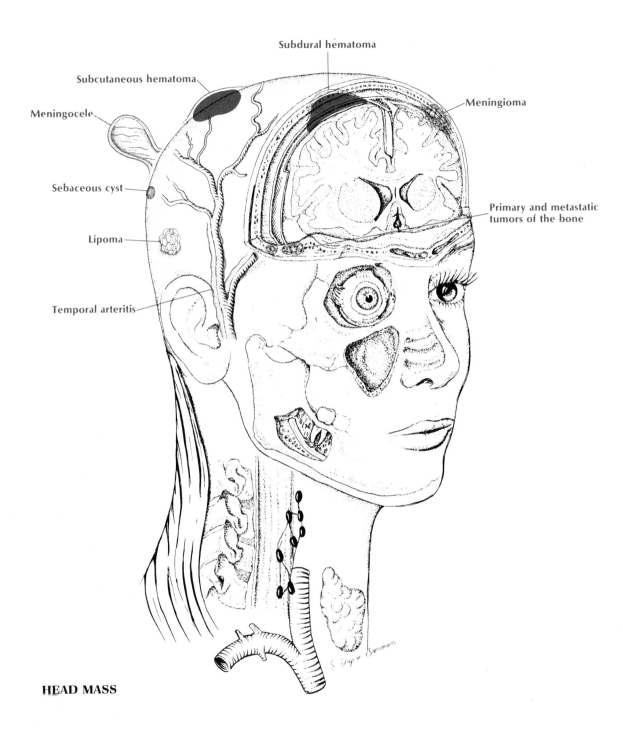

Subdural hematoma

Subcutaneous hematoma

Meningioma

Meningocele

Sebaceous cyst

Primary and metastatic tumors of the bone

Lipoma

Temporal arteritis

HEAD MASS

HEPATOMEGALY

Two key words to think of here are **histology** and **obstruction.** The analysis of the differential diagnosis of hepatomegaly is best begun with a histological breakdown of the liver tissue (Table 2-11). Thus, there are **parenchymal cells** that can be involved by toxic or inflammatory hepatitis. A variety of drugs (*e.g.,* isoniazid) and toxins (*e.g.,* carbon tetrachlo-

ride) can cause toxic hepatitis. Infectious hepatitis is most commonly caused by a virus, types A or B (which is usually tranfusion-transmitted but may be transmitted by fecal-oral route), or to infectious mononucleosis.

Beginning with the smallest organism (virus) and working up to the largest, one must consider brucellosis, tuberculosis (bacteria), syphilis, leptospirosis, (spirochetal) amebiasis, amebic abscess, schistosomiasis, hydatid cysts (parasites), and histoplasmosis, actino-

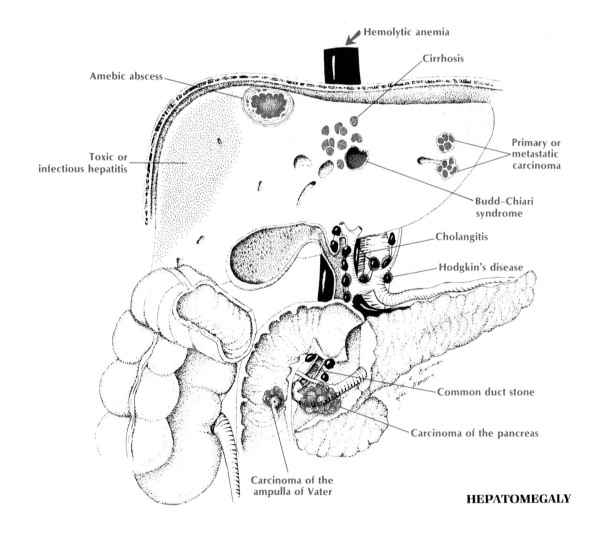

HEPATOMEGALY

mycosis, and other systemic mycoses (fungi). When considering the **supporting tissue,** do not forget lupoid hepatitis, periarteritis nodosa, sarcoidosis, and cirrhosis. Also, because the liver contains von Kupffer's cells, any disease causing proliferation of the reticuloendothelial system may produce hepatomegaly. Myeloid metaplasia and Gaucher's disease are good examples of this.

The **hepatic veins** may be involved with a thrombosis and lead to hepatomegaly (Budd–Chiari syndrome). The **portal veins** may be obstructed by a thrombophlebitis (pyelophlebitis) usually secondary to infection elsewhere in the gut. **Portal lymphatics** involved in Hodgkin's disease may cause hepatomegaly. From the **bile canaliculi** down to the hepatic and common bile ducts, obstruction may occur from stones, neoplasms (pancreatic or ampullary), infection (cholangitis), or parasites (*e.g.,* clonorchis sinensis). Chlorpromazine and related drugs cause obstruction of the small canaliculi and present an obstructive picture. Pancreatitis may cause the pancreas to swell and produce bile duct obstruction and hepatomegaly.

The **parenchymal cells** can respond in other ways to various etiologic agents to cause hepatomegaly. In diabetes and alcoholism, they may undergo fatty degeneration and in-

TABLE 2-11.   HEPATOMEGALY

	V Vascular	I Infection	N Neoplasm	D Degenerative
Parenchyma		Viral hepatitis Infectious mononu- cleosis Amebiasis	Hepatoma Metastatic carcinoma	Fatty liver
Supporting Tissue			Sarcoma	
Veins	Hepatic vein thrombosis	Pyelophlebitis		
Arteries	Hepatic artery ligation			
Lymphatics			Hodgkin's disease	
Bile Ducts		Cholangitis Clonorchis Sinensis	Papilloma Ampullary carcinoma Pancreatic carcinoma	
Cholangioles		Bacterial cholangitis	Cholangioma	

filtration. They may become hyperplastic in cirrhosis or neoplasm causing hepatomas. Metastatic carcinoma is a common cause of hepatomegaly. Supporting tissue may proliferate to form a sarcoma. Edema of the liver with hepatomegaly results from chronic congestive heart failure. Infiltration with amyloid or glycogen may cause hepatomegaly. CHF and infectious hepatitis cause a tender liver, which distinguishes them from other forms of hepatomegaly. Extrinsic conditions causing apparent hepatomegaly but which are really only displacement of the liver are diaphragmatic abscess and pulmonary emphysema. In hemolytic anemias the liver may be enlarged because of the increased load on the reticuloendothelial tissue (both in liver and spleen) to dispose of the damaged red cells.

Approach to the Diagnosis

When there is no jaundice, a liver scan and biopsy are useful in determining the cause of hepatomegaly. Congestive heart failure should be excluded with a venous pressure and circulation time. In the presence of jaundice, a careful laboratory workup (Appendix I) to rule out obstruction must be done before a biopsy is entertained.

I Intoxication	C Congenital	A Autoimmune	T Trauma	E Endocrine
Alcoholism Carbon tetrachloride Drugs	Cystic disease Hamartoma	Lupoid Hepatitis	Contusion Laceration	Hyperthyroidism
	Gaucher's disease Hemolytic anemias	Periarteritis nodosa Myeloid metaplasia		
			Hepatic artery ligation	
Milk causing bile inspissation	Biliary atresia		Stones	Stones (diabetes)
Thorazine Birth control pills	Dubin–Johnson syndrome			Pregnancy

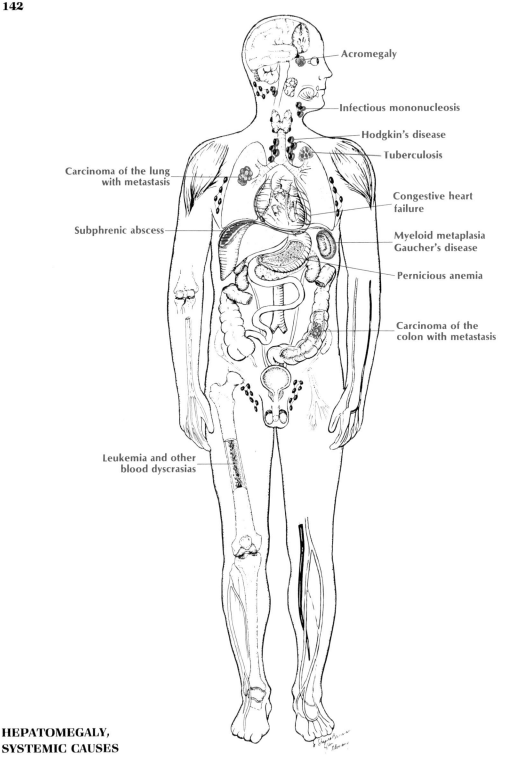

Acromegaly

Infectious mononucleosis

Hodgkin's disease

Tuberculosis

Carcinoma of the lung
with metastasis

Congestive heart
failure

Myeloid metaplasia
Gaucher's disease

Subphrenic abscess

Pernicious anemia

Carcinoma of the
colon with metastasis

Leukemia and other
blood dyscrasias

**HEPATOMEGALY,
SYSTEMIC CAUSES**

JAW SWELLING ■

Applying **anatomy** one can quickly ascertain that a lump in the jaw may come from the skin and subcutaneous tissues, glands, or bones.

1. **Skin and subcutaneous tissue.** This will remind one of lipomas, fibromas, and sebaceous cysts, although cellulitis and carbuncles may occur too. Other skin masses are discussed on page 166.
2. **Parotid gland.** Important lesions here are mumps, Mikulicz's syndrome in Hodgkin's disease, Behçet's disease of uveoparotid fever, and mixed tumors of the salivary gland. A stone in Stensen's duct may cause an intermittent swelling of the parotid gland.
3. **Jaw bone.** These are best divided into etiologic groups using the mnemonic **MINT.**
   M—Malformations include congenital protrusions of the jaw, acquired protrusion from acromegaly, and thickening of the jaw in Paget's disease.
   I—Inflammation suggests alveolar abscesses, osteomyelitis, actinomycosis and tuberculosis, or syphilis.
   N—Neoplasms include osteomas, adamantomas, sarcomas, myelomas, metastatic carcinomas, and odontomas.
   T—Trauma obviously can cause severe fracture dislocations, subperiosteal hematomas, and dislocation of the jaw. It is worthwhile to mention that hyperparathyroidism may cause cystic lesions of the jaw (generalized osteitis fibrosa cystica).

Approach to the Diagnosis

The approach to the diagnosis is to obtain roentgenograms of the jaw and teeth, and calcium, phosphorus, and alkaline phosphatase determinations and to perform biopsy and excision when indicated. Sialography and bone scans may be useful in selected cases.

(Text continues on p. 146)

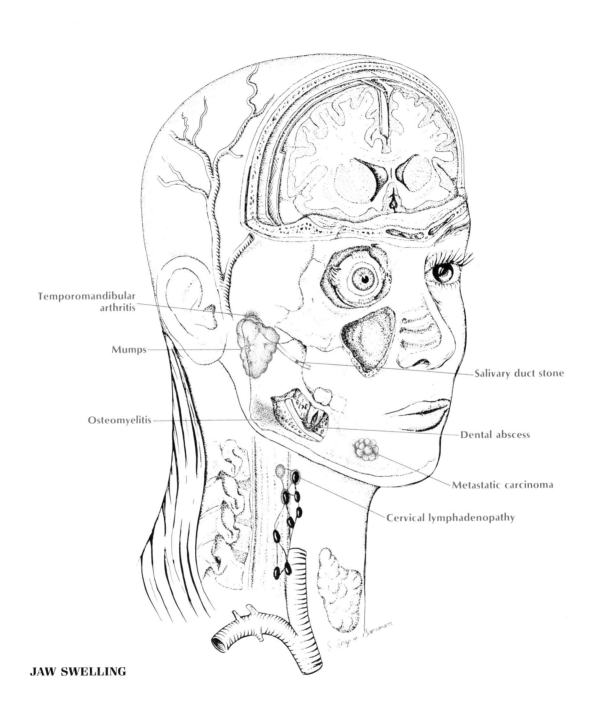

Temporomandibular
arthritis

Mumps

Osteomyelitis

Salivary duct stone

Dental abscess

Metastatic carcinoma

Cervical lymphadenopathy

JAW SWELLING

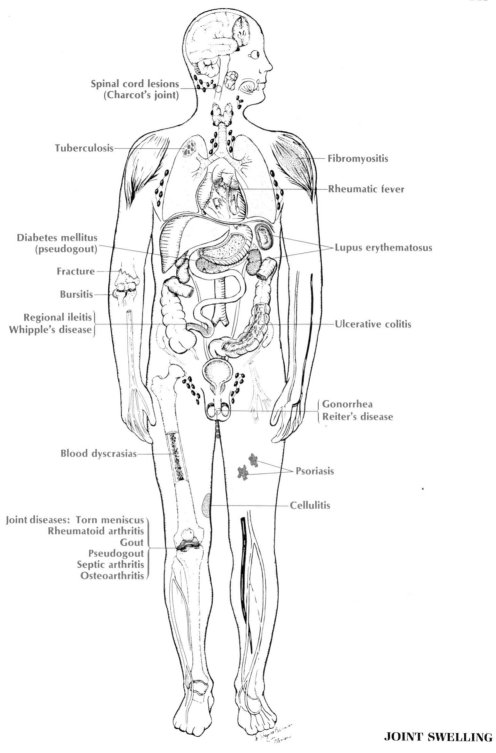

Spinal cord lesions
(Charcot's joint)

Tuberculosis

Diabetes mellitus
(pseudogout)

Fracture

Bursitis

Regional ileitis
Whipple's disease

Blood dyscrasias

Joint diseases: Torn meniscus
Rheumatoid arthritis
Gout
Pseudogout
Septic arthritis
Osteoarthritis

Fibromyositis

Rheumatic fever

Lupus erythematosus

Ulcerative colitis

Gonorrhea
Reiter's disease

Psoriasis

Cellulitis

JOINT SWELLING

JOINT SWELLING ■

The best approach to analysis of this symptom is **anatomical** and **histological** (Table 2-12). However, if one remembers the biochemical causes of joint disease, gout, pseudogout, and ochronosis immediately come to mind.

Let us discuss the conditions to be considered in an anatomical and histological breakdown of the joint. In the **skin** an abscess or hematoma is a possibility. Subcutaneous lipoma and pretibial myxedema may involve

the area of the joint as may edema, particularly in phlebitis. Around all joints are **bursae** which can become inflamed and swollen, especially when torn ligaments constantly rub against them.

Next let us consider the **ligaments** of the joint, especially those in the knee. Weak collateral ligaments will lead to recurrent swelling from fluid accumulation in the knee. Ruptured anterior or posterior cruciate ligaments will also create intermittent pain and swelling. To diagnose this condition, bend the knee and pull the tibia and lower leg forward and

TABLE 2-12.   JOINT SWELLING

	V Vascular	I Infection	N Neoplasm	D Degenerative
Skin		Carbuncle		
Subcutaneous Tissue		Cellulitis	Lipoma	
Bursa		Bursitis		
Synovium		Gonococcal arthritis Tuberculous arthritis Streptococcal arthritis	Synovioma	
Ligaments of Joint				
Joint Space				"Joint mice"
Cartilage				Degenerative osteoarthritis
Bone	Aseptic bone necrosis	Staphylococcal osteo- myelitis Tuberculous osteo- myelitis		
Blood Vessels	Sickle cell anemia	Phlebitis		

backward like opening and closing a drawer. Finally, if the meniscus is ruptured a distinct popping or locking of the joint will occur when the joint is flexed and then extended under pressure, especially with internal or external rotation of the lower leg.

The **synovium** is the site of most pathological conditions of the knee. Rheumatic fever, rheumatoid arthritis, lupus erythematosus, and Reiter's disease are classical collagen diseases affecting the synovium. The most common infectious diseases are gonorrhea and streptococcus, but tuberculosis and brucellosis should not be forgotten. Trauma to the synovium produces hemarthrosis, but it does not take much to cause hemarthrosis in hemophilia and occasionally in other coagulation disorders.

Moving on to the bone, osteomyelitis and syphilis must be considered; staphylococcus and tuberculosis are also common offenders. Aseptic bone necrosis (e.g., Osgood–Schlatter disease of the knee) is another condition of the bone that causes apparent joint swelling.

Idiopathic degeneration of the cartilage is a common cause of joint disease in the form of

I Intoxication	C Congenital or Collagen	A Allergic Autoimmune	T Trauma	E Endocrine
			Hematoma	
	Lupus Rheumatoid arthritis	Reiter's disease Serum sickness	Hemarthrosis	
			Ruptured ligaments	
Gout pseudogout	Rheumatic fever		Hemarthrosis	Intermittent hydrarthrosis
	Ochronosis		Torn meniscus	
	Hemophilia			

osteoarthritis. Ochronosis may lead to degeneration, but there is usually calcification of the
cartilage on roentgenograms.

Approach to the Diagnosis

The most important diagnostic procedure is
to aspirate the joint. The differential diagnosis
of joint fluid may be found on page 503, Appendix I. Multiple joint involvement is more
common in collagen diseases, while gonorrhea and gout classically affect one joint at a
time, but this is not a hard and fast rule. Migratory arthritis is classically seen in rheumatic fever. Osteoarthritis usually affects the
distal phalanges (Heberden's nodes), whereas
rheumatoid arthritis affects the metacarpo-
phalangeal joints most frequently. These and
other methods of narrowing the differential
diagnosis are more appropriately discussed
in physical diagnosis texts. Other diagnostic
tests are listed in Appendix I.

LYMPHADENOPATHY, GENERALIZED ■

Many of the conditions that cause splenomegaly also cause generalized lymphadenopathy. They are best recalled with the use of
the mnemonic **MINT.**

M—Malformations include sickle cell anemia and other congenital hemolytic
  anemias, the reticuloendothelioses (Niemann–Pick disease, Hand–Schüller–Christian disease, and Gaucher's disease), and
  lymphangiomas.
I—Inflammatory disorders constitute the
  largest group of lymphadenopathies. Breaking them down into subgroups according
  to the size of the organism further assists
  the recall.
  1. **Viral illnesses** include infectious mono-
     nucleosis, lymphogranuloma venereum,

German measles, chickenpox, and viral
     upper respiratory illnesses. There are
     also many other conditions in this cate-
     gory.
  2. **Rickettsial diseases** include typhus
     and Rocky Mountain spotted fever.
  3. **Bacterial diseases** include typhoid,
     plague, tuberculosis, skin infections, tu-
     laremia, meningococcemia, and brucel-
     losis.
  4. **Spirochetes** includes syphilis and
     Borelia vincentii.
  5. **Parasites** include malaria, filariasis, and
     trypanosomiasis.
  6. **Fungi** include histoplasmosis, dissemi-
     nated coccidiomycosis, and blastomy-
     cosis.
N—Neoplasms. Dissemination of almost
  every malignancy may cause a generalized
  lymphadenopathy. The most likely ones to
  present with generalized lymphadenopathy, however, are lymphatic leukemia,
  monocytic leukemia, Hodgkin's disease,
  and lymphosarcoma. Myelophthisic anemia must be considered too.
T—Toxic disorders that cause generalized
  lymphadenopathy are numerous. Dilantin
  toxicity may mimic Hodgkin's disease. Drug
  allergies from sulfonamides, hydralazine,
  and iodides are just a few of the others.

In addition to the conditions listed above,
systemic diseases that may cause lymphadenopathy include the autoimmune disorders such as lupus erythematosus (50% of the
cases with lupus erythematosus are associated with lymphadenopathy), dermatomyositis, sarcoidosis, and Still's disease.

Approach to the Diagnosis

Obviously it is tempting simply to do a lymph
node biopsy, but certain other procedures
should be done first. If the patient is febrile,
febrile agglutinins, Monospot test, blood cultures, and cultures of any other suspicious

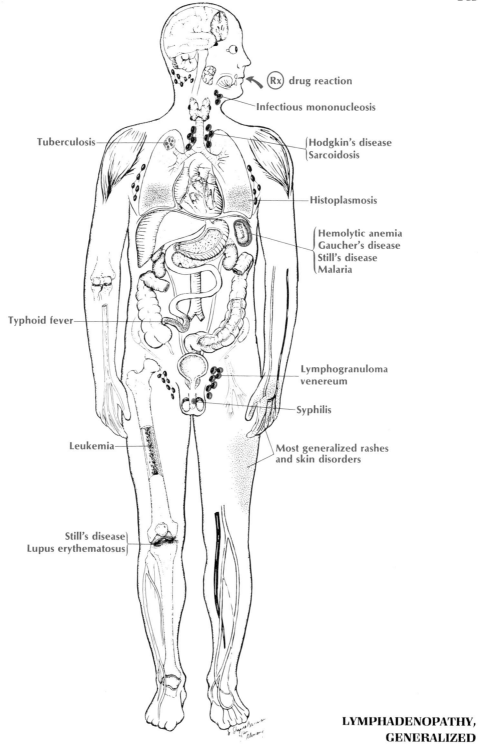

(Rx) drug reaction

Infectious mononucleosis

Tuberculosis

Hodgkin's disease
Sarcoidosis

Histoplasmosis

Hemolytic anemia
Gaucher's disease
Still's disease
Malaria

Typhoid fever

Lymphogranuloma
venereum

Syphilis

Most generalized rashes
and skin disorders

Leukemia

Still's disease
Lupus erythematosus

**LYMPHADENOPATHY,
GENERALIZED**

body fluid should be made. A fluorescent treponemal antibody absorption test (FTA–ABS) should be done as well as a chest roentgenogram and tuberculin test to rule out tuberculosis. A blood count usually shows leukemia, but a bone marrow may be necessary to diagnose leukemia and Hodgkin's disease as well as the reticuloendothelioses. Other roentgenograms, skin tests, and special diagnostic procedures that may be necessary are listed in Appendix I.

NASAL MASS OR SWELLING ■

Although anatomy may assist somewhat in developing the differential here, it is probably an unnecessary exercise because the mnemonic **MINT** will bring virtually all the etiologies to mind.

M—Malformation reminds one of the broad nose of cretinism, mongolism, gargoylism, myxedema, and acromegaly.

I—Inflammation suggests caruncles, cellulitis, syphilis, acne, rosacea with rhinophyma, Wegener's midline granuloma, and granulomas from tuberculosis, aspergillosis, rhinosporidiosis, mucormycosis, and other chronic infections.

N—Neoplasms suggest carcinomas of the external nares, and also squamous cell carcinoma of the nasal mucosa (such as Schmincke tumors), and nasal polyps secondary to allergic rhinitis.

T—Trauma reminds one of fractures, dislocations, and contusions, even though these diagnoses are usually obvious.

Approach to the Diagnosis

The diagnosis is not difficult except in the case of granulomas and carcinomas, when skillful biopsy and culturing are necessary. In Wegener's midline granuloma a search for alveolitis and glomerulonephritis will help determine the diagnosis. Appendix I provides additional tests that may be used in difficult diagnostic problems.

NECK MASS ■

Anatomy is the most important basic science used in developing the differential diagnosis in the case of a neck mass. **Histology** is then applied to each anatomical structure to further develop the list. As with any mass, a neck mass may be due to the proliferation of tissues in any of the anatomical structures, a displacement or malposition of tissues or anatomical structures, or the presence of fluid, air, bleeding, or other substance foreign to the neck.

Visualize the anatomy of the neck and think of the skin, thyroid, lymph nodes, trachea, esophagus, jugular veins, carotid arteries, brachial plexus, cervical spine, and muscles. Thus, taking **thyroid** enlargement, hypertrophy and cystic formation (endemic goiter), hyperplasia (Grave's disease), neoplasm (adenomas and carcinomas), thyroiditis (subacute or Hashimoto's), cysts (colloid type), and hemorrhage come to mind. Thyroglossal duct cysts also occur.

Lymph nodes may be enlarged by many inflammatory diseases, but when they present as an isolated mass they are usually infiltrated with Hodgkin's disease or a metastatic carcinoma from the thyroid, lungs, breast, or stomach. Tuberculosis, actinomycosis, and other chronic inflammatory diseases may present this way. **Tracheal** enlargement is rarely a problem in differential diagnosis, but bronchial cleft cysts may present as a mass. Pulsion diverticuli are the main masses of **esophageal** origin but carcinoma of the esophagus

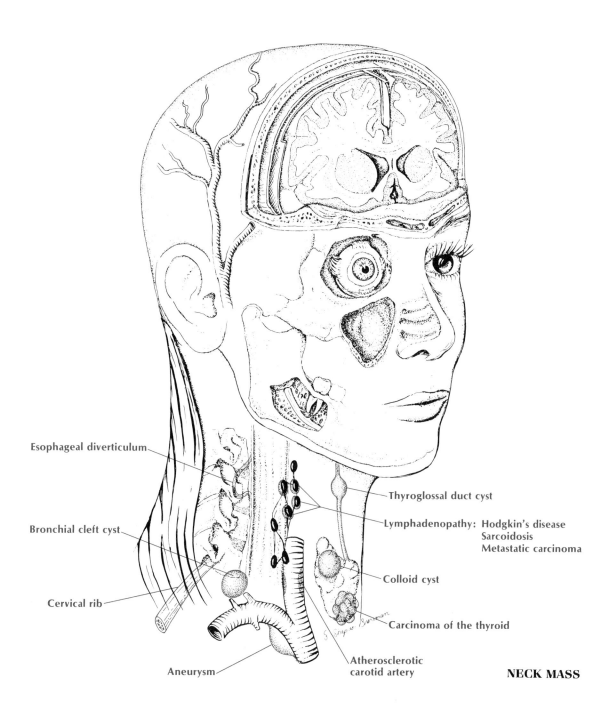

Esophageal diverticulum

Bronchial cleft cyst

Cervical rib

Aneurysm

Thyroglossal duct cyst

Lymphadenopathy: **Hodgkin's disease**
Sarcoidosis
Metastatic carcinoma

Colloid cyst

Carcinoma of the thyroid

Atherosclerotic carotid artery

NECK MASS

may involve the upper third on rare occasions. There is rarely a problem distinguishing **jugular veins** from a mass of other origin. **Carotid artery** aneurysms are distinguished by their pulsatile nature; occasionally, an aortic aneurysm may be felt in the neck. When there is severe atherosclerotic disease of the carotids, one or both may be felt as a "lead pipe" in the neck. Neuofibromas of the **brachial plexus** are rare but must be considered. Any neoplasm that metastasizes to the **cervical spine** may spread out into the neck; a plasmacytoma is likely to do this in multiple myeloma. A cervical rib may occasionally be

TABLE 2-13.   NECK MASS

	V Vascular	**I** Inflammatory	**N** Neoplasm	**D** Degenerative
Skin		Subcutaneous emphysema	Lipoma Angioma Carcinoma	
Thyroid		Cysts (colloid type) Thyroiditis	Adenomas Carcinomas	Endemic goiter
Lymph Nodes		Tuberculosis Actinomycosis Lymphadenitis	Hodgkin's disease Metastatic carcinoma	
Trachea		Bronchial cleft cyst		
Esophagus			Carcinoma of esophagus	
Jugular Veins	Thrombosis Varicocele Obstruction		Hemangiomas	
Carotid Arteries	Aneurysms			Atherosclerotic disease
Brachial Plexus			Neurofibromas	
Cervical Spine		Tuberculosis	Multiple myeloma Metastatic carcinoma	
Muscles of Neck		Myositis	Rhabdomyosarcoma	

felt in the neck. Finally, a large scalenus anterior muscle may be felt as a mass in the neck.

Neoplasms of the *skin* present here, as elsewhere (*e.g.,* lipoma). Abnormal accumulations of fluid, air, or other substances in colloid cyst and bronchial cleft cysts have already been mentioned, but what about carbuncles, sebaceous cysts, and angioneurotic edema? Cystic hygromas present from birth contain a serous or mucoid material and may be huge. Finally, subcutaneous emphysema must not be forgotten. These conditions are illustrated in Table 2-13.

I Intoxication	C Congenital	A Allergic and Autoimmune	T Trauma	E Endocrine
	Cystic hygroma	Angioneurotic edema	Contusion Fractured rib	
				Grave's disease Thyroid carcinoma
		Sarcoidosis		
	Diverticulum of esophagus		Surgical esophageal bypass	
			Hemorrhage	
			Contusion	
	Cervical rib		Fracture Sprain Contusions	
	Scalenus anticus			

Approach to the Diagnosis

If it can be determined that the mass is an enlarged lymph node, exploration and biopsy might best facilitate the diagnosis if a chest roentgenogram and an upper GI series fail to reveal a source for metastasis. Roentgenograms of the cervical spine, tuberculin skin test, arteriography, and bronchoscopy are all indicated in selected cases. A CT scan may disclose an unsuspected mediastinal mass. Appendix I lists these and other useful tests for the workup of the mass in the neck.

ORAL OR LINGUAL MASS   ■

Most of these lesions are tumors, but because some are caused by other etiologies it is well to use the mnemonic **MINT** to review the possibilities.

M—Malformations include dermoid cysts, ranula, Wharton's duct cysts or stones, mucous cysts, and thyroglossal cysts.

I—Inflammation should suggest peritonsillar abscesses, tonsillitis, sialadenitis, Ludwig's angina, and actinomycosis. Alveolar abscesses and granulomas may present as a mass inside the mouth.

N—Neoplasms are most commonly squamous cell carcinomas and are usually ulcerated. Angiomas, lipomas, papillomas, and sarcomas also occur.

T—Trauma suggest subperiosteal hematomas and submucosal hematomas, and also fracture-dislocations.

Approach to the Diagnosis

Most of these lesions are referred to the oral surgeon for diagnosis and treatment, so an elaborate discussion of the workup is unnecessary in a text of this scope. Obviously, cultures should be made in cases of suspected infectious granulomas, whereas biopsy or excision is the main diagnostic tool for neoplasms.

ORBITAL MASS   ■

Because most orbital masses cause exophthalmos, the differential diagnosis of the two is very similar (for illustration see Exophthalmos, p. 130). The best method to use to arrive at the causes is to visualize the **anatomy** of the orbit and then to think of the mnemonic **MINT.**

1. **Subcutaneous tissue.** Subcutaneous tissue proliferation in the orbit occurs in hyperthyroidism. There may be an orbital cellulitis or orbital hemorrhage into the subcutaneous tissue. Wegener's granulomatosis, orbital cysts, sarcomas, and metastatic carcinomas may occur here.
2. **Eyeballs.** An orbital echinococcal cyst may occur. Tumors, infections, and trauma to the eyeball may occasionally spread to the orbit.
3. **Veins.** These are distended in cavernous sinus thrombosis, carotid-cavernous fistulas, and hemangiomas.
4. **Arteries.** Aneurysms of the ophthalmic artery are rare but they may cause an orbital mass.
5. **Lacrimal gland.** Tumors and inflammation of this gland (*e.g.,* in Boeck's sarcoid) should be remembered.
6. **Sinuses.** Inflammatory lesions and tumors of the sinuses may spread to the orbit.
7. **Bone.** Sphenoid ridge meningiomas, metastatic carcinomas, tuberculous or syphilitic orbital periosteitis, and Hodgkin's disease may involve the bones of the orbit. Orbital fractures and hematomas may result from trauma.

The workup of these lesions is similar to the workup for exophthalmos (see p. 472).

PAPILLEDEMA

No anatomical analysis of this condition is necessary because most cases of papilledema are caused by intracranial pathology. Three notable extracranial conditions are optic neuritis, hypertension, and pseudotumor cerebri. The polycythemia and right heart failure of chronic pulmonary emphysema may combine to produce papilledema, but this is uncommon.

Analysis of the intracranial causes of papilledema is performed using the mnemonic **VINDICATE.**

V—Vascular lesions are aneurysms and arteriovenous malformations that cause subarachnoid hemorrhages. Severe hypertension may lead to an intracerebral hemorrhage or hypertensive encephalopathy, thus causing papilledema. Cerebral thrombosis and emboli rarely lead to papilledema.

I—Infection is not a common cause of papilledema unless a space-occupying lesion is produced or the condition persists. Thus a brain abscess is often associated with papilledema whereas acute bacterial meningitis is not. Chronic cryptococcal meningitis, syphilitic meningitis, and tuberculous meningitis, on the other hand, are not infrequently associated with some degree of papilledema. Viral encephalitis may occasionally be associated with papilledema. Cavernous sinus thrombosis and septic thrombosis of the other venous sinuses may produce papilledema.

N—Neoplasms, primary and metastic, are the most common cause of papilledema.

D—Degenerative diseases are rarely the cause.

I—Intoxication brings to mind lead encephalopathy, but other toxins and drugs rarely cause papilledema.

C—Congenital malformations that cause papilledema include the aneurysms and arteriovenous malformations already mentioned plus the various types of hydrocephalus, skull deformities (oxycephaly), hemophilia (because of intracranial hemorrhages), and occasionally Schilder's disease and other congenital encephalopathies.

A—Autoimmune recalls lupus cerebritis and periarteritis nodosa (when associated with severe hypertension).

T—Trauma does not usually produce papilledema in the early stages of concussions or epidural or subdural hematomas, but in chronic subdural hematomas it is the rule.

E—Endocrine disorders bring to mind the papilledema of malignant pheochromocytomas (with hypertension), and the fact that pseudotumor cerebri occurs in obese, amenorrheic, and emotionally disturbed women.

Approach to the Diagnosis

The approach to the diagnosis of papilledema in someone without hypertension or hypertensive retinopathy must include a thorough neurological examination and a CT scan. If focal signs are present or the CT scan is positive, referral to a neurosurgeon is indicated. A spinal tap is contraindicated. If there are no focal signs it may be worthwhile to differentiate papilledema from optic neuritis by having an ophthalmologist perform a visual field. This may also be helpful in differentiating pseudotumor cerebri because there may be bilateral visual defects in the inferior nasal quadrants. Papilledema from increased intracranial pressure will show only an enlarged blind spot (unless there is a tumor of the optic tracts, radiations, or occipital cortex), whereas

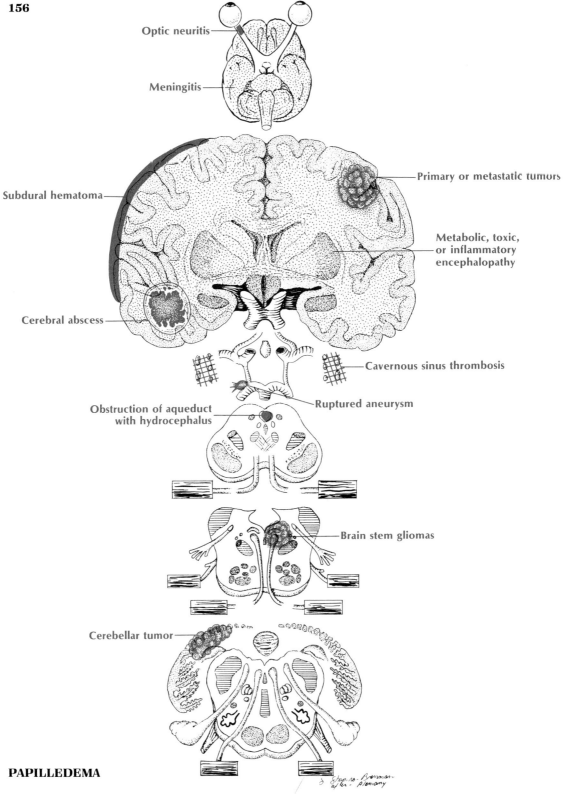

Optic neuritis

Meningitis

Primary or metastatic tumors

Subdural hematoma

Metabolic, toxic, or inflammatory encephalopathy

Cerebral abscess

Cavernous sinus thrombosis

Obstruction of aqueduct with hydrocephalus

Ruptured aneurysm

Brain stem gliomas

Cerebellar tumor

PAPILLEDEMA

optic neuritis will show scotomata peripheral to the blind spot (disc). Appendix I lists several other procedures that may be useful in the workup of papilledema. Appendix II will be useful to confirm the diagnosis of a specific disease.

PELVIC MASS

A mass in the pelvis is usually but not always a neoplasm. Is there a quick way to recall all the various causes while examining the pelvis? **Anatomy** is the key. Apply the mnemonic **MINT** to develop a list of the many possibilities (Table 2-14).

Anatomically, there are three major groups of structures: the urinary tract, the female genital tract, and the lower intestinal tract. Breaking these down into their components, there are the bladder and ureters, the vagina, cervix, uterus, fallopian tubes and ovaries, and the rectum and sigmoid colon. In addition to these structures, the diseases of the aorta and iliac vessels, spine, and surrounding muscles and fascia must be considered. Other structures fill the pelvis from above. The small intestines, the omentum, and the appendix may

(Text continues on p. 160)

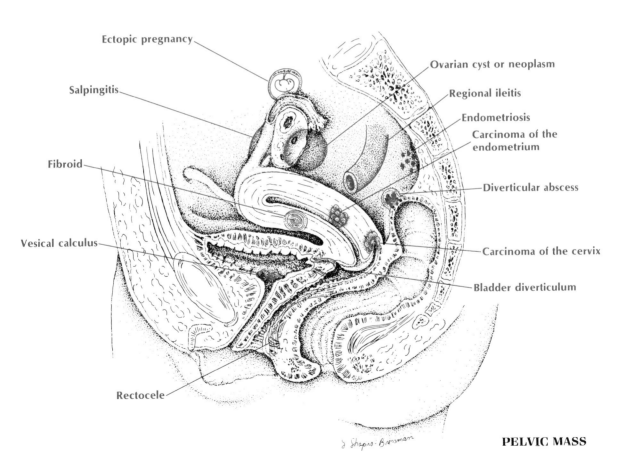

PELVIC MASS

TABLE 2-14.   PELVIC MASS

Anatomy	M Malformation	I Inflammation
Bladder	Obstruction with diverticuli Calculi	Hunner's ulcer
Urethra	Urethrocele Cystocele	
Ureters	Double ureter Calculi Ureterocele	
Vagina	Prolapsed cervix Rectocele	Bartholinitis fistula with rectum or bladder
Cervix		Cervicitis (rarely)
Uterus	Bicornuate uterus Retroversion	Endometritis
Fallopian Tubes	Ectopic pregnancy Endometriosis	Salpingitis
Ovary	Benign congenital ovarian cysts (*e.g.,* Morgagni)	Oophoritis
Rectum	Prolapse Rectocele	Inflamed hemorrhoids Rectal abscess Fistula
Sigmoid	Diverticulum	Diverticulitis Granulomatous colitis Ulcerative colitis
Arteries	Aneurysms	
Spine	Lordosis Scoliosis	Rheumatoid arthritis Spondylosis Tuberculosis
Miscellaneous	Pelvic kidney Omental cysts and adhesions	Appendicitis Regional ileitis

N **Neoplasms**	T **Trauma**
Carcinoma Polyps	Rupture of the bladder
Papilloma	
Carcinoma	Foreign body Tear
Carcinoma Polyps	
Endometrial carcinoma Choriocarcinoma Fibroids	Rupture during pregnancy
Carcinoma (rarely)	
Cystadenomas Cystadenocarcinomas Follicular and granulosa cell cysts	
Rectal carcinoma	
Carcinoma of polyps	Foreign body
Metastatic carcinoma Myeloma Hodgkin's disease	Fracture Ruptured disc
Pelvic metastasis from stomach, *e.g.*	Blood clots in cul-de-sac Surgical abscess

be felt; even the kidney may drop into the pelvis.

1. **Bladder.** Prominent conditions that must be considered here are stones, diverticuli, Hunner's ulcer, and carcinomas. A distended bladder is deceptive.
2. **Urethra.** A cystocele and urethrocele are felt easily during a pelvic examination, but if they are not, have the patient strain or stand up.
3. **Ureters.** A ureteral calculus or ureterocele may be felt.
4. **Vagina.** Vaginal carcinomas, prolapsed cervix or procidentia, rectocele, and Bartholin's cysts may be felt. A foreign body (*e.g.,* a pessary) should be considered.
5. **Cervix.** Carcinoma or polyps are the main considerations here, because an inflamed cervix does not usually cause a mass.
6. **Uterus.** Fibroids are the most likely tumor to be felt, but pregnancy, chronic endometritis and choriocarcinoma, and endometrial carcinomas all present as a mass. A retroverted uterus may masquerade as a mass in the cul-de-sac.
7. **Fallopian tubes.** Tubo-ovarian abscesses and endometriosis of these structures account for most cases. Ectopic pregnancy is always possible.
8. **Ovary.** Ovarian cysts and carcinomas must be considered as well as endometriosis.
9. **Rectum.** Carcinoma, abscesses and diverticulum, and prolapse are good possibilities here. Feces may masquerade as a mass.
10. **Sigmoid colon.** Again the disorders mentioned under Rectum (p. 165) must be considered. Granulomatous or ulcerative colitis may present as a mass.
11. **Arteries.** It is unusual for an aortic aneu-

rysm or an iliac aneurysm to be felt here, but they should be kept in mind.
12. **Spine.** Deformities of the spine (*e.g.,* lordosis), tuberculosis (Pott's disease), and metastatic or primary malignancies of the spine (*e.g.,* myeloma) may present as a pelvic mass.
13. **Miscellaneous.** A pelvic kidney may be felt. An inflamed segment of ileum (regional ileitis) or the appendix should be considered, as should omental cysts and adhesions.

Approach to the Diagnosis

The association with other symptoms is the key to the clinical diagnosis. A painless mass is likely to be a neoplasm, whereas a tender mass with fever suggests pelvic inflammatory disease (PID) or a diverticular abscess. Obviously, an ectopic pregnancy should be associated with tender breasts, frequency of urination, and morning sickness. The next logical step is ultrasonography.

Laboratory tests include urinalysis and culture, pregnancy test, stool for blood and parasites, and vaginal cultures. A proctoscopy and barium enema may be useful. Colonoscopy, culdoscopy, or peritoneoscopy and cystoscopy may all need to be done before an exploratory laparotomy is done.

PERIORBITAL AND FACIAL EDEMA

The mechanism for periorbital and facial edema is similar to that for edema of the extremities. Thus increased back pressure of the veins will cause periorbital edema in right heart failure, constrictive pericarditis, advanced pulmonary emphysema, and thrombosis or extrinsic obstruction of the superior

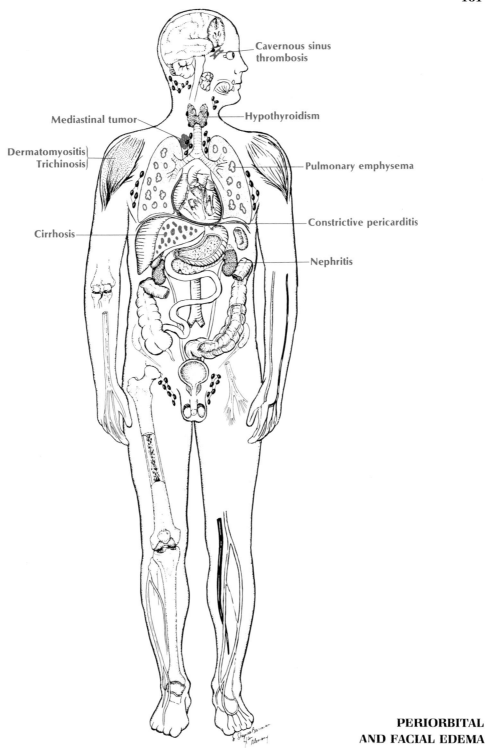

Cavernous sinus
thrombosis

Mediastinal tumor

Hypothyroidism

Dermatomyositis
Trichinosis

Pulmonary emphysema

Constrictive pericarditis

Cirrhosis

Nephritis

**PERIORBITAL
AND FACIAL EDEMA**

vena cava (as in mediastinal tumors). High blood pressure from acute glomerulonephritis and malignant hypertension will cause periorbital and facial edema. Low serum albumin will lead to periorbital and facial edema in nephrosis and cirrhosis. Mucoprotein in the subcutaneous tissue will cause periorbital edema in hypothyroidism.

Other causes for periorbital edema are not associated as frequently with edema in the extremities. Allergic or inflammatory dilatation of the capillaries around the eyelids will cause periorbital edema in dermatomyositis and trichinosis. A thrombosed cavernous sinus will also cause periorbital edema, but this is similar to thrombophlebitis of an extremity. Local causes for periorbital edema include orbital cellulitis, urticaria, angioneurotic edema, contusions, and other orbital trauma.

The workup of periorbital edema is similar to that for edema of the extremities (p. 128).

POPLITEAL SWELLING ■

The key to recalling the causes of a popliteal swelling is **anatomy**. Each structure in the popliteal space may be involved by one or two conditions that cause a mass or swelling. In visualizing the anatomy one encounters the skin, subcutaneous tissue, muscle, bursae, veins, arteries, lymphatics, nerves, and bones.

1. **Skin.** The skin may be involved by urticaria, sebaceous cysts, carbuncles, lipomas, hemangiomas, and various other skin masses.
2. **Subcutaneous tissue.** Lipomas, sarcomas, and cellulitis are the main lesions encountered.
3. **Muscle.** Contusions of the gastrocnemius

and semimembranous muscles may cause a mass in the popliteal fossa.

4. **Bursae.** Popliteal cysts (Baker's cysts) may result from filling of the bursa between the gastrocnemius and semimembranous muscles with a gelatinous or serous substance.
5. **Veins.** The veins may enlarge from a varicocele or thrombophlebitis.
6. **Artery.** An aneurysm of the popliteal artery may result from atherosclerosis or a gunshot wound. When there is a loud bruit over the artery and distention of the veins, an arteriovenous fistula should be considered.
7. **Lymphatics.** Enlarged popliteal nodes may result from infections in the distal portion of the extremity, tuberculous adenopathy, or metastatic malignancy.
8. **Nerves.** Traumatic neuromas or neurofibromas may involve the nerves here.
9. **Bone.** Exostosis arising from the epiphyseal cartilage of the femur is a well-defined tumor of children or young adults. Medullary giant cell tumors, fibrosarcomas of the periosteum, and osteomyelitis may present as a mass in this area also. Fractures and periosteal hematomas should present no problem in diagnosis.

Approach to the Diagnosis

A roentgenogram of the bones and joints in the area is the first step. If the mass is thought to be a varicocele it should disappear on elevation of the leg. If a Baker's cyst is suspected, aspiration will be helpful in diagnosis. Bone scans may be useful in diagnosing early primary or metastatic tumors. Arteriography, phlebography, and a lymphangiogram may be useful. Exploration and biopsy may be the only way to establish a definitive diagnosis in some cases.

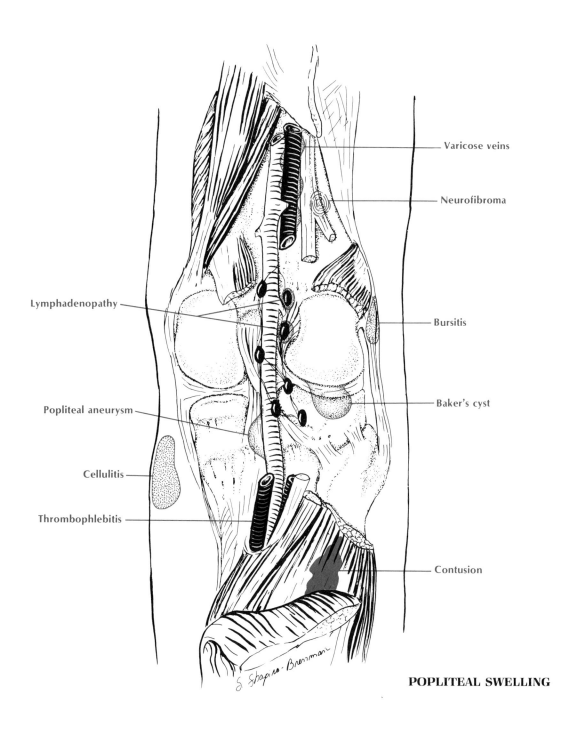

Varicose veins

Neurofibroma

Lymphadenopathy

Bursitis

Popliteal aneurysm

Baker's cyst

Cellulitis

Thrombophlebitis

Contusion

S. Shapiro-Brennan

POPLITEAL SWELLING

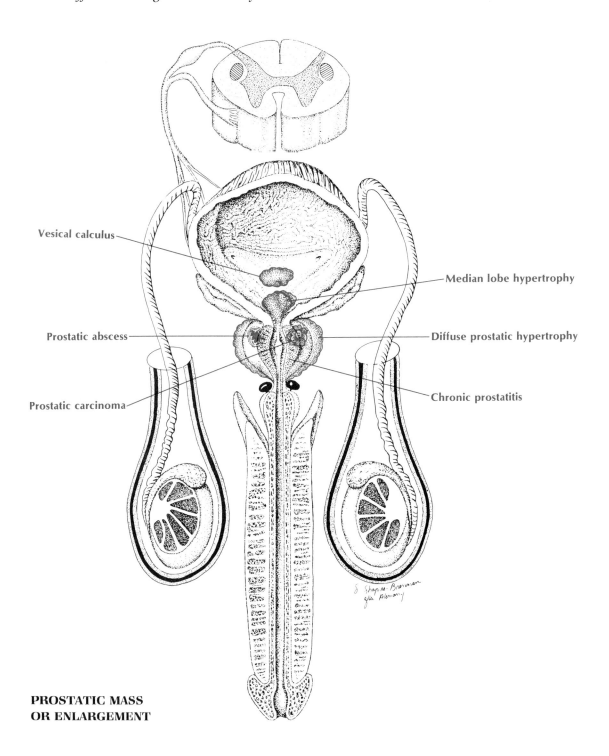

Vesical calculus

Median lobe hypertrophy

Prostatic abscess

Diffuse prostatic hypertrophy

Prostatic carcinoma

Chronic prostatitis

**PROSTATIC MASS
OR ENLARGEMENT**

PROSTATIC MASS OR ENLARGEMENT ▪

When the physician examines the rectum and prostate in a routine physical, generally there are only two conditions that he is looking for—benign prostatic hypertrophy and prostatic carcinoma. The former presents a diffuse enlargement, soft in consistency, and the prostate varies in size from a plum to an orange. Prostatic carcinomas, on the other hand, present as a stony, hard nodule in the lateral superior or inferior areas in the early stages or as a diffuse, hard nodular enlargement in the more advanced stage. The approach is different for the patient presenting with a urethral discharge or difficulty voiding, because then one must include **acute** and **chronic prostatitis** and also **prostatic abscess** in the differential.

In brief, that is the differential diagnosis of an enlarged prostate. The only trick that might be useful in remembering it is to keep in mind the ages 20–40–60–80. In general, the 20-year-old male will usually have acute prostatitis from gonorrhea or other bacteria. The 40-year-old males would probably have chronic prostatitis from previous gonorrhea or from nonspecific prostatitis. The 60-year-old males may have prostatic hypertrophy, and the 80-year-old males would most likely have prostatic carcinoma. It is important to remember that any one of these diseases may appear at the ages of 40, 60, and 80.

Approach to the Diagnosis

The approach to the diagnosis is first to massage to see if a urethral discharge can be elicited (not wise in acute prostatic abscess), then to do a smear and culture of the discharge. Order a urine culture (and catheterization for residual urine if obstruction is suspected), an IVP, and a voiding cystogram for further con-

firmation of obstruction or infection. Finally, cystoscopy and prostatic biopsy may be necessary. One of the rewarding things about the speciality of urology is that diagnosis can be almost 100% accurate if all the special procedures are judiciously applied (Appendix I).

RECTAL MASS ▪

Of course the physician is looking for a rectal carcinoma when he does a routine rectal examination, but what else might he find? Use the mnemonic **VINDICATE** in order to have a list of possibilities clearly in mind before the examination.

V—Vascular suggests internal and external hemorrhoids.

I—Inflammation includes submucous and perirectal abscesses.

N—Neoplasms most often manifest as rectal polyps and carcinomas. Other conditions to be remembered include the Blummer's shelf of metastatic carcinoma from many sites into the pouch of Douglas, and prostatic hypertrophy and carcinomas.

D—Degenerative conditions are not associated with a rectal mass.

I—Intoxication signifies a fecal impaction, particularly from a hunk of barium after a barium enema.

C—Congenital and **acquired anomalies** should remind one of diverticuli that may become abscessed and create a mass in the cul-de-sac. They may also recall a pelvic appendix and rectal prolapse.

A—Autoimmune conditions include regional ileitis, which may lodge in the cul-de-sac and create a fistula with the rectum.

T—Trauma signifies a ruptured bladder.

E—Endocrine recalls the various ovarian tumors and ruptured ectopic pregnancy that will produce a mass in the cul-de-sac.

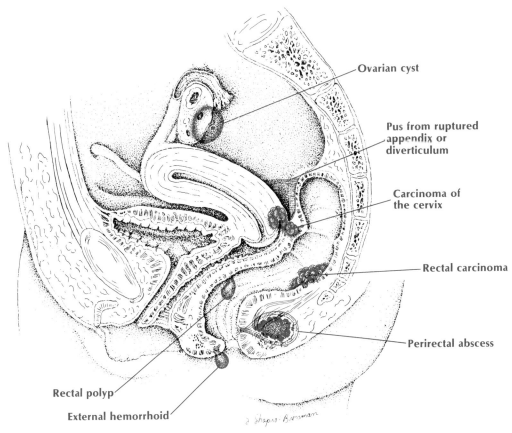

Ovarian cyst

Pus from ruptured appendix or diverticulum

Carcinoma of the cervix

Rectal carcinoma

Perirectal abscess

Rectal polyp

External hemorrhoid

RECTAL MASS

There are, therefore, numerous disorders to keep in mind when examining the rectum.

Approach to the Diagnosis

Anoscopy, sigmoidoscopy and a barium enema are the most significant tools in the proctologist's armamentarium. Biopsy or excision of polyps is routine. When one polyp is found a barium enema or colonoscopy is always done to look for others. Appendix I lists other important tests.

SKIN MASS ▪

Masses of the skin may be better termed nodules if they are greater than 0.5 cm and are not just neoplastic in origin. The term **VINDI-CATE** serves as a useful mnemonic to recall the important skin masses. When the physician is considering the cause of a mass in any part of the body, he must include a possible skin mass in the differential. Therefore, although I have limited the discussion of skin

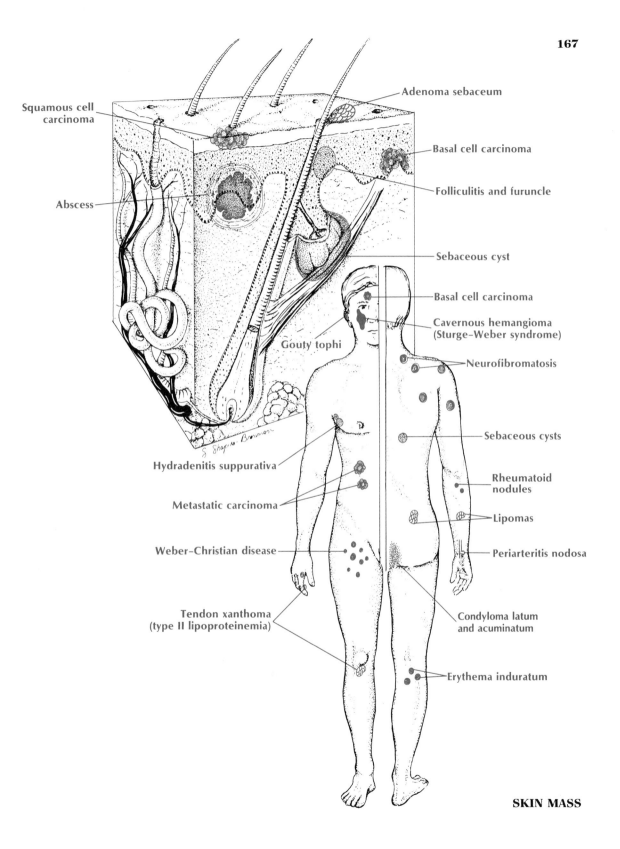

Squamous cell carcinoma

Abscess

Adenoma sebaceum

Basal cell carcinoma

Folliculitis and furuncle

Sebaceous cyst

Basal cell carcinoma

Cavernous hemangioma (Sturge-Weber syndrome)

Neurofibromatosis

Gouty tophi

Sebaceous cysts

Hydradenitis suppurativa

Rheumatoid nodules

Metastatic carcinoma

Lipomas

Weber-Christian disease

Periarteritis nodosa

Tendon xanthoma (type II lipoproteinemia)

Condyloma latum and acuminatum

Erythema induratum

SKIN MASS

lesions in other sections, the reader should turn to this section if the mass is thought to originate in the skin.

V—Vascular lesions include cavernous hemangiomas, varicose veins, hemorrhages from scurvy or coagulation disorders, and emboli from subacute bacterial endocarditis (Osler's nodules).

I—Inflammatory masses include caruncles, furuncles, warts, condyloma latum and acuminatum, molluscum contagiosum, tuberculomas, gummas, and granulomas from coccidiomycosis, sporotrichosis, and other fungi.

N—Neoplasms constitute the largest group of skin masses. The important ones to remember are basal cell and squamous cell carcinomas, melanomas, nevi, sarcomas, metastatic nodules, Kaposi's sarcomas, lipomas, neurofibromatosis, dermoid cysts, leiomyomas, lymphangiomas, and mycosis fungoides. Leukemic infiltration and Hodgkin's disease may cause skin nodules or plaques.

D—Degenerative diseases do not produce any skin masses worthy of mention but predispose to pressure sores. Heberden's nodes of osteoarthritis should be considered here.

I—Intoxication suggests the lesions of bromism.

C—Cystic lesions of the skin include sebaceous cysts, epithelial cysts, and dermoid cysts. Congenital lesions such as eosinophilic granulomas of the skin, tuberous sclerosis, and neurofibromatosis should not be overlooked.

A—Autoimmune disease includes the aneurysms of periarteritis nodosa, rheumatoid and rheumatic nodules, localized lupus or amyloidosis, and Weber–Christian disease.

T—Trauma induces contusions and edema of the skin.

E—Endocrine and metabolic diseases that cause skin masses are diabetes mellitus (ab-

scesses, *necrobiosis lipoidica diabeticorum*), hyperthyroidism (pretibial myxedema, acromegaly (tufting of the distal phalanges), gout (tophaceous deposits), hyperlipemia and hypercholesterolemia with multiple xanthomas, and calcinosis in hypercalcemic states.

Approach to the Diagnosis

A biopsy or excision is the best approach to the diagnosis. If a systemic disease is suspected because of a lesion, appropriate studies for these may be found in Appendix I.

SPLENOMEGALY

The patient is lying on the table and there is a palpable mass in the left upper quadrant. The mass has a hard smooth surface with a notch on the edge and descends on inspiration. The patient has an enlarged spleen. What can be done about it? What is causing it?

The key word is **histology.** Think about the histological components: parenchyma, supporting tissue, arteries, veins, and a capsule. What is the parenchyma? It is nothing more than the components of the blood: red cells, white cells, lymph tissue, and platelets. Now it is possible to form a differential. Increased numbers of red cells recall polycythemia; increased numbers of white cells recall leukemia and infection. Increased lymph tissue suggests Hodgkin's disease, whereas increased supporting tissue indicates reticuloendotheliosis and acromegaly. Increased size of the veins occurs in obstruction of the portal vein as in cirrhosis, thrombosis of the portal vein, and congestive heart failure. If the artery has a local increase in size an aneurysm forms, compressing the splenic veins.

A differential is at hand, but it is still incomplete. Now think of **physiology.** The spleen is

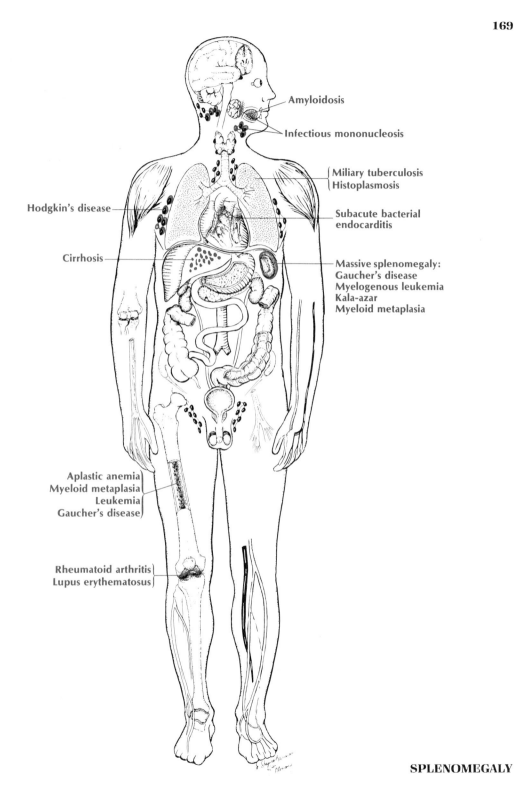

Amyloidosis

Infectious mononucleosis

Miliary tuberculosis
Histoplasmosis

Hodgkin's disease

Subacute bacterial
endocarditis

Cirrhosis

Massive splenomegaly:
Gaucher's disease
Myelogenous leukemia
Kala-azar
Myeloid metaplasia

Aplastic anemia
Myeloid metaplasia
Leukemia
Gaucher's disease

Rheumatoid arthritis
Lupus erythematosus

SPLENOMEGALY

a reserve for blood storage. It is also able to form red cells and other components of the blood when the bone marrow is atrophied, as in extramedullary erythropoiesis. More important, it is involved in the destruction of old or damaged red cells and platelets. Finally, it hypertrophies to fight infection just like the lymph glands. Extramedullary erythropoiesis recalls the splenomegaly of aplastic anemia and myeloid metaplasia, just as destruction or sequestration of cells brings to mind the splenomegaly of hemolytic anemias (*e.g.,* hereditary sphenocytosis, malaria, and lupus erythematosus) and thrombocytopenic purpura. The hypertrophy to fight infection or diffuse inflammation of the body should suggest the splenomegaly of bacterial endocarditis, kala-azar, infectious mononucleosis, miliary tuberculosis, and rheumatoid arthritis. Almost anything that causes general-

TABLE 2-15.   SPLENOMEGALY

	Increased Production	Neoplasia
Red Cells	Aplastic anemia Myelophthisic anemia	Polycythemia
White Cells	Myeloid metaplasia Infection	Leukemia
Platelets		
Lymph Tissue	Infectious mononucleosis	Hodgkin's disease Lymphangioma
Supporting Tissue		Metastatic carcinoma (rare)
Arteries		
Veins		Hemangioma

ized lymphadenopathy can cause splenomegaly.

Only one category of splenomegaly is not brought to mind by this approach, but it is easily remembered because it is an exception—infiltration of inert material. Thus in gargoylism there is a foreign mucopolysaccharide in the spleen. Numerous mucopolysaccharidoses are now described in the literature. There is a buildup of lipids in the reticuloendotheliosis of Gaucher's disease, Niemann–Pick disease and Hand–Shüller–Christian disease, but these are intracellular. Amyloid may infiltrate the spleen. Metastatic carcinoma of the spleen is rare.

Table 2-15 summarizes the above discussion and gives additional causes of splenomegaly to consider in the differential. One final diagnosis to consider is traumatic splenomegaly.

Increased Destruction	Obstruction	Infiltration
Hemolytic anemia Lupus erythematosus Pernicious anemia		
Agranulocytosis		
Idiopathic thrombocytopenic purpura (ITP)		
Lupus erythematosus Collagen disease		Hemochromatosis Reticuloendotheliosis Hurler's disease Amyloidosis Sarcoidosis
	Embolism Aneurysm	
	Congestive heart failure Cirrhosis Thrombosis Banti's disease Carcinoma of the tail of the pancreas	

Approach to the Diagnosis

How does one go about pinning down the diagnosis? First of all, there are several clinical clues. One looks in the physical examination for jaundice, lymphadenopathy, a rash, sore throat, hepatomegaly, and a positive Rumpel–Leede test. The combination of symptoms and signs will eliminate certain causes and make others more plausible. For example, splenomegaly with jaundice but no hepatomegaly suggests hemolytic anemia. The size of the spleen is also an important differential feature. If the spleen is very large it should suggest myeloid metaplasia, chronic myelogenous leukemia, Gaucher's disease, and kala-azar.

The laboratory is the principal aid from this point on (Appendix I). Smears for red cell morphology, malaria, and other parasites are invaluable. Blood cultures and a lymph node and bone biopsy may be useful. If a specific disease is strongly suspected Appendix II should be consulted to order appropriate tests.

SWOLLEN GUMS AND GUM MASS

The number of conditions causing focal or diffuse swelling of the gums is far out of proportion to the size of this organ and the fact that physicians frequently pay little attention to it unless the patient mentions it. The best approach is to apply the mnemonic **VINDI-CATE** to the gums and the list of possible causes will quickly come to mind.

V—Vascular disorders are not a significant cause of swollen gums.

I—Inflammatory lesions include gingivitis, whether viral (aphthous stomatitis), or fusospirochetal ("trench mouth"), or due to moniliasis. Focal abscesses of the gums are common. Alveolar abscesses also cause focal swelling of the gums.

N—Neoplasms remind one of monocytic leukemia and multiple myeloma, which are associated with diffuse hypertrophy and local tumors such as a sarcoma, papilloma, odontoma, and squamous cell carcinoma.

D—Deficiency diseases include scurvy and most vitamin deficiencies.

I—Intoxication suggests the common diffuse hyperplasia in epileptics on diphenylhydantoin and related drugs, including barbiturates.

C—Congenital or acquired malformations remind one of the gingivitis secondary to malocclusion, poor-fitting crowns or orthodontal appliances, and periodontal cysts, secondary to chronic periapical granuloma.

A—Autoimmune and **allergic** diseases include the hypertrophy of thrombocytopenic purpura and the contact gingivitis from dentures, mouth washes, and tooth pastes.

T—Trauma to the gums may cause local hematomas and fractures.

E—Endocrine disorders suggest several conditions that may cause gum hypertrophy. Gingival hyperplasia in pregnancy, the giant cell granulomas of hyperparathyroidism, juvenile hypothyroidism, pituitary dysfunction, and diabetes mellitus are the most important.

Approach to the Diagnosis

The approach to the diagnosis is to rule out systemic disease by checking other organs by physical examination and laboratory tests (Appendix I) and then refer the patient to a periodontist. When making a referral, it is wise to have the patient return or call back with the results of the examination after seeing the specialist. In this way one can be ready to do a further diagnostic workup should periodontal examination be negative.

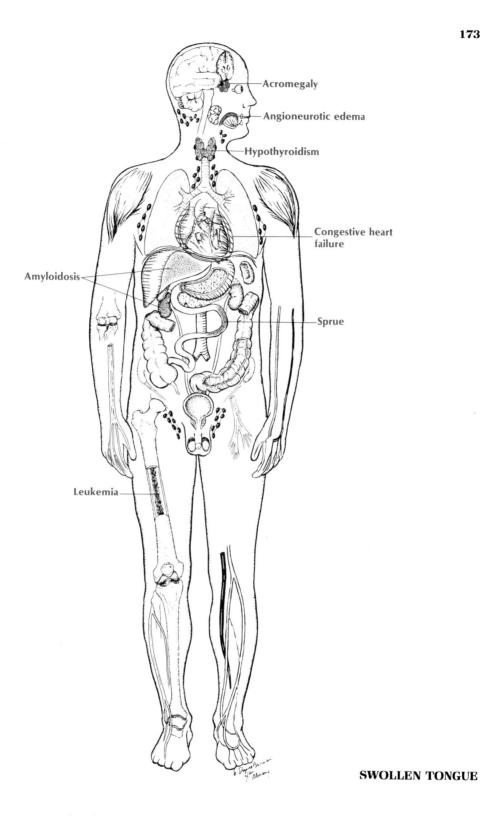

Acromegaly

Angioneurotic edema

Hypothyroidism

Congestive heart
failure

Amyloidosis

Sprue

Leukemia

SWOLLEN TONGUE

SWOLLEN TONGUE

Swollen tongue (macroglossia) is an uncommon complaint, yet on examination, it is not infrequently found. Is it possible to think of more than two or three causes? In most instances this is difficult, yet there is a key to recalling the many causes.

This symptom affords the opportunity to introduce yet another method of arriving at a differential diagnosis, the **histopathological** method. First of all, analyze the tissues of the tongue and then decide what can happen to enlarge them. There are mucosa, submucosal tissue, muscle, supporting tissue, blood ves-sels, and nerves. What pathologic process can enlarge each of these? Increase in size and number of the cells; infusion of serous fluids, pus, or blood; infiltration of a foreign protein or fat, and infiltration of foreign cells could cause such enlargement. These are all included in Table 2-16.

The **mucosa** can increase the number of cells in carcinoma of the tongue. It is swollen with a serous fluid in reaction to things put in the mouth such as hot food, mercury, and aspirin. Other less well-understood sources of fluid in the mucosa are erythema multiforme and pemphigus. The **submucosal** and **supporting tissue** may be enlarged by a serous fluid in angioneurotic edema, by a purulent

TABLE 2-16.   SWOLLEN TONGUE

	Serous Fluid	Pus
Mucosa	Mercury Aspirin Burns Erythema multiforme Pemphigus	
Submucosa and Supporting Tissue	Angioneurotic edema Insect bite	Acute diffuse glossitis Ludwig's angina
Muscle		
Blood Vessels	Dermatomyositis	

fluid in acute diffuse glossitis (usually caused by streptococcus organisms), or by a hemorrhagic fluid in leukemia, scurvy, and other hemorrhage disorders. The **subcutaneous** and **supporting tissue** can also be infiltrated by a mucoprotein in myxedema and cretinism and by amyloid in primary amyloidosis. There may be infiltration of neoplastic cells in leukemia and lymphoma.

The **muscle** hypertrophies in acromegaly. Distention of the **blood vessels** may cause macroglossia in congestive heart failure and pulmonary emphysema. A few conditions may be left out by this approach. The tongue, for example, seems large in mongolian idiocy but this is caused by the fact that it hangs out and appears larger than it really is. The tongue is large and smooth in both riboflavin deficiency and sprue.

If the clinician prefers, he can arrive at an excellent differential by using the mnemonic **VINDICATE.**

Approach to the Diagnosis

The diagnosis of macroglossia depends on the presence of other physical findings (almost invariably present) associated with the disorders mentioned above, and, in most cases, the results of systematic workup. A lingual biopsy is valuable in primary amyloidosis.

Blood	Foreign Protein	Increase In Cells	Hypertrophy
		Carinoma of the tongue	
Leukemia Scurvy Thrombocytopenia	Myxedema Cretinism Primary amyloidosis	Lymphoma Leukemic infiltrate	Acromegaly
			Acromegaly
Congestive heart failure Pulmonary emphysema			

TESTICULAR MASS ■

Like that of most masses, the differential diagnosis of testicular masses is the best analyzed by the **anatomical** and **histological** approach (Table 2-17). The **skin** may be involved by many inflammatory conditions leading to swelling, including carbuncle, cellulitis, and dermatitis of various types. The tunica vaginalis is involved with hernias and hydroceles, which may be differentiated by using hydrocele transilluminates. The **venous plexus** of the scrotum and testes is involved by varicoceles and phlebitis (usually of the left venous plexus), and a varicocele may be the sign of a carcinoma of the kidney when the left spermatic vein is obstructed. Thus one readily sees how frequently obstruction is a pathophysiological mechanism in tumors here or elsewhere.

The **testis** is swollen in carcinomas (e.g.,

TABLE 2-17. TESTICULAR MASS

	Vascular	Inflammation	Neoplasm	Degenerative
Skin		Carbuncle	Carcinoma	
Subcutaneous Tissue		Cellulitis		
Tunica Vaginalis				
Venous Plexus		Phlebitis	Obstruction from renal carcinoma	
Testis		Orchitis Syphilis	Seminoma Chorioepithelioma	
Epididymis		Bacterial epididymitis Tuberculosis		
Artery	Torsion			
Vas Deferens			Secondary to obstruction by carcinoma of prostate	
Lymphatics		Filariasis		

seminomas, choriocarcinomas, teratomas, Leydig's cell tumors) and in orchitis (secondary to mumps, bacterial diseases, syphilis, or tuberculosis). The **epididymis** is frequently inflamed and swollen when there is orchitis and only rarely is inflamed by itself. It may also be enlarged from a spermatocele or from a *vas deferens* obstruction caused by prostatic disease (inflammation or neoplasm). Finally,

arterial occlusion caused by torsion of the testicle may cause a testicular mass.

Approach to the Diagnosis

Testicular masses may be differentiated by **transillumination** (hydroceles and spermatoceles transilluminate whereas hernias and tumors do not). Hernias may also be differen-

Intoxication	Congenital	Allergic-Autoimmune	Trauma	Endocrine	Obstruction
		Urticaria	Contusion		Subaceous cyst
			Direct inguinal hernia		
	Indirect inguinal hernia Hydrocele		Hematoma		
	Varicocele				
	Teratoma Hydatid cyst of Morgagni				
	Cyst				Spermatocele
	Torsion				
					Prostatic disease

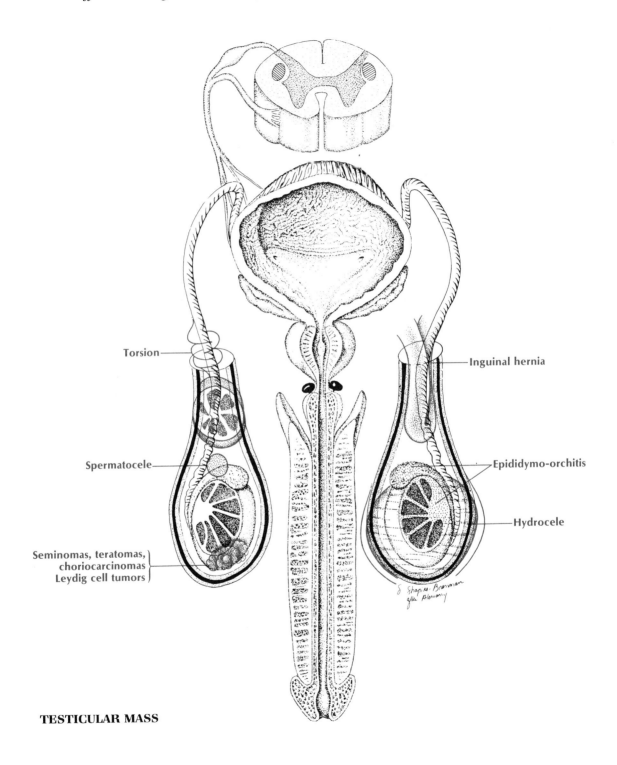

Torsion

Inguinal hernia

Spermatocele

Epididymo-orchitis

Hydrocele

Seminomas, teratomas,
choriocarcinomas
Leydig cell tumors

TESTICULAR MASS

tiated by reducing them (some will not reduce, however, if they are incarcerated) and auscultation may reveal bowel sounds. In noncommunicating hydroceles and testicular tumors, one may get above the swelling, whereas in torsion and hernias one cannot. In torsion, the tenderness is increased by elevation of the testicle, whereas in orchitis the tenderness is relieved if elevation is done for an hour or more. Surgery may be the only way to differentiate the cause of the mass. Other tests are listed in Appendix I.

BLOODY DISCHARGE

Chapter 3

GENERAL DISCUSSION

Any body orifice may be the site of a bloody discharge. It is usually the cause of great alarm on the part of the patient, as well it should be in most cases. That is because a bloody discharge often signifies malignancy, trauma, or a vascular disease, all of which are potentially lethal or disabling. Outside of de-generative and endocrine diseases, however, every etiology suggested by the mnemonic **VINDICATE** comes into play. Thus, this mnemonic is applied frequently in this section. Many systemic diseases may also cause a bloody discharge.

The basic science most helpful in developing a differential diagnosis here is **anatomy,** and the key word in recalling the components of the anatomy is "**tree.**" Thus bloody sputum is from lesions of the respiratory tree, hematemesis is caused by lesions of the gastrointestinal (GI) tree, and hematuria is caused by lesions along the genitourinary tree. A table is used in most cases to cross-index the various anatomical components with the etiologies. Biochemistry is an additional basic science that must be applied because of the coagulation mechanism.

Once a list of possibilities is recalled the exact diagnosis can be established by performing the history and physical examination with these possibilities in mind, linking the symptoms and signs to an appropriate laboratory workup, Appendix I or Appendix II.

Before undertaking expensive laboratory tests, group symptoms and signs together to eliminate the need for at least some of these. For example, painless hematuria usually requires an intravenous pyelogram and cystoscopy, whereas painful hematuria is often caused by cystitis and may merely require a urine culture and sensitivity, especially in women. Hemoptysis with fever and evidence of phlebitis would suggest a pulmonary infarct and thus indicate a lung scan, whereas hemoptysis in a smoker without fever or other signs suggests a neoplasm, thus bronchoscopy might be more appropriate. These are just a few examples of the application of this method.

The laboratory procedures most useful in the diagnosis of a bloody discharge are cytological examination of the fluid, culture for tuberculosis and other organisms, endoscopy, x-ray film of the tree involved, especially with contrast material and angiography. The availability of CT scans has obviated these studies in many cases and also the need for exploratory surgery. It is well to order coagulation studies in all but the most obvious cases. Further discussion of the studies that are useful in specific cases are taken up under each symptom.

BLEEDING UNDER THE SKIN ■

Conditions of the skin, subcutaneous tissue, vascular wall, and blood may all be associated with bleeding under the skin or purpura, thus both **anatomy** and **physiology** must be used to develop this differential (Table 3-1). The **skin** may hemorrhage from infections such as smallpox, scabies, chickenpox, and measles, especially when the patient traumatizes the area to relieve the itching. A bug bite may cause hemorrhage by this means. Focal and metastatic neoplasms may cause hemorrhage in the skin, whereas degeneration of the skin may lead to senile purpura. Trauma is by far the most common cause of hemorrhage of the skin.

The **subcutaneous tissue** is distinguished separately, so that one will recall the Ehlers-Danlos syndrome and pseudoxanthoma elasticum. The **vascular wall** may be damaged by numerous etiologies. The most important infectious etiologies are subacute bacterial endocarditis and meningococcemia, but typhoid fever, Weil's disease, and Rocky Mountain spotted fever should not be forgotten. Systemic neoplasms that infiltrate the vascular wall (such as leukemia) are significant causes, but these usually cause purpura by inducing a thrombocytopenia. Vascular degeneration and deficiency diseases such as scurvy are uncommon causes of purpura. Toxic conditions are more likely to be related to bone marrow suppression of platelets. Congenital lesions such as hereditary telangiectasias are important to remember.

Most important of all are the allergic and autoimmune disorders because something can be done to alleviate the condition (*e.g.*, steroids or immunosuppressants). Henoch–Schönlein purpura is a significant form of allergic vasculitis, but periarteritis nodosa is important too. Trauma is just as important here

as in the skin. Thus a ruptured varicose vein, crush injury, whooping cough, or contusions are important causes of purpura. Endocrine disorders also cause vascular purpura (as in Cushing's syndrome).

Disorders of the **blood** figure prominently in purpura. Significant among these are the numerous disorders that cause suppression or increased destruction of platelets. Toxic disorders such as gold injections, salicylate ingestion, potassium iodide, quinidine, ergot and chloral hydrate are just a few of these. It is best to assume that any drug may cause purpura until proven otherwise. Leukemic overgrowth of the bone marrow may cause purpura because of thrombocytopenia, but any neoplasm that infiltrates the marrow (myelophthisic anemia) must be considered. Autoimmune disease suggests the purpura of idiopathic thrombocytopenic purpura (ITP) and lupus erythematosus.

Degenerative disorders bring to mind aplastic anemia, although this is often caused by drug suppression of the bone marrow. Congenital disorders are more often the cause of coagulation disorders such as hemophilia, but coagulation disorders are often associated with heparin and dicoumarin therapy as well. Trauma and endocrine disorders do not figure as prominently here. There may still be a platelet disorder even though the platelet count is normal. Thus, one should investigate for hereditary thrombasthenia and salicylate toxicity, among other things, by doing a clot retraction test as a screen.

Approach to the Diagnosis

The clinical approach to purpura involves taking a drug history and a good family history, and ordering appropriate coagulation studies, tourniquet testing, and other tests (see p. 496). Referral to a hematologist is wise in obscure cases.

(Text continues on p. 186)

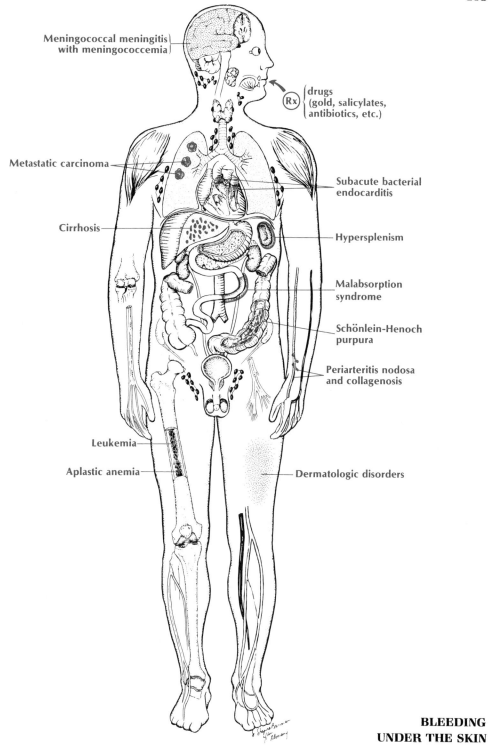

Meningococcal meningitis
with meningococcemia

Rx { drugs
(gold, salicylates,
antibiotics, etc.)

Metastatic carcinoma

Subacute bacterial
endocarditis

Cirrhosis

Hypersplenism

Malabsorption
syndrome

Schönlein-Henoch
purpura

Periarteritis nodosa
and collagenosis

Leukemia

Aplastic anemia

Dermatologic disorders

**BLEEDING
UNDER THE SKIN**

TABLE 3-1.   BLEEDING UNDER THE SKIN (PURPURA)

	V Vascular	I Inflammatory	N Neoplasm	D Degenerative

Skin		Smallpox
		Scabies
		Chickenpox
		Measles
			Focal and
			  metastatic
			  neoplasms
				Senile
				  purpura

Subcutaneous Tissue				

Vascular Wall		Subacute bacterial
		  endocarditis
		Meningococcemia
		Typhoid fever
		Weil's disease
		Rocky Mountain
		  spotted fever
			Leukemia
			  (systemic
			  neoplasms)
				Scurvy

Blood			Leukemia
			Overgrowth
			Myelophthisic
			  anemia
				Aplastic
				  anemia

I Intoxication	C Congenital	A Allergic and Autoimmune	T Trauma	E Endocrine
			Bug bite Scratching (most common causes)	
	Ehlers–Danlos syndrome Pseudo- xanthoma elasticum			
Telangiectasis (hereditary) von Wille- brand's disease	Henoch– Schönlein purpura Periarteritis nodosa		Ruptured varicose vein Crush injury Whooping cough Contusions	Cushing's syndrome Waterhouse– Friderichson syndrome
Gold injec- tions Salicylate ingestion Potassium iodide, quinidine Ergot, Hepa- rin, and Dicumarol therapy Salicylate toxicity	Hemophilia von Willebrand's disease Hereditary throm- basthenia	Idiopathic thrombocy- topenia Lupus erythem- atosus		

EPISTAXIS

The differential diagnostic approach to epistaxis is **anatomical** and **histological.** Table 3-2 breaks the nasal passages into anatomical and histological components and cross-indexes them with the various etiologies.

By far, the most common cause of epistaxis is **trauma** from nose picking. Many people are particularly vulnerable to this because of the closeness of Kiesselbach's plexus of veins and capillaries to the surface of the septal mucosa. This cause can quickly be ruled out by nasoscopic examination of the anterior portion of the septum. This same area may be

TABLE 3-2. EPISTAXIS

	V Vascular	**I** Inflammation	**N** Neoplasm	**D** Deficiency
Anterior Septal Mucosa		Rhinitis Syphilis Leprosy Mucormycosis Tuberculosis	Carcinoma (rarely)	
Sinuses		Tuberculosis Mucormycosis Viral sinusitis	Polyps Carcinomas	
Nasopharynx			Schmincke tumor Adenoids	
Veins and Capillaries	Venous obstruction from emphysema, asthma, and congestive heart failure		Hemangiomas	
Arteries	Hypertension			
Blood			Leukemia Polycythemia	Aplastic anemia

inflamed or ulcerated by various infections, particularly syphilis, tuberculosis, leprosy, and mucormycosis. Carcinomas in this area are uncommon, but the Schmincke tumor of the nasopharynx should not be forgotten; more important are allergic polyps, which usually do not bleed unless traumatized. Wegener's midline granulomatosis is an autoimmune disease that may present with a bloody or nonbloody nasal discharge. It usually involves the sinuses, however, and must be differentiated from mucormycosis.

Other systemic diseases are prominent causes of epistaxis. Back pressure from obstructed veins in emphysema, asthma, and right heart failure must be considered. Arte-

I Intoxication	C Collagen or Congenital	A Allergic and Autoimmune	T Trauma	E Endocrine
		Midline granuloma and polyps Rhinitis	Nose- picking Foreign body	Menopause Menstruation
		Midline granuloma and polyps Sinusitis		
		Rheumatic fever	Skull fracture Foreign body	
	Kiesselbach's plexus Telangiec- tasis			
Heparin and Warfarin therapy	Hemophilia and other coagulation defects	Thrombo- cytopenia		

rial hypertension, from whatever etiology, is a common cause from middle-age onwards. Rheumatic fever and blood dyscrasias round out the picture.

Other miscellaneous causes of epistaxis are skull fracture and menopause. In most cases, adequate examination of the nasal septum discloses the diagnosis and coagulation or nasal packing will suffice in treatment. The blood pressure should always be checked and, in recurrent cases, nasopharyngoscopy, coagulation studies, and a search for systemic disease must be made. Appendix I lists these and other important tests.

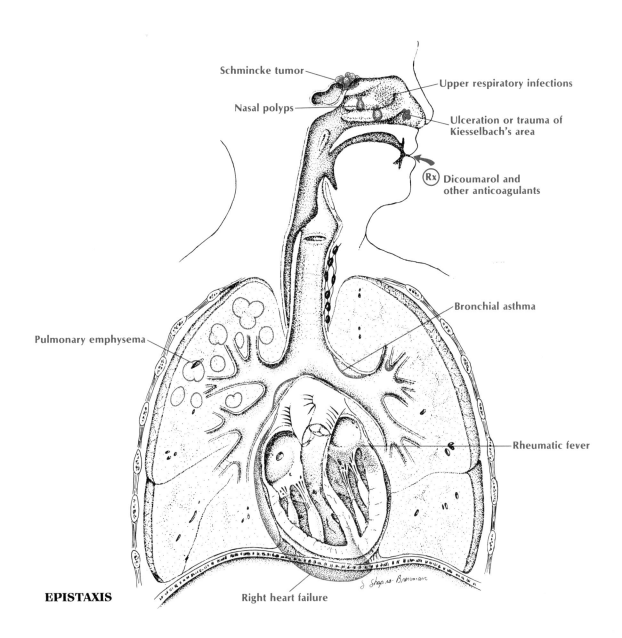

Schmincke tumor

Upper respiratory infections

Nasal polyps

Ulceration or trauma of Kiesselbach's area

(Rx) Dicoumarol and other anticoagulants

Pulmonary emphysema

Bronchial asthma

Rheumatic fever

EPISTAXIS

Right heart failure

HEMATEMESIS AND MELENA ■

Hematemesis means vomiting or regurgitation of frank bright red blood or coffee ground material that is positive for occult blood. It may be differentiated from hemoptysis because it usually gives an acidic reaction to nitrazine paper. It may be swallowed blood from any site in the oral cavity or nasophar-

ynx, thus careful examination of these areas must be done.

The differential of hematemesis, like that for bleeding from other body orifices, is best developed with the use of **anatomy.** Thus, beginning with the esophagus and working down to the ligament of Treitz and at the same time cross-indexing each structure with the various etiologies, one can make a chart like Table 3-3.

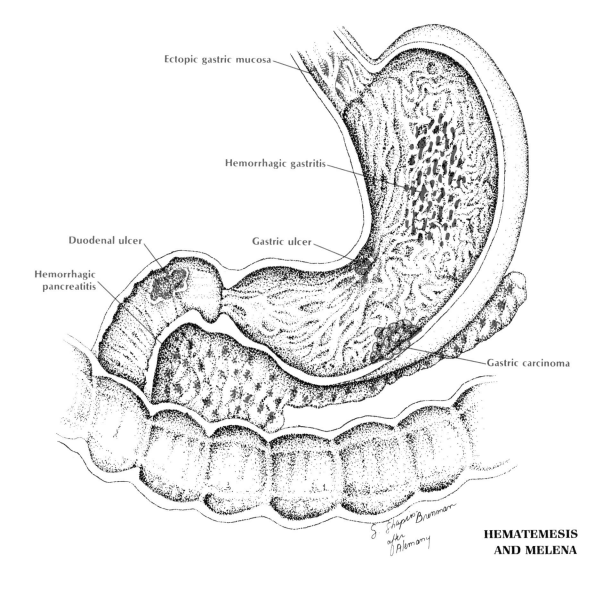

Ectopic gastric mucosa

Hemorrhagic gastritis

Duodenal ulcer

Gastric ulcer

Hemorrhagic pancreatitis

Gastric carcinoma

HEMATEMESIS AND MELENA

The major causes are illustrated on pages 189 and 192. In the esophagus the most common causes are varices, reflux esophagitis, carcinoma, and the Mallory–Weiss syndrome. One should not forget foreign bodies or irritants such as lye, especially in children. Barrett's esophagitis and ulcers caused by ectopic gastric mucosa are rare congenital causes of hematemesis. Finally, aortic aneurysms, mediastinal tumors, and carcinomas of the lung may ulcerate through the esophagus and bleed.

In the **stomach** inflammation, especially gastritis and ulcers, is a prominent cause. Aspirin or alcohol, however, is often the cause. Varices of the cardia of the stomach may bleed. Carcinomas and **hereditary telangiectasis** are less common causes. Duodenal ulcers are almost always the cause of bleeding from the duodenum, but occasionally neoplasms and regional ileitis may be involved. Ulceration of gallstones through the gallbladder and duodenal wall is another rare cause of bleeding from this site. The pancreas is in-

TABLE 3-3.   HEMATEMESIS AND MELENA

	V Vascular	I Inflammatory	N Neoplasm	D Degenerative and Deficiency
Esophagus	Esophageal varices Aortic aneurysm	Reflux esopha- titis Ulcer T. Cruzi	Carcinomas of esophagus and lung	
Stomach	Cardiac varices Ruptured aneurysm	Gastritis Gastric ulcers	Carcinomas	Atrophic gastritis
Duodenum		Ulcers		
Pancreas		Acute pancreatitis (hemorrhagic)		
Blood			Leukemia Polycythemia	Aplastic anemia Vitamin K deficiency

cluded in the drawing because occasionally one encounters gross hematemesis during acute hemorrhagic pancreatitis when blood pours out of the duct and is vomited.

Trauma is an important cause of bleeding from all the aforementioned sites, especially following entubation or surgery. Blood dyscrasias associated with coagulation disorders should be looked for immediately whenever a focal cause of hematemesis cannot be found, especially if bleeding is massive.

Approach to the Diagnosis

When confronted with solid evidence of hematemesis, the clinician should not waste valuable time on a thorough history and physical examination when endoscopy is more important in both diagnosis and therapy. Ordering a type and cross for multiple units of blood, coagulation studies, and the other tests listed in Appendix I should also be done immediately in most cases. The history of alco-

I Intoxication	C Congenital	A Autoimmune Allergic	T Trauma	E Endocrine
Lye and other irritants Foreign bodies	Hiatal hernias and esophagitis	Scleroderma	Foreign body Nasogastric tube Mallory–Weiss syndrome	
Alcoholic gastritis, aspirin, and other drugs (*e.g.*, arsenic)	Hereditary telangiectasis		Perforation and laceration surgery	Zollinger–Ellison syndrome
		Regional ileitis	Perforation and laceration surgery	Zollinger–Ellison syndrome
Warfarin Heparin Other drugs	Hemophilia and other hereditary coagulation disorders	ITP Collagen disease and other causes of thrombocytopenia		

192

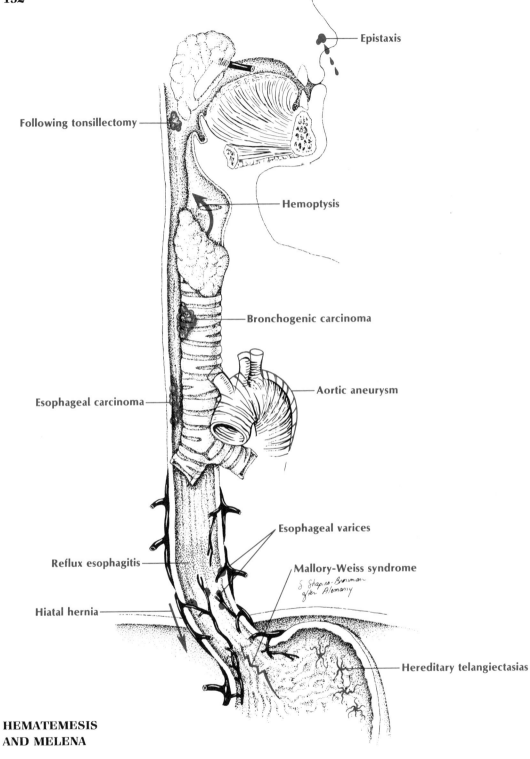

Epistaxis

Following tonsillectomy

Hemoptysis

Bronchogenic carcinoma

Aortic aneurysm

Esophageal carcinoma

Esophageal varices

Mallory-Weiss syndrome

Reflux esophagitis

S. Shapiro-Bronman
after Alemany

Hiatal hernia

Hereditary telangiectasias

**HEMATEMESIS
AND MELENA**

holism, use of aspirin and other drugs, and previous ulcers or esophageal disease is important to get while preparing for endoscopy and other emergency procedures. Patients without massive or recent acute hematemesis may be approached with traditional methods. A history of vomiting nonhemorrhagic gastric fluid prior to the onset of hematemesis is helpful in diagnosing a Mallory–Weiss syndrome.

HEMATURIA ■

Utilizing the **anatomical** approach, the physician can arrive at most of the causes of hematuria (Table 3–4). One need only visualize the urinary tract and proceed from the kidney on down to get a differential list. Let us apply the mnemonic **VINDICATE** to the kidney:

V—Vascular diseases make one think of embolic glomerulonephritis, renal vein thrombosis, and subacute bacterial endocarditis.

I—Infectious causes of hematuria are pyelonephritis (infrequently) and renal tuberculosis.

N—Neoplasms that may present with hematuria are hypernephromas and papillomas and carcinomas of the renal pelvis. Wilm's tumors present with hematuria less frequently.

D—Degenerative diseases rarely present with hematuria as in other organ systems.

I—Intoxicants such as sulfa drugs (that lead to nephrocalcinosis), mercury poisoning, and blood transfusion reactions are common causes of hematuria, gross or microscopic.

C—Congenital lesions such as polycystic kidneys and medullary sponge kidneys cause hematuria and also predispose to stones and infections that may present with hematuria.

A—Autoimmune conditions such as acute and chronic glomerulonephritis, Goodpasture's disease, Wegener's midline granulomatosis, and lupus erythematosus commonly present with hematuria.

T—Trauma to any organ causes hemorrhages and the kidney is no exception. Hematuria after automobile or other accidents should signal the need for hospitalization, IVP, and close observation of vital signs. Hematuria may present with a crush injury to any muscle or a burn.

E—Endocrine–metabolic diseases caused by stones. Most calcium stones are not caused by hyperparathyroidism, but it should always be considered a possibility. Urate stones are usually caused by gout and cystine stones are always associated with congenital cystinuria.

Ureter. Stones, papillomas, and congenital defects (contributing to stones) are the most likely causes here.

Bladder. Vascular disease is infrequently a cause but cystitis (especially acute or "honeymoon" type) is a common cause. Stones, neoplasms (papillomas and transitional cell cardinomas), and foreign bodies are the next most likely causes. Trauma should not be forgotten, especially because of the numerous instances of various instruments being introduced into the bladder.

Prostate. Neoplasms of the prostate occasionally cause hematuria, but most other etiological conditions (prostatitis) are rarely associated with gross or microscopic hematuria.

Urethra. Stones, neoplasms, and infections of the urethra may all cause hematuria, but very infrequently.

Utilizing **biochemistry** as the basic chemistry, do not forget the coagulation disorders that may cause hematuria. Thus hematuria is often found in idiopathic thrombocytopenia purpura and in almost any disorder in which the platelet count drops below 40,000 cells per cu mm. Hemophiliacs may present with hematuria. Patients given too much warfarin (Coumadin) will often get hematuria. Fibrinolysins and afibrinogenemia will also cause hematuria.

From this exercise, it should be evident that arriving at the causes of hematuria is not difficult if one visualizes the anatomy of the urinary tree and then considers each etiological category in this light.

TABLE 3-4. HEMATURIA

	V Vascular	I Inflammatory	N Neoplasm	D Degenerative and Deficiency
Kidney	Embolic glomerulone- phritis Renal vein thrombosis Subacute bacterial endocarditis	Pyelonephritis Renal tubercu- losis	Hypernephromas Papillomas Carcinomas Wilm's tumor	
Ureters			Papillomas	
Bladder		Cystitis Hunner's ulcer Foreign body	Papillomas Transitional cell carcinomas	
Prostate		Prostatitis	Carcinomas	
Urethra		Infections of urethra, *e.g.,* gonorrhea	Neoplasm	

Approach to the Diagnosis

Urinalysis, urine cultures, urine cytology, IVP, and cystoscopy and retrograde pyelography will establish the diagnosis in most cases. A CT scan will disclose obscure renal tumors or cysts. Blood cultures for subacute bacterial endocarditis, an antinuclear antibody (ANA) test, and a search for other systemic diseases is necessary in some cases. Appendix I provides many useful tests for the difficult diagnostic problem.

I Intoxication	C Congenital	A Autoimmune Allergic	T Trauma	E Endocrine and Metabolic
Sulfa drugs Mercury poisoning Blood trans- fusion reactions	Polycystic kidneys Medullary sponge kidneys Congenital lesions	Acute and chronic glomerulone- phritis Goodpasture's disease Wegener's midline granuloma- tosis Lupus erythe- matosus	Accidents auto; crush injury to muscle, burn, laceration	Stones (uric acid, cal- cium phosphate, cystine)
	Congenital bands, *e.g.*, aberrant vessels			Stones (see above)
			Ruptured bladder (*e.g.*, from instruments)	Stones (see above)
				Stones (see above)

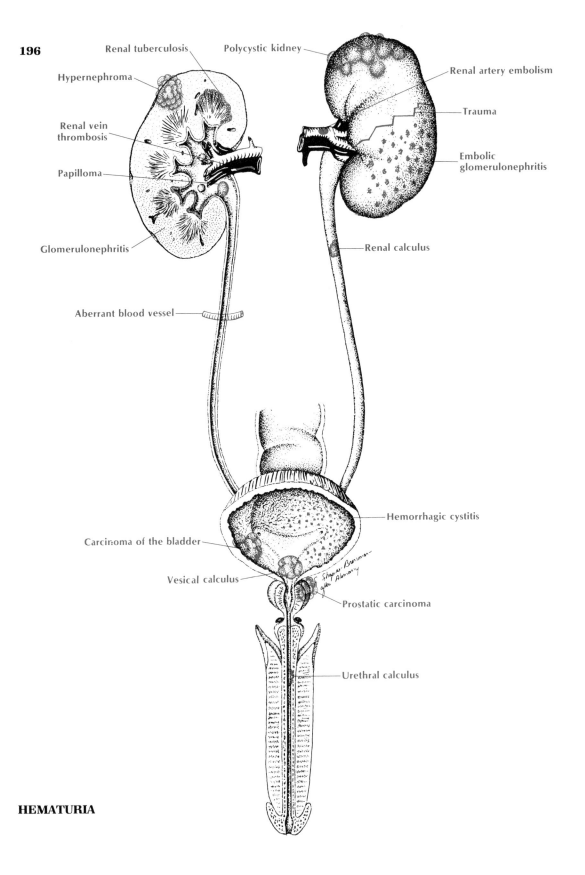

Renal tuberculosis

Polycystic kidney

Hypernephroma

Renal artery embolism

Trauma

Renal vein thrombosis

Embolic glomerulonephritis

Papilloma

Glomerulonephritis

Renal calculus

Aberrant blood vessel

Hemorrhagic cystitis

Carcinoma of the bladder

Vesical calculus

Prostatic carcinoma

Urethral calculus

HEMATURIA

HEMOPTYSIS

True **hemoptysis** must be distinguished from **epistaxis** (see p. 186) and hematemesis (see p. 189). If the blood is bright red and alkaline (use nitrazine paper to test) and the nasal passages and posterior pharynx are clear, then it is probably hemoptysis.

Anatomy is the basic science to apply to develop a differential diagnosis of hemoptysis. Beginning at the **larynx** and working down

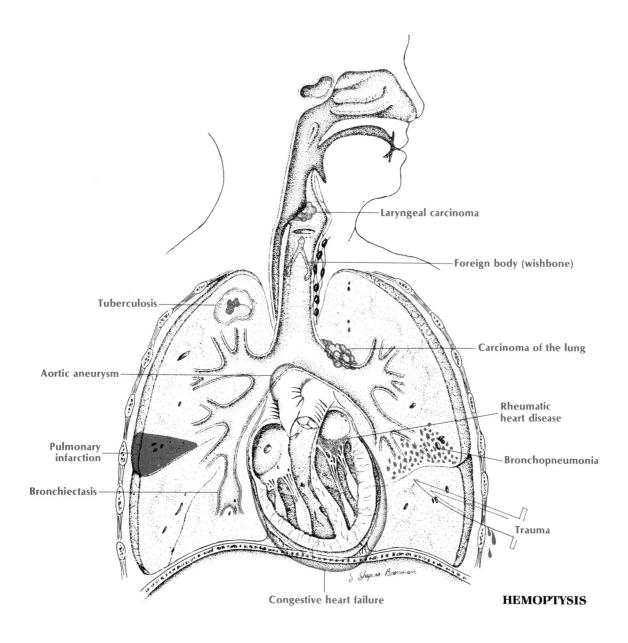

Laryngeal carcinoma

Foreign body (wishbone)

Tuberculosis

Carcinoma of the lung

Aortic aneurysm

Rheumatic heart disease

Pulmonary infarction

Bronchopneumonia

Bronchiectasis

Trauma

Congestive heart failure

HEMOPTYSIS

the trachea, bronchi, and alveoli, one can quickly recall the major causes of hemopytysis using the cross-index of the various etiologies as in Table 3-5. Laryngitis is an infrequent cause of hemoptysis but laryngeal carcinoma may cause it. Tuberculosis of the larynx used to be a common cause but it is not often seen today. A foreign body such as a chicken bone lodged in the larynx or **trachea** should al-

ways be considered, especially in children. Additional etiologies of hemoptysis that one might encounter in the trachea are ulceration and rupture of an aortic aneurysm or a carcinoma of the esophagus with a tracheoesophageal fistula. Hereditary telangiectasia may lead to hemoptysis anywhere along the tracheo-bronchial tree. In the **bronchi**, carcinoma, tuberculosis, and bronchiectasis become prom-

TABLE 3-5. HEMOPTYSIS

	V Vascular	I Inflammatory	N Neoplasm	D Degenerative and Deficiency
Larynx		Laryngitis especially tuberculosis	Carcinomas Polyps	
Trachea	Aortic aneurysm	Tracheitis	Carcinoma and adenomas Esophageal carcinoma	
Bronchi	Ruptured bronchial vein	Chronic bronchitis and tuberculosis Viral influenza	Carcinoma and bronchial adenomas	
Alveoli	Pulmonary embolism Congestive heart failure	Tuberculosis Pneumonia Fungi Parasites	Carcinomas, primary and metastatic	Pulmonary fibrosis Scurvy
Blood		Sepsis with disseminated intravascular coagulopathy (DIC)	Leukemia Polycythemia Lymphoma	Aplastic anemia Vitamin K deficiency

inent causes. These are probably the most common causes of chronic hemoptysis in the adult.

In the **alveoli** the acute causes of hemoptysis—pneumonia (pneumococcal and Friedländer's, especially), and pulmonary embolism or infarctions—are encountered. Congestive heart failure may cause a foamy hemoptysis. Carcinoma, tuberculosis, fungi, parasites, and trauma are also important. Collagen diseases, Goodpasture's syndrome, and primary hemosiderosis should be looked for in the elusive cases.

As in all cases of bleeding from a body orifice, blood dyscrasias may be a cause (Table 3-5). One should always rule out a coagulation disorder or leukemia when the hemoptysis persists and a focal cause is not found. Ap-

I Intoxication and Idiopathic	**C** Congenital	**A** Autoimmune Allergic	**T** Trauma	**E** Endocrine Metabolic
Laryngitis Smoke			Foreign body	
Tracheitis from smoke	Hereditary telangiectasis		Foreign body	
	Bronchiectasis		Foreign body	Carcinoid
Sarcoidosis	Sickle cell anemia Kartagener's syndrome Primary hemosiderosis	Collagen disease Wegener's granuloma Goodpasture's disease	Biopsy, fracture Perforation and contusion	
Drugs Warfarin sodium Heparin	Coagulation defects (hemophilia)	Thrombocytopenia		

pendix I lists the important tests that should be ordered in the workup of hemoptysis.

MISCELLANEOUS SITES OF BLEEDING ▪

Bleeding from the Ear. This is not usually a serious condition. **Anatomy** is again applied to formulate a diagnosis. The blood may be from the external or middle ear and usually is caused by diseases of the skin or drum. Trauma is the most significant cause and is usually related to self-inflicted lacerations from digging at wax with hairpins or pencils, for example, which may occasionally rupture the ear drum. Children are prone to lodge foreign bodies in their ears. Skull fractures of the posterior fossa may present with bleeding from the ear. External otitis and otitis media may cause a bloody discharge, but this is not common. If the drum is ruptured by infection, there is usually bleeding from the ear. Carcinomas of the skin of the external canal may cause a bloody discharge and cholesteatomas will cause bleeding when they ulcerate through the tympanic membrane. Coagulation disorders rarely present with bleeding from the ear, in contrast to epistaxis and bleeding from the gums.

Bleeding from the Gums. No anatomical breakdown is necessary here. The causes may be divided into local and systemic categories but by using the word **VINDICATE** one can cover all the etiological categories adequately.

V—Vascular includes the hemorrhagic disorders, especially hemophilia, thrombocytopenia, heparin and warfarin (Coumadin) therapy, and fibrinogenopenia, as in disseminated intravascular coagulopathy (DIC).

I—Inflammatory includes acute gingivitis, dental abscesses, pyorrhea, actinomycosis, or syphilis.

N—Neoplasms suggest both local neoplasms (*e.g.,* odontoma, papillomas, and epulis) and systemic neoplasms (Hodgkin's disease and leukemia).

D—Degenerative disorders include aplastic anemia and deficiencies such as scurvy and vitamin K deficiencies.

I—Intoxication recalls mercury, phosphorus, and diphenylhydantoin intoxication, in which the gums are usually severely hypertrophied as well.

C—Congenital conditions, other than congenital blood dyscrasias (*e.g.,* sickle cell anemia) include erythema bullosum.

A—Autoimmune suggests thrombocytopenic purpura, Henoch's purpura, and lupus erythematosus.

T—Trauma indicates bleeding from vigorous brushing or picking with a toothpick.

E—Endocrine disorders are not likely to cause bleeding except secondarily, as in diabetic-induced pyorrhea or the alveolar bone degeneration or dysplasia (osteotic) of hyperparathyroidism.

Gingivitis as part of a diffuse stomatitis may be seen in pemphigus, Stevens–Johnson's syndrome, Vincent's stomatitis (spirilla and bacilli fusiformis), and various other bacterial forms. The job of the clinician is to exclude the systemic causes and then refer the patient to a periodontist for evaluation and treatment of the local causes.

Bleeding from the Breast, Hemorrhagic Discharge. Suspect a neoplasm, such as a ductal carcinoma (Paget's disease), fibroadenosis, and ductal papillomas unless proven otherwise. With a magnifying glass one may be able to tell which of the 20 or so ducts is bleeding, but expressing one small segment at a time, working spirally, is also helpful.

RECTAL BLEEDING

This discussion considers the causes of bright red or maroon stools. (The causes of melena or black stools are the same as the causes of hematemesis; the differential diagnosis is given on page 189.) Bright red blood may occasionaly result from an upper GI lesion if there is associated diarrhea.

A list of the causes of rectal bleeding of fresh blood is best developed with the use of the mnemonic **VINDICATE.**

V—Vascular prompts the recall of hemorrhoids, but one cannot forget mesenteric infarctions.

I—Inflammation suggests perirectal abscess, anal fissure or ulcer, and amebic colitis or condyloma latum and acuminatum.

N—Neoplasms call to mind polyps and carcinomas of the rectum and anus.

D—Degenerative does not suggest anything in particular.

I—Intoxication suggests pseudomembranous colitis complicating gentamicin, clindamycin, and other antibiotic therapy. Jejunal ulcers from potassium chloride tablets should be considered here.

C—Congenital and **acquired** anomalies suggest fistula in ano, bleeding Meckel's diverticulum, and bleeding colon diverticuli, among other congenital conditions. Intussusception would fall in this category also.

A—Autoimmune recalls granulomatous colitis and ulcerative colitis.

T—Trauma suggests the bleeding from any foreign body inserted into the rectum, including the male organ.

E—Endocrine does not suggest anything other than the Zollinger–Ellison syndrome, which, because it causes ulceration of the jejunum, may be associated with maroon stools.

In disorders of the upper colon and small intestines the blood is older and thus a maroon color is likely. In addition, the blood is mixed with the stool and may indeed be so well mixed that it will not be discovered without a test for occult blood. Other features are more prominent in bacillary dysentery and salmonellosis.

Approach to the Diagnosis

Armed with a more comprehensive list of causes of rectal bleeding, the clinician is ready to eliminate some of them as he asks appropriate questions during the history and performs the examination with all the causes in mind. The diagnosis may be pinned down by the presence or absence of other symptoms and signs (see p. 80). The principal diagnostic procedures are stool cultures, stool examination for ova and parasites, proctoscopy, barium enema, and colonoscopy. Others are listed in Appendix I.

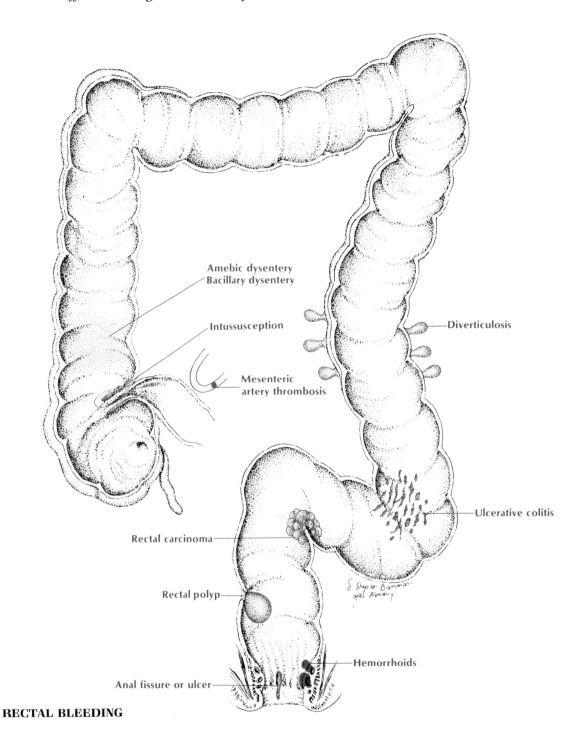

Amebic dysentery
Bacillary dysentery

Intussusception

Mesenteric
artery thrombosis

Diverticulosis

Ulcerative colitis

Rectal carcinoma

Rectal polyp

Hemorrhoids

Anal fissure or ulcer

RECTAL BLEEDING

VAGINAL BLEEDING

As with most hemorrhages from body orifices, vaginal bleeding is best approached by the **anatomical** method. Thus, the important structures of the female genital tract are cross-indexed with etiologic categories as in Table 3-6. In all bleeding symptoms, one must include blood vessels and the blood as part of the anatomical breakdown. Histological breakdown is of little importance anywhere except in the uterus and in making certain one does not forget the many types of ovarian tumors (e.g., fibromas, polycystic ovaries, corpus leuteum, follicular cysts, and arrheno-

blastoma). In the uterus, histology reminds one of endometriosis and adenomyosis and also fibroids.

Physiology should bring to mind the most common cause of uterine bleeding—dysfunctional bleeding. Thus, when the normal sequence of follicle-stimulating hormone (FSH) stimulating estrogen production and luteinizing hormone (LH) stimulating progesterone production from the corpus luteum is interrupted, by whatever cause, the resulting poorly formed endometrium will bleed at an inappropriate time (metrorrhagia) or excessively during the appropriate time (menorrhagia). Aside from the many neoplasms, cysts, and inflammatory conditions of the ovary

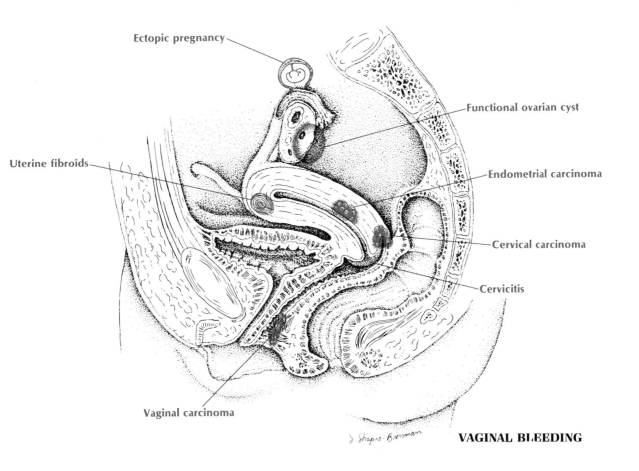

VAGINAL BLEEDING

(listed in Table 3-6), one must consider other endocrine disorders such as adrenal neoplasms, hyper- and hypothyroidism, hypopituitarism, and acromegaly.

Although the differential diagnosis is developed adequately in Table 3-6, a description of most important causes is provided here. The most important vaginal conditions are a rup-

TABLE 3-6.   VAGINAL BLEEDING

	V Vascular	I Inflammatory	N Neoplasm	D Degenerative or Deficiencies
Introitus	Varicosities	Syphilitic ulcer Warts	Granulomatous polyp	
Vagina		Vaginitis	Carcinoma Extension of rectal carci- noma	Atrophic vaginitis
Cervix		Chronic cervi- citis Herpes	Carcinoma Polyps	
Uterus		Endometritis	Endometriosis Carcinoma Polyps Fibroids Pregnancy	Menopause Scurvy Vitamin K deficiency
Fallopian *Tubes*		Pelvic inflam- matory disease	Ectopic preg- nancy	
Ovaries		Oophoritis Tuberculosis	Carcinoma and adenoma Corpus luteum cysts	
Blood *Vessels* *and* *Blood*			Leukemia	Anemia Aplastic ane- mia
Others			Hydatidiform mole	

tured hymen, atrophic vaginitis, and carcinoma. Cervical carcinoma is the most important cause of bleeding of the cervix. Fibroids may be a more common cause of uterine bleeding than endometrial carcinoma, but both are superceded by pregnancy and dysfunctional uterine bleeding. Proceeding to the fallopian tubes, one must not forget ectopic

I Intoxication	C Congenital Malformation	A Allergic or Autoimmune	T Trauma	E Endocrine Disorders
			Intercourse Trauma to hymen	
			Foreign bodies	
	Placenta previa		Laceration	
Birth control pills Estrogens and other hormones	Anteversion of uterus Retroversion or flexion	ITP	Foreign bodies Abortion induced	Menopause Dysfunctional bleeding Abruptio pla- centa
				Hypopituitarism Hypothyroidism Stein Leventhal ovaries
Toxic sup- pression of platelets Heparin Warfarin		Lupus erythe- matosus	Surgery	

pregnancy and pelvic inflammatory disease as causes of vaginal bleeding. Ovarian cysts and tumors are common causes of dysfunctional bleeding, but the serous cystadenoma and carcinomas present that way only infrequently.

Approach to the Diagnosis

A careful vaginal examination with the patient fully relaxed is most important. A rectovaginal examination must be performed also in order to palpate masses in the cul-de-sac. Any vaginal discharge must be cultured to rule out pelvic inflammatory disease. A pregnancy test and ultrasonography are needed to exclude an ectopic pregnancy. Cervical lesions must be biopsied. A D & C and examination under anesthesia may be necessary. In some cases, culdoscopy, peritoneoscopy, or an exploratory laparotomy will be indicated, but the clinician usually prescribes a trial of cyclical estrogen and progesterone therapy first (a "medical D & C"), unless other findings dictate these examinations. Other tests that may be indicated in the workup of vaginal bleeding are presented in Appendix I.

NONBLOODY DISCHARGE

Chapter 4

GENERAL DISCUSSION

Just as any body orifice may exude a bloody discharge, so may it exude a nonbloody discharge. Whereas bloody discharges often signify malignancy, nonbloody discharges usually signify **inflammation,** particularly that of an infectious nature. It should be kept in mind, however, that chronic discharges are usually caused by an additional etiologic factor. This is where the mnemonic **MINT** comes into play in this section. A chronic nonbloody discharge is often caused by a **malformation** (such as a fistula), a **neoplasm** with superimposed infection, or **trauma** induced by a foreign body (such as calculus) with superimposed infection. All of these conditions may produce an obstruction and cause infection by this pathophysiological mechanism.

Like that for bloody discharge, the basic science most useful in developing a differential list is **anatomy.** A key word that will suggest the anatomical components in each case is "**tree.**" Thus in the analysis of sputum one would visualize the respiratory tree, whereas in analyzing the causes of a vaginal discharge one would visualize the female genital tree. Once a list of conditions is recalled, pinning down the exact diagnosis depends on a thorough history and physical examination with these possibilities in mind, a linking together the presence or absence of other key symptoms, and a laboratory workup.

For example, a nonbloody discharge from a swollen, tender breast most certainly signifies mastitis or breast abscess, whereas a nonbloody discharge from a nontender, normal size breast would suggest galactorrhea of endocrine origin.

The laboratory workup for all forms of discharge includes an examination of a fresh preparation of the discharge **by the physician himself,** a smear and culture, and appropriate roentgenograms of the tree involved. Endoscopy is not as frequently indicated as in bloody discharge but it still has its place. Exploratory surgery is also not as frequently necessary to establish the diagnosis. There is no substitute for careful follow-up lest the condition become chronic and intractible.

In all cases of nonbloody discharge that defy diagnosis, one should consider syphilis, tuberculosis, fungi, and parasites, as well as all the conditions suggested above by the mnemonic **MINT** which, of course, may cause **obstruction.**

AURAL DISCHARGE (OTORRHEA)

The differential diagnosis of a nonbloody discharge of the ear can best be done by using **anatomy.** Visualize the components of the ear apparatus. A discharge may arise from the external canal, the middle ear, the mastoids and petrous bone, the inner ear, or the cere-

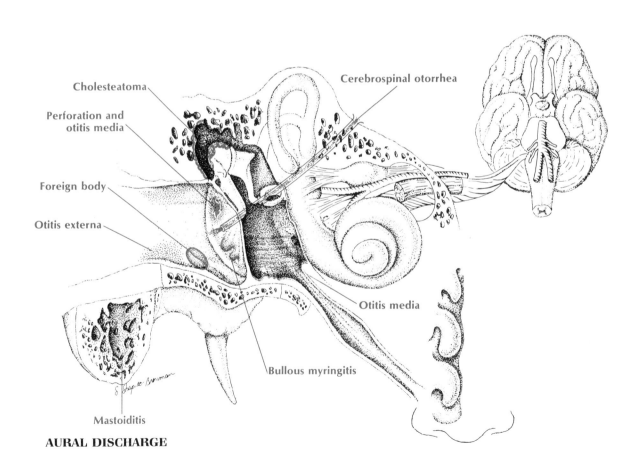

AURAL DISCHARGE

brospinal fluid. As elsewhere in the body, nonbloody discharge signifies inflammation and infectious or allergic conditions, but foreign bodies and malignancies can trigger an infection by causing an obstruction or lowering resistance.

The **external canal** may be involved by bacterial infection as in furunculosis, diffuse otitis externa, and Eaton agent pneumonitis; and by **viral infection** in herpes zoster (Ramsay Hunt syndrome). Fungi may infest the external canal, particularly when wax or a foreign body accumulates. Atopic, contact, or seborrheic dermatitis may also involve the external canal.

In the **middle ear,** bacterial infections may produce an acute or chronic purulent otitis media with or without rupture of the drum, but a serous otitis media from allergy, viral infections, or obstruction of the eustachian tube does not usually cause otorrhea. In addition to perforation, otitis media may lead to mastoiditis, petrositis, and ultimately to a chronic granuloma called a cholesteatoma. All of these are usually associated with a chronic continuous or intermittent nonbloody discharge.

Conditions arising in the **inner ear** (e.g., labyrinthitis) are rarely associated with otorrhea, but a basilar skull fracture may lead to cerebrospinal otorrhea. This is usually bloody at onset, but if it goes unrecognized it may become clear or, when infected, purulent.

Approach to the Diagnosis

The approach to the diagnosis of an aural discharge is similar to the approach for discharges from any body orifice (Appendices I and II). After careful examination for a foreign body or obstruction, the discharge is cultured and appropriate therapy begun. A Gram's stain of the material often allows more specific antibiotic therapy. If the discharge is chronic, roentgenograms of the mastoids and

petrous bones may be necessary, as well as tomography. Obviously, referral to an otolaryngologist is wise at this point.

BREAST DISCHARGE

A purulent discharge from the breast, just like a purulent discharge from any other body orifice, should signify inflammation (a mastitis or breast abscess), yet this is not the most common cause of a nonbloody discharge from the breast. Obviously, the most common cause is lactation. This is, of course, physiological in the postpartum period, but what about other periods of a woman's life? The cause in these cases is usually a pituitary, hypothalamic, or ovarian disturbance causing excessive production of prolactin. Among these are pituitary tumor, Chiari–Frommel syndrome, and ovarian atrophy or tumors. Hyperthyroidism may occasionally be responsible. Certain drugs such as chlorpromazine HCl (Thorazine) and methyldopa (Aldomet) may also cause galactorrhea. Certainly malignancy, particularly papillomas or carcinomas of the ducts, should be considered here, but they usually produce a bloody discharge.

Approach to the Diagnosis

The workup of purulent breast discharge is usually simply a smear and culture and occasionally a white blood cell count (WBC) and differential. When these are fruitless, an acid-fast smear and culture may be indicated but rarely nowadays; it concerns me that tuberculosis is almost invariably given too much space in other differential diagnosis textbooks. Mammography is ordered next. For an endocrine workup, skull x-ray films, a CT scan and serum prolactin levels may be done, but it is wise to refer the patient to an endocrinolo-

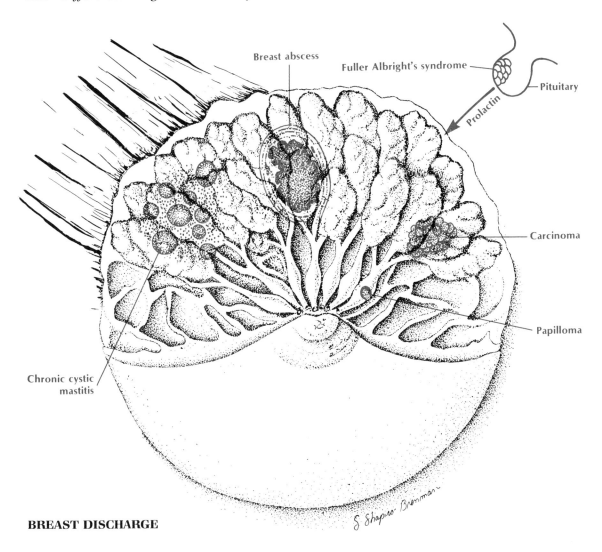

Breast abscess

Fuller Albright's syndrome

Pituitary

Prolactin

Carcinoma

Papilloma

Chronic cystic mastitis

S. Shapiro Brennan

BREAST DISCHARGE

NASAL DISCHARGE ■

gist to let him handle this and the numerous other tests that are indicated.

With nasal discharge (rhinorrhea and postnasal drip), **anatomy** is the key. In visualizing the structure from outside in, one encounters the external nares, the choana with the turbi-nates, the maxillary, ethmoid, frontal and sphenoid sinuses, and the nasopharynx with the openings of the eustachian tubes surrounded by the adenoids. In addition, the inferior meatus provides the opening for the nasolacrimal ducts. The etiologies of a nonbloody discharge of the nose are almost invariably inflammatory (infectious or allergic), but a fracture of the sinuses or cribriform plate may cause a cerebrospinal fluid rhinor-rhea. As in nonbloody discharges elsewhere, it is incumbent on the diagnostician to keep

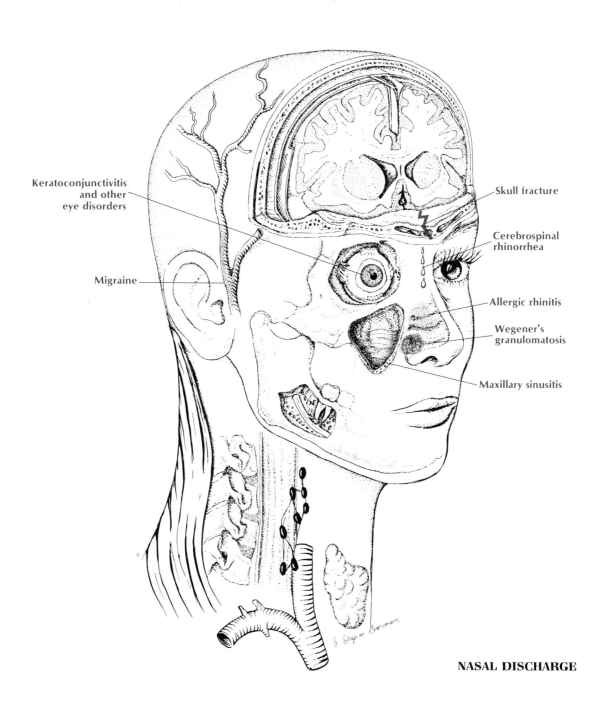

Keratoconjunctivitis and other eye disorders

Migraine

Skull fracture

Cerebrospinal rhinorrhea

Allergic rhinitis

Wegener's granulomatosis

Maxillary sinusitis

NASAL DISCHARGE

the possibility of neoplasm and foreign body and other causes of obstruction in mind as these may set the stage for infection.

Nasal conditions causing acute nonbloody rhinorrhea include the common cold (due to any one of at least 60 viruses), viral influenza, pertussis, measles, and allergic rhinitis (hayfever). The discharge is at first clear, but after a few hours of obstruction secondary bacterial infection may set in and the discharge often becomes purulent. Chronic rhinitis is usually allergic, bacterial, or fungal (as in mucormycosis), but it can be on an autoimmune basis (Wegener's granulomatosis). Toxins in the environment, (*e.g.,* smoke) may cause serous rhinorrhea. Too frequent use of nasal sprays should always be considered.

The **sinuses** may be inflamed in the same conditions that involve the nose. However, concern about whether or not a discharge is coming from the sinuses arises when the discharge becomes purulent, when there is associated pain over the sinus, or when the discharge becomes chronic. In chronic sinusitis the discharge may frequently be a postnasal drip.

The **nasopharynx** is also involved by the same viral, bacterial, and fungal conditions as the rest of the nasal passages, but, in addition, diphtheria may begin here, and if the **adenoids** become large enough they may obstruct the nasal canals and produce a secondary bacterial rhinitis with discharge.

Since the **nasolacrimal ducts** open into the inferior meatus, any eye condition that may cause excessive tearing may also produce a rhinorrhea. The unilateral rhinorrhea of histamine headaches is, at least in part, related to this mechanism, as is trigeminal neuralgia.

Approach to the Diagnosis

The diagnosis of nonbloody rhinorrhea is not usually necessary in the acute cases because it is frequently due to the "common cold" or allergic rhinitis (in which case the history will be helpful). When the rhinorrhea persists, a smear for eosinophils and appropriate skin testing are useful if the discharge is nonpurulent; a Gram's stain, a culture for bacteria and fungi, and roentgenograms of the sinuses will be valuable if the discharge is purulent. Cerebrospinal rhinorrhea is a possibility. Other useful tests may be found in Appendix I.

ORBITAL DISCHARGE

A clear on purulent discharge from the eye is usually due to allergy or infection, but a few notable exceptions exist. In addition to using **anatomy** to formulate the list of diagnostic possibilities, it is well to apply the mnemonic **MINT** to the various anatomical components.

Beginning with the **eyelids,** one should recall the following:

M—Malformations like a chalazion, ectropion, and entropion

I—Inflammatory conditions like blepharitis, a hordeolum (stye), and allergic or infectious conjunctivitis

N—Neoplasms such as squamous cell carcinoma and angiomas

T—Traumatic conditions, especially foreign bodies

The **nasolacrimal duct** may become inflamed and obstructed (dacryocystitis). The **bulbar conjuctiva** may be involved by malformations like a pterygium or a pingueculae and cause a clear discharge. Inflammatory and traumatic conditions here are similar to those of the palpebral conjunctiva. It is well to mention toxic causes of a nonbloody discharge, such as irritation from tobacco smoke, cold, and irritating gases; chronic alcoholism, arsenic poisoning, and iodism may cause a clear discharge.

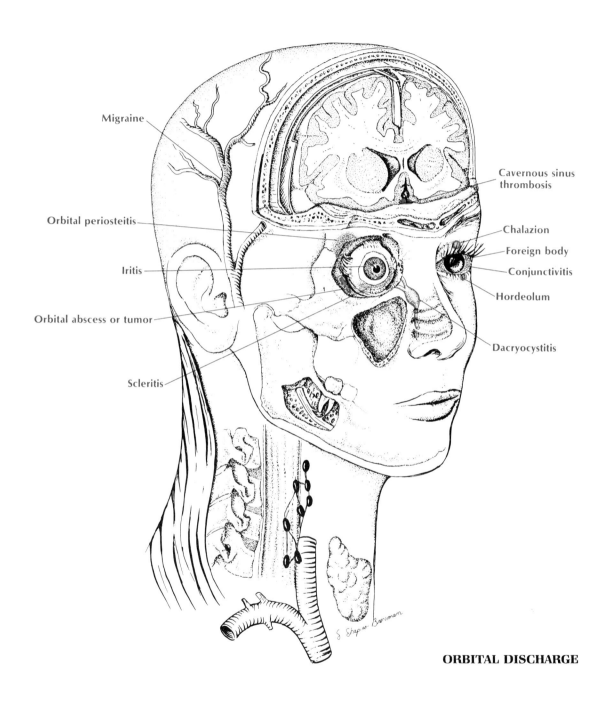

Migraine

Orbital periosteitis

Iritis

Orbital abscess or tumor

Scleritis

Cavernous sinus thrombosis

Chalazion

Foreign body

Conjunctivitis

Hordeolum

Dacryocystitis

ORBITAL DISCHARGE

Breaking down the **eyeball** into its various components, one recalls the **cornea** and immediately one should think of a foreign body of the cornea or of a laceration, a keratitis, and malformations like keratoconus. Next the **iris** suggests iritis as a cause of discharge, but by using the mnemonic one will not forget albinism as a cause of excessive tearing. Also the iris angle should remind one of acute glaucoma, which often presents with lacrimation as well as with pain. The **lens** should suggest refractive errors as a major cause of a clear discharge and predisposition to infection of the lids. Finally, the **sclera** is the site of episcleritis and scleritis, which are frequently associated with a nonbloody discharge.

Turning to the **lacrimal gland** one should remember mumps of this gland and other infections. The **vascular supply** to the eye should suggest the tearful discharge of histamine cephalalgia and obstruction of the venous drainage by a cavernous sinus thrombosis. Paralysis of the **muscles** of the eye, especially the facial nerve, creates a discharge by excessive exposure to dust and air.

Approach to the Diagnosis

Anatomy has served us well in developing a differential, although the cause of a discharge from the eye is often easy to establish. Foreign bodies, trauma, toxins, and conjunctivitis are the conditions most commonly responsible. That is why in the approach to the diagnosis one will first examine the eye carefully under magnification and use fluorescein to rule out a foreign body or laceration. Then a careful history of exposure to toxins (*e.g.*, industrial) is in order. Finally if the discharge is unilateral, a smear and culture of specific bacteria are valuable before treatment. If it is bilateral, allergy should be considered, as well as refractive errors. Tenometry should be performed. Referral to an opthalmologist may be appropriate at any one of these stages (when in doubt, refer it out).

PYURIA

Pyuria is included in the section on non-bloody discharges even though it is not a symptom or a definitive finding on physical examination. Examination of the urine, however, is so frequently a part of every physical examination that the causes of pyuria should be available for immediate recall for all primary-care physicians.

As in other cases of purulent discharge, inflammation is the cause of pyuria in most cases, thus an etiologic mnemonic would seem unnecessary. However, the mnemonic **MINT** must be considered at the outset so that one recalls the malformations, neoplasms, and traumatic foreign bodies that may cause an obstruction or provide a fruitful soil for bacterial growth. Unlike a nonbloody discharge elsewhere, pyuria is rarely associated with inflammation of a noninfectious nature; more than that, it is almost invariably due to bacteria. What is more the bacteria are usually gram-negative bacilli, particularly *E. coli, Aerobacter, Proteus*, or *Pseudomonas*.

With this in mind, let us visualize the **anatomy** of the genitourinary tree and develop a system for ready recall of the diagnostic possibilities. The **urethra** brings to mind all the various causes of urethritis (see p. 223). The **prostate** reminds one of prostatitis and prostatic abscess. The **bladder** suggests cystitis, stricture, Hunner's ulcers, calculi, and papillomas that may initiate infection. Some urologists may recall finding a vesicovaginal fistula or rectovesical fistula in patient who have had previous abdominal surgery; a fistula may also form in regional ileitis. The ureters suggest the numerous congenital anomalies (*e.g.*, stricture, congenital band, and aberrant vessel) that may cause obstruction and infection. The **renal pelvis** and **kidney** recall pyelitis and pyelonephritis, as well as renal carcinoma, calculi, and congenital

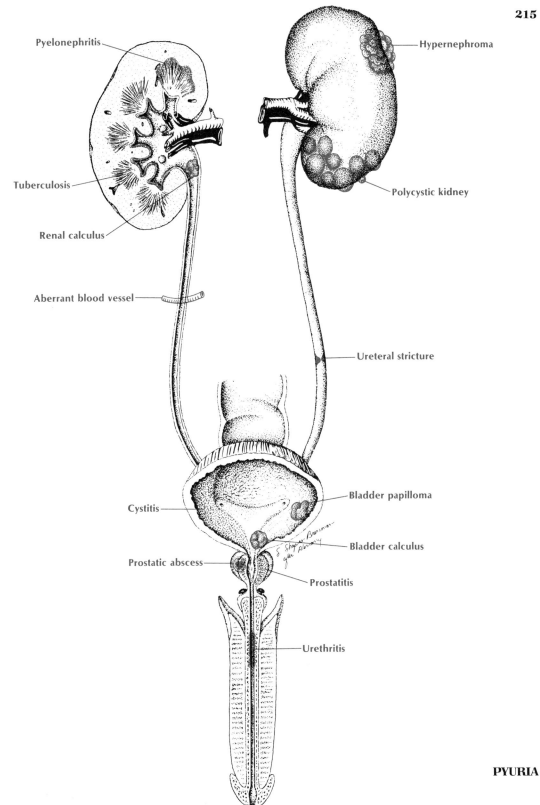

Pyelonephritis

Hypernephroma

Tuberculosis

Polycystic kidney

Renal calculus

Aberrant blood vessel

Ureteral stricture

Bladder papilloma

Cystitis

Bladder calculus

Prostatic abscess

Prostatitis

Urethritis

PYURIA

anomalies, all of which may contribute to infection.

The rare causes of pyuria must be considered. Tuberculosis of the kidney should be mentioned, because when routine cultures are negative this is one of the conditions to look for. Even actinomycosis can cause pyuria, thus a culture on Sabouraud's media is not unwarranted. Although Bilharzia hematobium parasites usually cause hematuria, pyuria is occasionally the initial finding. An interstitial nephritis of toxic or autoimmune origin may occasionally cause a "shower" of eosinophils into the urine. Finally, there is probably not a surgeon alive who has not been fooled by the pyuria of an acute appendicitis, salpingitis, or diverticulitis.

Approach to the Diagnosis

How does one track down the cause of pyuria? First it must be determined that the cloudy urine is really pyuria. Amorphous phosphates and other inert material will disappear on treating the urine with dilute acetic acid. Then, just as for other nonbloody discharges, one must do a smear and culture for the offending organism; an examination of the urine, especially the unspun specimen, is axiomatic. If one finds clumps of leukocytes, renal gitter cells, or WBC casts, the infection almost certainly comes from the kidney. Motile bacteria in an unspun specimen examined under high power microscopy signify infection and a colony count of over 100,000 per ml. A three-glass test may be helpful in localizing the site of origin of the pyuria. Anaerobic cultures and cultures for chlamydia may be needed. Look for eosinophils on a Wright's stain of the urine if toxic nephritis is suspected.

Vaginal examination and culture may disclose a source for the infection. In the male one episode of pyuria should be sufficient indication for an intravenous pyelogram; a female should have one after her second episode, especially if no cause can be found on physical examination. Cystoscopy and a voiding cystogram are often indicated at this time. Other tests for the workup of pyuria are listed in Appendix I.

RECTAL DISCHARGE ■

Rectal discharges are usually bloody, but the two notable exceptions to this are a **ruptured perirectal abscess** and an **anal fistula** (really the end result of the former). Use the mnemonic **MINT** and a few other conditions that might otherwise be overlooked come to mind.

M—Malformation that creates a nonbloody rectal discharge is loss of sphincter control, often due to rectal surgery or a deep midline episiotomy, but perhaps even more frequently due to neurological disturbances such as spinal cord injury or stroke (really fecal incontinence). A **pilonidal sinus,** although not specifically related to the rectum, may suggest to the patient that he has a rectal discharge.

I—Inflammation, in addition to those disorders already mentioned, recalls an anal fissure or ulcer that not only causes purulent material to weep on its own but also often permits fecal material to leak onto the underclothes of the patient. The fistulous tracts from regional ileitis and lymphogranuloma venereum must be considered here. Condyloma latum and acuminatum, although not causing a discharge themselves, may prevent complete closure of the anal canal and permit fecal material to leak through.

N—Neoplasms of the rectum and anus and even thrombosed hemorrhoids can behave in a similar manner.

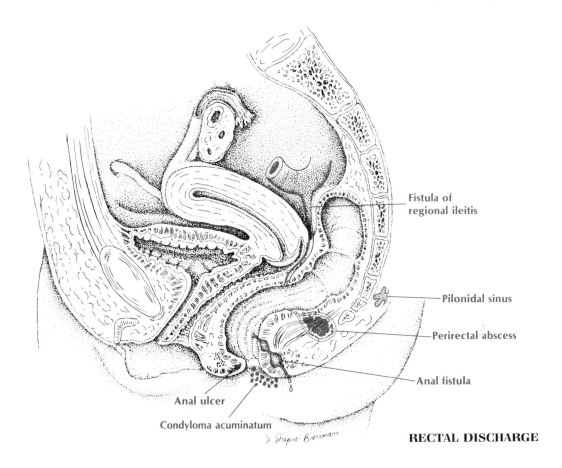

Fistula of
regional ileitis

Pilonidal sinus

Perirectal abscess

Anal fistula

Anal ulcer

Condyloma acuminatum

J. Shapiro-Brennman

RECTAL DISCHARGE

T—Trauma is mentioned merely to remind one again of episiotomies and rectal surgery that may create poor control and allow chronic escape of feces, especially the liquid form.

Approach to the Diagnosis

Smear and culture of the discharge are axiomatic. Visualization of the lesion with the anoscope or sigmoidoscope is usually necessary. A Frei test should be done if lymphogranuloma venereum is suspected. Other tests are listed in Appendix I.

SKIN DISCHARGE ■

The differential diagnosis of a weeping skin lesion is covered well under rash (see p. 433), but certain conditions should be mentioned here. In all nonbloody discharges infection (usually bacterial) is the most prominent etiology; the staphylococcus and streptococcus are the most common offenders in the skin. In working up from the smallest organism to the largest, however, one will not forget the weeping blisters of herpes zoster and simplex, smallpox and chickenpox; the ulcers and bullae of syphilis the draining sinuses and ulcers of actinomycosis, sporotrichosis, and other cutaneous mycosis; the weeping ulcers of *leishmaniasis americana* and *amebiasis cutis*. There are many more—but decidedly rare—infections in all these categories.

By recalling the anatomy of the skin, the infected hair follicles and sebaceous cysts (furunculosis and carbuncles), infected apocrine glands (hidradenitis suppurativa), and inflamed sweat glands (milariasis) come to mind.

Finally, using the mnemonic **VITAMIN** one will recall the following:

V—Vascular conditions of the skin like postphlebitic ulcers that cause a discharge

I—Inflammatory conditions of a noninfectious nature like erythema multiforme, pyoderma gangrenosum, and pemphigus that produce weeping

T—Traumatic conditions such as third degree burns

A—Autoimmune and **allergic** disorders associated with weeping vesicles and ulcers like periarteritis nodosa and contact dermatitis

M—Malformations such as bronchial clefts and urachal sinus tracts

I—Intoxicating lesions like a vesicular or bullous drug eruption

N—Neoplasms such as basal cell carcinoma and mycosis fungoides that produce weeping ulcers

Approach to the Diagnosis

Smear and culture of the lesion are most important, although a skin biopsy is sometimes necessary. Serological tests or cultures on special media are necessary to diagnose fungi and parasites.

SPUTUM

The approach to obtaining a differential is simply to visualize the various anatomical components as one travels down the respiratory tree and then consider the etiologies of each. A nonbloody discharge is almost invariably due to inflammation, infection, or allergy, but a few important exceptions are worth mentioning here.

Congestive heart failure from any cause (see p. 116) produces a frothy sputum that is occasionally bloodstained. Many toxic substances can produce severe acute inflammation or moderate-to-severe chronic inflammation and fibrosis. Most notable of these are pneumoconiosis, silicosis, beryllosis and asbestosis. Lipoid pneumonia is mentioned in most text books of differential diagnosis but is seldom seen. Adult respiratory distress syndrome may result from injection of heroin, shock, and septicemia. This condition is associated with a frothy sputum also. A few additional exceptions are mentioned as the respiratory tree is traversed.

In diseases of the **larynx** and **trachea,** sputum production is usually scanty, but several viruses (*e.g.,* influenza) and bacteria (Haemophilus influenza, pertussis, and diphtheria) may cause a productive sputum. Allergic laryngotracheitis does not usually produce sputum.

The **bronchi** may be inflamed by viruses (*e.g.,* influenza and measles), bacteria, and particularly by bronchial asthma. In bacterial infection the sputum is usually yellow, whereas in bronchial asthma it is white, thick, and mucoid. Chronic bronchitis is usually associated with cigarette smoking or exposure to some other irritating inhalant (such as silicosis). Bronchiectasis may result from acute or chronic bronchitis, or from a congenital lesion (*e.g.,* cystic fibrosis). The sputum in this condition is especially copious (one cup or more a day) and separates into three layers: a frothy layer (saliva); a greenish layer (white cells and bacteria); and a brown layer (yellow bodies, elastic fibers, or Dittrich's plugs).

The **bronchioles** and **alveoli** are the seat of numerous forms of pneumonia. The commonest by far are bacterial, particularly *Streptococcus pneumoniae*, but staphylococcal, Klebsiellae, and H. influenzal forms are not unusual. Gram-negative pneumonia is more common in hospitalized patients, especially

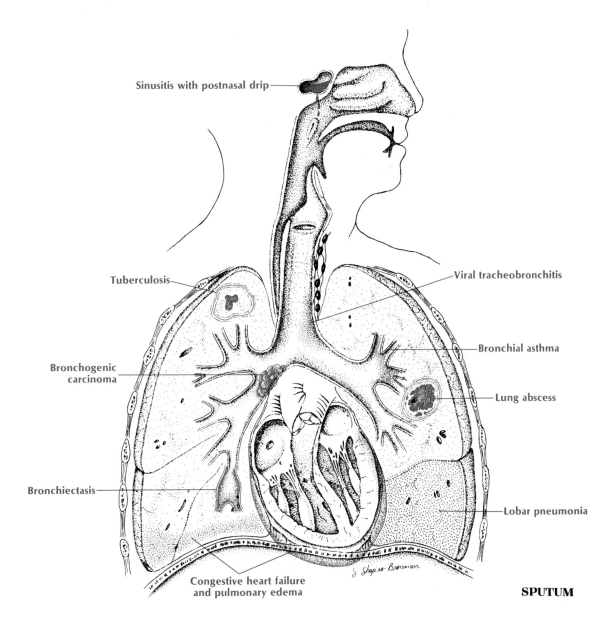

Sinusitis with postnasal drip

Tuberculosis

Viral tracheobronchitis

Bronchial asthma

Bronchogenic carcinoma

Lung abscess

Bronchiectasis

Lobar pneumonia

Congestive heart failure and pulmonary edema

SPUTUM

those who are debilitated or those who have pre-existing lung disease or malignancy. Viral pneumonias are also frequent and include psittacosis, mycoplasma, and even influenza or measles.

One cannot bypass either the miliary or the cavitary form of tuberculosis as a frequent cause of a chronic persistent cough that produces a grayish-yellow sputum. Lung abscesses are important causes of nonbloody sputum; the sputum is usually foul-smelling (one can barely stand to walk in the room)

because of the many anaerobes in the abscess. Histoplasmosis and other fungi must be looked for.

Allergic and autoimmune diseases that involve the alveoli and may produce a nonbloody sputum include Leoffler's pneumonitis, Wegener's granuloma, rheumatoid arthritis, scleroderma, and lupus erythematosus. Even rheumatic fever can produce a pneumonitis. A more extensive display of the conditions that may produce a nonbloody sputum is demonstrated in Table 4-1.

TABLE 4-1.   SPUTUM

	V Vascular	I Inflammatory	N Neoplasm
Larynx and Trachea		Laryngotracheitis Viral or bacterial infection Diphtheria	
Bronchi		Bronchitis, acute and chronic	Carcinoma of the lung Bronchial adenoma
Alveoli	Pulmonary infarct (rarely) Congestive heart failure	Pneumonia viral, bacterial Tuberculosis Fungus Parasites Rickettsiae	Alveolar carcinoma Metastasis
Capillaries			Hemangioma

Approach to the Diagnosis

Obviously the approach to the diagnosis begins with examination of the sputum. In acute cases, a Gram's stain often shows pneumococci or other bacteria. The laboratory should examine a 24-hour sputum for Curschmann's spirals (of bronchial asthma), eosinophils, and elastic fibers, but so should the physician (to differentiate bronchiectasis and lung abscess).

A routine and acid-fast bacillus (AFB) culture is usually necessary. The chest roentgenogram (posterior–anterior and both laterals) plus proper examination of the sputum and culture is usually all that is necessary. Spirometry and a circulation time will help rule out congestive heart failure. Bronchoscopy, bronchography, and lung scans may be necessary in the chronic or subacute cases. Repeated cultures and smears are often rewarding. Lung aspiration and biopsy may also be necessary. Appendix I provides a more extensive list of the various tests that might be useful in individual cases.

D Degenerative and Deficiency	I Intoxication	C Congenital	A Autoimmune Allergic	T Trauma	E Endocrine
	Aspiration Alcohol Tobacco	Tracheoesophageal fistula	Allergic laryngitis and epiglottitis		
	Turpentine aspiration Pneumoconosis Tobacco Poisonous gas	Bronchiectasis Cystic fibrosis Alpha 1 antitrypsin deficiency	Asthmatic bronchitis		
Pulmonary emphysema Pulmonary fibrosis	Lipoid pneumonia	Alveolar proteinosis	Wegener's granuloma		
		Goodpasture's syndrome Vasculitis Lupus			

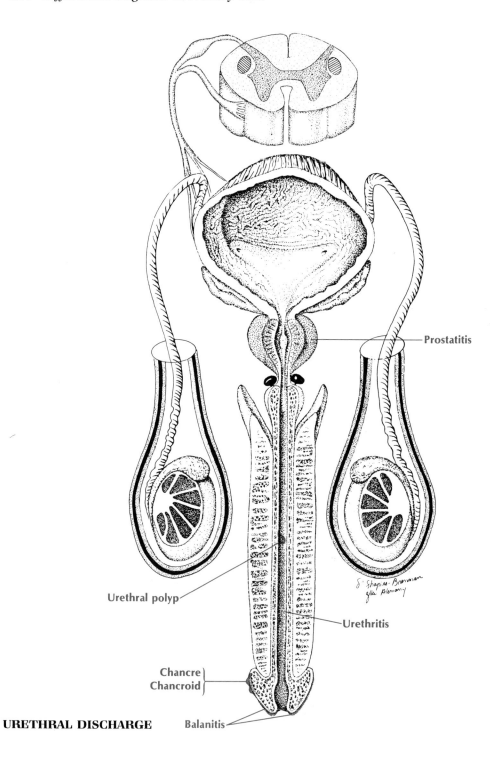

Prostatitis

Urethral polyp

Urethritis

Chancre
Chancroid

URETHRAL DISCHARGE   Balanitis

URETHRAL DISCHARGE ■

A significant purulent urethral discharge invariably signals the diagnosis of gonorrhea, and until a Gram's stain is done little consideration is given to the other causes of a nonbloody urethral discharge; however, one should also consider other etiological agents (staphylococcus, *E. coli*, herpes, mima polymorpha and especially *Chlamydia trachomatis*). Furthermore, the **anatomy** of the urogenital tree should be visualized so that inflammation of all the components can be carefully considered in the resistant case.

Beginning with the **prepuce,** the physician should consider balanitis of either infectious or autoimmune origin (*e.g.*, Reiter's disease). An ulcer from lues, chancroid, or lymphogranuloma inguinale or venereum must be looked for. The **urethra** suggests the urethritis of gonorrhea, chlamydia, and numerous other organisms, whereas autoimmune disorders like Reiter's disease precipitate a nonspecific urethritis and nonbloody discharge. Again, chancres and chanchroids, as well as herpes, may involve the anterior urethra. Trichomonas rarely produce a discharge in the male. In the female the Skene's glands may be infected by gonorrhea or other organisms. A urethral caruncle can easily be recognized as a small cherry-red mass at the urethral orifice.

Further up, the **prostate** is encountered and acute and chronic prostatitis and prostatic abscess are immediately suggested. Inflammation of Cowper's glands or of the seminal vesicles should be remembered as a possible cause of a discharge in resistant cases. In the female urethrovaginal fistula (most frequently from surgery or from a cervical carcinoma) should be considered.

As elsewhere, a purulent discharge does not necessarily signify inflammation alone. There may be a foreign body, a papilloma, and occasionally a carcinoma that precipitates a superimposed infection.

Approach to the Diagnosis

The association of other symptoms and signs is helpful in narrowing the list of possibilities. The discharge of acute urethritis is usually associated with severe pain on micturation whereas the discharge of prostatitis is often not. The discharge of chronic prostatitis is usually painless and occurs most frequently on arising. Urethral caruncles, papillomas, and carcinomas frequently have a bloody discharge, at least intermittently. On examination, the physician can detect enduration of a urethral chancre and the erythema of a balanitis is obvious when the prepuce is retracted. The presence of arthritis or conjunctivitis makes Reiter's syndrome a distinct possibility, although gonorrhea may do the same. The boggy prostate of prostatitis and the increase of the discharge on massage will assist greatly in this diagnosis.

In the laboratory, a smear and culture are axiomatic in diagnosis, and one must massage the prostate and milk the urethra if little discharge is found on simple inspection. After massaging the prostate, the first portion of a voided specimen should be examined, smeared, and cultured if no discharge is apparent. Culture for chlamydia if routine cultures are negative. Cystoscopy and cystograms may be necessary but the indications for these will be at the discretion of the urologist.

VAGINAL DISCHARGE ■

Again the female genital tract can be infected by all sizes of organisms, thus a useful method for recalling the causes of a purulent vaginal discharge is to work from the smallest to the largest organism. Thus we begin with herpes progenitalia and proceed to gonorrhea and nonspecific bacterial infection (now known as *Gardnerella vaginalis*), trichomoniasis, and finally moniliasis. This, however, does not cover all the causes of a nonbloody vaginal discharge. Consequently, **anatomy** is applied as well.

At the **vulva,** one encounters vulvitis, bartholinitis, and vulval carcinoma. In the **vagina** the conditions mentioned above are formed in addition to senile vaginitis, foreign bodies, and vaginal carcinomas. One should also not forget vesicovaginal and rectovaginal fistulas as well as enteric fistulas. At the **cervix,** cervicitis and endocervicitis (gonorrheal or non-

specific), cervical polyps, and carcinomas need to be mentioned. In the uterus, endometritis, polyps and carcinomas are recalled, but the latter two conditions are usually associated with a bloody discharge. Finally, salpingitis produces a mucopurulent discharge.

Approach to the Diagnosis

To workup a vaginal discharge, simply examining a fresh wet saline and potassium hydroxide (10%) preparation will expose the

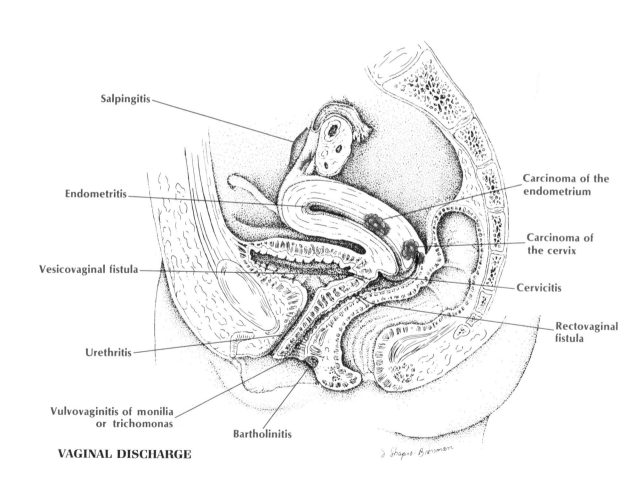

VAGINAL DISCHARGE

most common offenders, namely trichomonas and moniliasis. Some physicians treat all those patients with negative findings on these examinations as a nonspecific bacterial vaginitis, but this is not a particularly scientific procedure. It is best to do a smear and culture (especially for gonococci). Cultures are also available for trichomonas and monilia. If gonorrhea is suspected, material from the endocervix should be cultured. Chlamydia cultures are routinely done in some clinics.

Obviously, if the cervix is eroded and the discharge seems to be coming from there, biopsy and conization may be indicated. Referral to a gynecologist is preferred if this procedure is deemed necessary. Of course, the primary physician may prefer to cauterize the superficial lesions himself. Patients with discharges thought to be due to lesions beyond the cervix should probably also be referred.

VOMITUS ■

The numerous causes of vomiting are discussed under functional changes (see p. 353). It is worthwhile, however, to discuss a few of the important causes of nonbloody vomitus here. Like other "discharges" simply by visualizing the anatomy of the "tree" one can assimilate the causes of nonbloody vomitus.

In the posterior **pharynx** and **larynx** mucus may be regurgitated from a postnasal drip of sinusitis or material that cannot be swallowed because of a stricture, myasthenia gravis, or bulbar palsy. There may also be drainage from a retropharyngeal abscess. In the **upper esophagus,** a foreign body, diverticulum stricture, or web of Plummer–Vinson syndrome may cause regurgitation of food, mucus, and saliva. In the **lower esophagus** lye strictures, esophagitis, cardiospasm, and carcinomas are responsible for regurgitation of food and mucus. Extrinsic pressure and the resulting obstruction from an aneurysm, cardiomegaly, or a mediastinal tumor may also cause a nonbloody "discharge."

Nonbloody vomitus from the **stomach** is usually due to gastritis, an ulcer, pyloric obstruction, or carcinoma of the stomach. When intestinal obstruction occurs beyond the pyloris or when there is ulceration or obstruction because of a gastrojejunostomy, the vomitus is often bile-stained. The many other causes of intestinal obstruction may produce a nonbloody vomitus. If there is a gastrocolic fistula the vomitus may be feculent.

Extrinsic causes of vomiting such as migraine, labyrinthitis, or glaucoma usually cause a nonbloody vomitus with or without bile stain. If it becomes bloody, one should consider a complicating Mallory–Weiss syndrome. The approach to the diagnosis of vomiting is discussed on page 358.

226

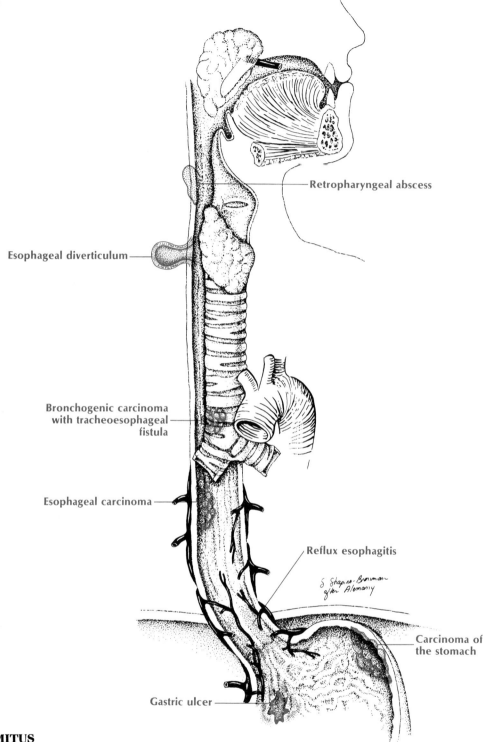

Retropharyngeal abscess

Esophageal diverticulum

Bronchogenic carcinoma
with tracheoesophageal
fistula

Esophageal carcinoma

Reflux esophagitis

S Shapiro-Brownman
after Alamony

Carcinoma of
the stomach

Gastric ulcer

VOMITUS

FUNCTIONAL CHANGES

Chapter 5

GENERAL DISCUSSION

The symptoms of functional changes may be classified into three groups.

1. Symptoms due to **decreased** function (*e.g.*, depression, bradycardia, and constipation)
2. Symptoms due to **increased** function (tachycardia, diarrhea, and polyphagia)
3. Symptoms due to an **alteration** in function (*e.g.*, chorea, tremors, and cardiac arrhythmias)

In most of these symptoms **physiology** and **biochemistry** are the basic sciences most useful in arriving at a differential diagnosis. Anatomy may provide one with the organs where the disease process takes place, but understanding why the symptom develops when that organ fails to function normally is the key to a differential diagnosis.

Jaundice, for example, is due to an increased bilirubin in the blood. Using pathophysiology one can appreciate that an increased serum bilirubin may result from an increased production of bilirubin (by increased hemolysis of red cells), a poor transport of bilirubin (congestive heart failure) to the liver for excretion, insufficient uptake and conversion of bilirubin for excretion (*e.g.*, hepatitis), and decreased excretion of the converted (conjugated) bilirubin due to obstruction of the bile ducts (*i.e.*, common duct stones or carcinoma of the head of the pancreas).

It is essential to do an effective review of systems for additional symptoms that may help the clinician eliminate some of the possibilities in the differential developed by the method above. This is done by thinking of each organ system and asking the patient about symptoms of increased function, decreased function, or altered function. Thus one can quickly run through possibilities by asking, "Do you have any palpitations, shortness of breath, diarrhea, or polyuria?" for increased function, or "Do you have anorexia, weakness, constipation or any difficulty swallowing?" for decreased function. With respect to jaundice one would ask about other symptoms that may be related to poor liver function: loss of appetite, malaise, fatigue, constipation, and itching.

Of course the clinician must ask about the other groups of symptoms (pain, bloody and nonbloody discharge, and mass). With a specific disease of the liver in mind (determined by using pathophysiology) the clinician will ask more meaningful questions to track down the diagnosis. For example, if viral hepatitis is suspected, he would ask about fever, dark urine, tenderness in the right upper quadrant, and blood transfusions. Narrowing or pinpointing the diagnosis can often be facilitated by grouping the signs and symptoms together.

Now one is ready to write appropriate orders to further pinpoint the diagnosis. If only two or three conditions are left in the differential diagnosis, Appendix II will be most useful because it provides orders for specific diseases. Appendix I should be consulted if a considerable number of diseases are still to be ruled out. The principles introduced here are elaborated further in the discussions of each symptom of dysfunction.

ANOREXIA

Physiology is the most appropriate basic science to use in developing a list of the causes of anorexia. A good appetite depends on a psychic desire for food; a happy GI tract that is secreting hydrochloric acid, pancreatic and intestinal enzymes, and bile in the proper amounts; a smooth absorption of food; a smooth transport of food and oxygen to the cell; and an adequate uptake of food and oxygen by the cells. Examining each of these physiological mechanisms provides a useful recall of the differential diagnosis of anorexia.

1. **Psychic desire for food.** This may be impaired in functional depression, psychosis, anorexia nervosa, and organic brain syndromes (*e.g.*, cerebral arteriosclerosis, senile dementia, and tumors).
2. **Gastrointestinal disease.** Esophagitis, esophageal carcinomas, gastritis, gastric and duodenal ulcers, gastric carcinomas, intestinal parasites, regional enteritis, intestinal obstruction, ulcerative colitis, diverticulitis, chronic appendicitis, and colon neoplasms are the most important diseases to consider here. Many drugs increase acid production (*e.g.*, caffeine) and cause gastritis (*e.g.*, aspirin, corticosteroids, and reserpine) or interfere with intestinal motility and cause anorexia.
3. **Decreased pancreatic enzymes.** Pancreatitis, fibrocystic disease, pancreatic carcinomas, and ampullary carcinomas are considered here.
4. **Proper bile secretion.** Gallstones, cholecystitis, cholangitis, liver disease, and carcinoma of the pancreas and bile ducts must be considered here.
5. **Smooth absorption of food.** Celiac disease and the many other causes of malabsorption are brought to mind in this category.
6. **Smooth transport of food and oxygen.** Anything that interferes with oxygen and food reaching the cell may be considered here. Pulmonary diseases that interfere with the intake of oxygen or release of carbon dioxide are recalled here, as are anemia and congestive heart failure.

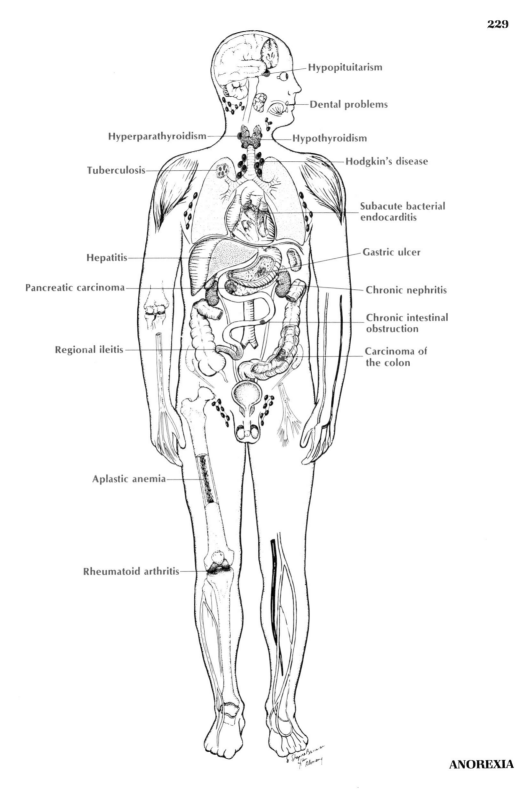

Hypopituitarism

Dental problems

Hyperparathyroidism

Hypothyroidism

Hodgkin's disease

Tuberculosis

Subacute bacterial endocarditis

Hepatitis

Gastric ulcer

Pancreatic carcinoma

Chronic nephritis

Chronic intestinal obstruction

Regional ileitis

Carcinoma of the colon

Aplastic anemia

Rheumatoid arthritis

ANOREXIA

7. Uptake of food and oxygen by the cell. This will be decreased in diabetes mellitus (when there is no insulin to provide the transfer of glucose across the cell membrane); in hypothyroidism (when the cell metabolism is slow so uptake of oxygen and food is also slowed down); in adrenal insufficiency, where the proper relation of Na^+, Cl^-, and K^+ is interfered with; in uremia, hepatic failure, and other toxic states from drugs that interfere with cell metabolism; and in histotoxic anoxia, where the uptake of oxygen by the cell is impaired (*e.g.,* cyanide poisoning). Chronic infections like pulmonary tuberculosis may also produce anorexia by this mechanism.

Approach to the Diagnosis

Again the association with other symptoms and signs narrows the diagnosis considerably. Anorexia with jaundice points to the liver as the cause. Anorexia with thickening of the hair and the nails and nonpitting edema suggests hypothyroidism. Anorexia with dysphagia suggests cardiospasm of the esophagus, esophagitis, or esophageal carcinoma. Laboratory tests include thyroid function studies, a gallbladder series, an upper GI series, esophagram, a barium enema, liver and kidney function tests, electrolytes, and blood sugar. Total body CT scans, ultrasound, and other special diagnostic procedures are useful in selected cases in which other symptoms warrant their need. FSH and LH levels are usually depressed in anorexia nervosa.

ANURIA AND OLIGURIA

Diminished output of urine (oliguria with less than 500 ml output in 24 hours) and no output of urine (anuria) are best understood using **pathophysiology.** The causes may be divided into prerenal (where less fluid is delivered to the kidney for filtration), renal (where the kidney is unable to produce urine because of intrinsic disease), and postrenal (where the kidney is obstructed and the urine cannot be excreted).

1. **Prerenal causes.** Anything that reduces the blood flow to the kidney may cause anuria. Thus shock from hemorrhage, myocardial infarction, dehydration, drugs, or septicemia may be the cause. Congestive heart failure in which the effective renal plasma flow is reduced is also a possibility. Intestinal obstruction or intense diarrhea may cause the loss of enormous amounts of fluid through vomiting or diarrhea and the accompanying shock results in anuria. Embolic glomerulonephritis, bilateral renal artery thrombosis, and dissecting aneurysms may cause renal shutdown.

2. **Renal causes.** These may be analyzed with the mnemonic **VINDICATE** so that none are missed.

   V—**Vascular** lesions include embolic glomerulonephritis and dissecting aneurysm; transfusion reactions are considered as well as intravascular hemolysis of any cause.

   I—**Inflammatory** lesions include pyelonephritis, necrotizing papillitis, and renal tuberculosis.

   N—**Neoplasms** of the kidney rarely cause anuria because only one kidney is affected at a time.

   D—**Degenerative** conditions are unlikely to cause anuria.

   I—**Intoxication** from numerous antibiotics (*e.g.,* gentamycin, sulfa, streptomycin) and from gold, arsenic, chloroform, carbon tetrachloride, or phenol, for example, is a common cause of anuria. Renal calculi and nephrocalcinosis should be considered here.

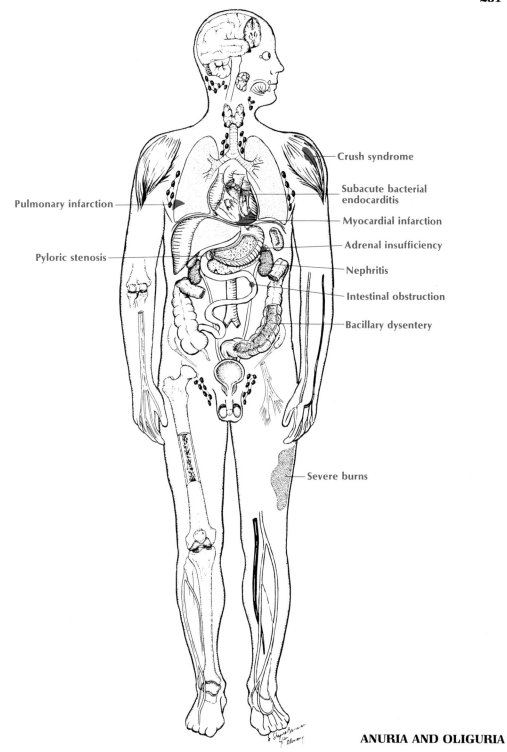

Crush syndrome

Subacute bacterial
endocarditis

Myocardial infarction

Adrenal insufficiency

Nephritis

Intestinal obstruction

Bacillary dysentery

Pulmonary infarction

Pyloric stenosis

Severe burns

ANURIA AND OLIGURIA

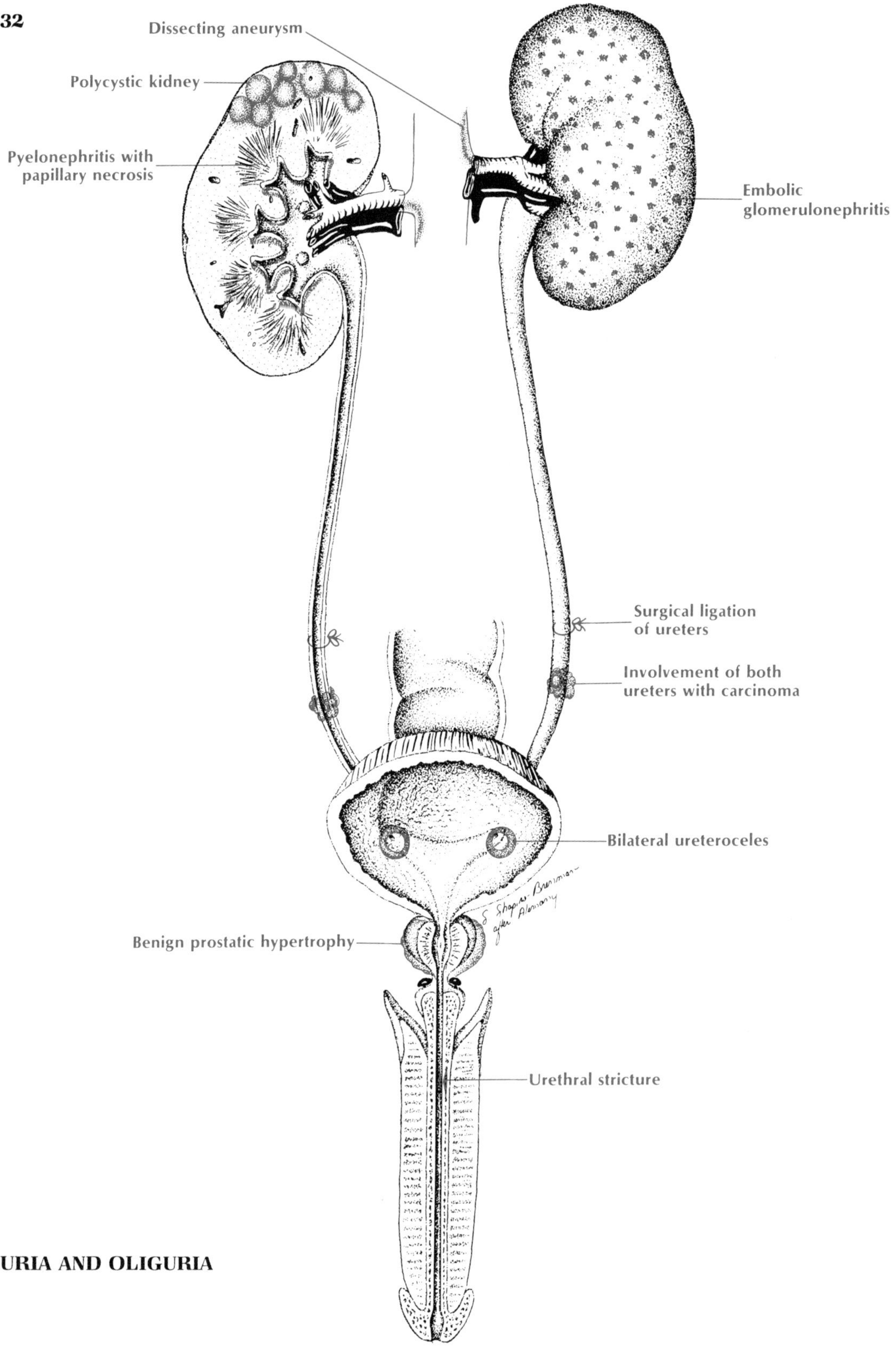

Dissecting aneurysm

Polycystic kidney

Pyelonephritis with
papillary necrosis

Embolic
glomerulonephritis

Surgical ligation
of ureters

Involvement of both
ureters with carcinoma

Bilateral ureteroceles

Benign prostatic hypertrophy

Urethral stricture

ANURIA AND OLIGURIA

C—Congenital disorders include polycystic kidneys and medullary sponge kidneys.

A—Autoimmune disorders form the largest group of renal causes of anuria. Lupus erythematosus, polyarteritis nodosa, acute glomerulonephritis, amyloidosis, Wegener's granulomatosis, and scleroderma are included here.

T—Trauma includes contusions and lacerations of the kidney for completeness; however, lower nephron nephrosis from crush injury or burns is not unusual.

E—Endocrine disorders include diabetic glomerulosclerosis, necrotizing papillitis from diabetes, and nephrocalcinosis from hyperparathyroidism and related disorders.

3. **Postrenal causes.** The mnemonic **MINT** will help recall this group of disorders that obstruct the kidneys and bladder.

M—Malformations may cause anuria; they include congenital bands, aberrant vessels over the ureters, horseshoe kidney, and ureteroceles.

I—Inflammation includes cystitis, urethritis, and prostatitis.

N—Neoplasms include carcinomas of the bladder obstructing both ureters, prostatic hypertrophy, and carcinomas of the uterus or cervix involving both ureters. "N" also signifies neurological disorders such as polio, multiple sclerosis, and acute trauma to the spinal cord that may cause anuria.

T—Trauma signifies surgical ligation of the ureters, ruptured bladder, and instrumentation of the urinary tract.

Approach to the Diagnosis

To work up a case of anuria, catheterize the bladder to rule out obstructions there; if there is any suspicion of an obstructive uropathy, cystoscopy and retrograde urography should be done. The urine is examined and cultured to exclude infection. If a prerenal cause is suspected, the blood volume is returned to normal or a test of a mannitol drip is begun and urine output monitored. If urine output does not rise to 40 ml an hour within 2 hours, a dose of furosemide is given; this may be doubled at intervals until either an output is established or 1000 mg have been given. If prerenal and postrenal causes have been effectively excluded, a nephrologist should be consulted and the long process of treating the renal causes and establishing renal dialysis is undertaken until the kidney regains its function.

AUSCULTATORY SIGNS OF PULMONARY DISEASE

It is questionable whether this topic should be included in a differential diagnosis book, but because it is important for the clinician to be able to recall a fairly complete list of possible causes for these signs while he is still examining the patient, a discussion is included here. Regardless of what the sign is, it almost invariably may be considered the result of local disease of the lung or heart. Infrequently, a disease of another organ has spread to the lung. Cross-indexing these topics with the mnemonic of etiologies, **VINDICATE,** will provide a useful list of possibilities.

Lung

V—Vascular diseases includes pulmonary embolism and infarction and Goodpasture's disease.

I—Inflammatory disease suggests viral, bacterial tuberculosis, parasitic and fungal pneumonia, and lung abscess. Pleurisy must also be considered.

N—Neoplasms remind one of carcinoma of the lungs (primary or metastatic) and bronchial adenomas.

D—Degenerative disease suggests emphysema and pulmonary fibrosis.

I—Intoxication brings to mind the pneumoconioses and changes from drugs such as nitrofurantoin.

C—Congenital disorders include cystic fibrosis, alpha 1 antitrypsin deficiency, bronchiectasis, alveolar proteinosis, atelectasis, and lung cysts.

A—Autoimmune diseases include rheumatoid arthritis, lupus, Wegener's granulomatosis, periarteritis nodosa and scleroderma. The "**A**" also stands for **Allergic** disease, including asthma and Löffler's syndrome.

T—Trauma should suggest pneumothorax and hemopneumothorax.

E—Endocrine disease suggests the bronchoconstriction of the carcinoid syndrome.

Heart

V—Vascular diseases of the heart that cause auscultatory signs include myocardial infarction and hypertension with congestive heart failure and the various arrhythmias associated with them.

I—Inflammatory diseases of the heart also affect the lungs. Subacute and acute bacterial endocarditis may shed emboli in the lung if they involve the right heart. Myocarditis may cause failure and pericarditis may cause pleural effusion.

N—Neoplasms of the heart rarely affect the lung.

D—Degenerative diseases include muscular dystrophy and other cardiomyopathies.

I—Intoxication reminds one of alcoholic myocardiopathy with congestive failure and arrhythmias that may lead to emboli. Digitalis and other cardiac drugs may do the same. Electrolyte disturbances must also be considered here.

C—Congenital heart diseases brings to mind a host of diseases that may cause failure.

A—Autoimmune diseases, especially lupus erythematosus, scleroderma, and amyloidosis, affect the heart and lung.

T—Traumatic hemopericardium or aneurysm of the heart may cause auscultatory changes of the lung.

E—Endocrine diseases like hyperthyroidism, hypothyroidism, acromegaly, and diabetes mellitus affect the heart and may ultimately lead to congestive heart failure and edema in the lungs. Endocrine causes of hypertension (aldosteronism and Cushing's syndrome) may lead to hypertensive cardiovascular disease (HCVD) and congestive heart failure.

Diseases of Other Organs

V—Vascular suggests pulmonary embolism from systemic phlebitis.

I—Inflammation includes embolic abscesses or pneumonitis of the lungs and pulmonary tuberculosis, tularemia, plague, *Echinococcus*, *Paragonimus westermani*, histoplasmosis, and so forth. Shock lung from septicemia is a possible cause.

N—Neoplasms suggest metastatic carcinoma from other organs. Meigs' syndrome is also suggested here.

D—Degenerative suggests nothing here, although pleural effusion may result from nephrosis and cirrhosis.

I—Intoxication may result from ingested turpentine and other products that subsequently affect the lung. Aspiration pneumonitis must be considered in this category.

C—Congenital disorders, especially neurological diseases and esophageal atresia, may lead to recurrent pneumonia.

A—Autoimmune diseases have been reviewed above.

T—Trauma and burns anywhere may result in pulmonary edema from shock lung.

E—Endocrine diseases have been discussed above.

Approach to the Diagnosis

Clinically, the grouping together of signs provides the best way of narrowing the differential diagnosis.

Rales

1. Bilateral crepitant rales, lack of dullness, and normal breath sounds suggest pulmonary edema or pneumonitis.
2. Focal crepitant rales, reduced alveolar breathing, dullness to percussion, and increased tactile and vocal fremitus suggest lobar pneumonia or pulmonary infarction.
3. Bilateral sibilant and sonorous rales without dullness and with increased bronchial breathing suggest asthma, chronic bronchitis and emphysema, acute bronchitis or bronchiolitis, and cardiac asthma.
4. Focal crepitant rales, amphoric breathing with dullness below and hyperresonance above suggest a lung abscess or cavitation.

Hyperresonance

1. Hyperresonance bilaterally with diminished breath sounds bilaterally and sibilant rales suggests pulmonary emphysema or asthma.
2. Focal hyperresonance with diminished or absent breath sounds and no rales suggests pneumothorax.
3. Focal hyperresonance with normal or only diminished breath sounds suggests a large bulla.

Dullness or Flatness

1. Dullness with diminished breath sounds and no rales suggests atelectasis or pleural effusion from empyema, congestive heart failure, or pulmonary infarct. In atelectasis there is no hyperresonance or egophony above the dullness.
2. Dullness with diminished breath sounds and crepitant rales suggests pneumonia or pulmonary infarct. If there is bronchophony as well there is probably no associated effusion. If there is no bronchophony but hyperresonance and egophony above the dullness, then an associated pleural effusion should be considered.

Laboratory Workup

Crepitant rales should prompt a sputum examination, smear and culture, possibly a tuberculin test, venous pressure and circulation time, chest roentgenogram, and ECG to secure the diagnosis. If the chest x-ray film shows no consolidation and the individual is in no acute distress, a pulmonary function study may help. If it shows a reduced vital capacity with a normal timed vital capacity, congestive heart failure is most likely diagnosis. In acute cases, shock lung or adult respiratory distress syndrome must always be considered. Other tests to work up pulmonary and cardiovascular disease are listed in Appendix I.

BALDNESS

A clever mnemonic to apply here is **HAIR.** The **H** stands for **hereditary baldness** and **hormonal** baldness, such as hypothyroidism and hyperthyroidism. The **A** stands for **alope-**

cia areata and **autoimmune** disease, such as lupus erythematosus. The **I** stands for **inflammatory** conditions, most notably tinea capitis, impetigo, and any condition associated with prolonged fever. The **I** also stands for **intoxication,** with arsenic and gold therapy most important here. Finally, the **R** stands for **radiation.** This is particularly significant today with so many victims of neoplasms being treated with this modality.

Approach to the Diagnosis

The Wood's lamp and scrapings of any scaly material are useful in distinguishing tinea capitis from lupus and other disorders, but a skin biopsy is wise in any unusual lesion. Referral to a dermatologist is best if fungus or other infections are ruled out and thyroid function studies are normal.

BLURRED VISION, BLINDNESS, AND SCOTOMATA ■

The causes of blurred vision and blindness can best be recalled with the use of **anatomy.** If the path of light is followed through the eye to the nervous system, the various components of the eye and nervous system that may be involved may be considered in terms of the common diseases that may affect them.

Conjunctiva. Chemical, allergic, and infectious conjuctivitis may cause blurred vision but it rarely causes blindness. A pterygium may grow across the cornea and impair vision. Trachoma may cause blindness if left untreated.

Cornea. Foreign bodies, keratitis, herpes ulcers, and keratoconus may cause blurred vision and blindness. Congenital syphilis forms an extensive progressive interstitial keratitis. Trachoma may cause corneal ulcers and blurred vision.

Canal of Schlemm. At the angle of the iris and cornea, the canal of Schlemm prompts the recall of glaucoma because obstruction of this area figures so prominently in the pathophysiology.

Iris. Iritis from sarcoid, tuberculosis, histoplasmosis, and other causes is considered here. Iridocyclitis occurs when both the lens and iris are involved.

Lens. The two most common causes of blurred vision, cataracts and refractive errors, are considered here. Cataracts may result from diabetes, myotonic dystrophy, galactosemia, and many systemic diseases. They are also congenital and senile, posttraumatic, and associated with various mental deficiency states. Refractive errors include myopia, hyperopia, and astigmatism. These are usually correctable.

Vitreous humor. Hemorrhages of the vitreous and precipitation of triglycerides (lipemia retinalis) may cause blurred vision.

Retina. Chorioretinitis causes blurred vision and blindness and may result from syphilis, tuberculosis, toxoplasmosis, retinitis pigmentosa, and proliferative retinitis in diabetes mellitus. Retinal detachment may result from all the above. Retinal hemorrhages and exudates of hypertension, diabetes, lupus erythematosis, aplastic anemia, and subacute bacterial endocarditis are all possible causes of blurred vision and blindness.

Retinal artery. Occlusion of the retinal artery is a prominent cause of blurred vision or blindness in older people. Emboli, thrombi, and vasculitis secondary to temporal arteritis are all possible causes of the occlusion. Migraine and birth control pills should be considered, and migraine, in particular, should be a prominent consideration in scintillating scotomas.

Retinal vein. A retinal vein thrombosis is a possibility here. Following the course of the vein, however, one encounters the cavernous sinus, and a thrombosis here may lead to bilateral blurred vision and blindness.

Optic nerve. Papilledema, optic neuritis, and optic atrophy are the most important conditions to consider. The papilledema is usually due to an intracranial space-occupying lesion, but hypertension and benign intracranial hypertension need attention in the differential. Optic neuritis requires the consideration of multiple sclerosis, neurosyphilis, tuberculosis, diabetes mellitus, sinusitis, and lead poisoning. Optic atrophy should suggest syphilis, methyl alcohol poisoning, hereditary optic atrophy, Foster Kennedy syndrome (frontal lobe tumors), and various congenital anomalies. It may be secondary to diseases of the retina. The optic nerve may be severed by an orbital fracture.

Optic chiasma. Pituitary tumors, sphenoid ridge meningiomas, colloid cysts of the

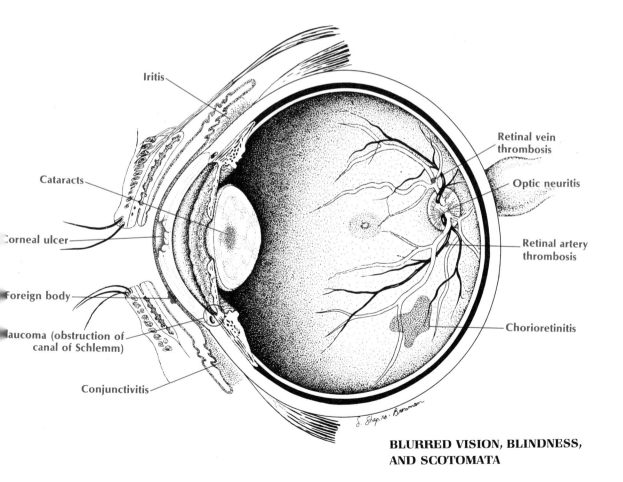

Iritis

Cataracts

Corneal ulcer

Foreign body

Glaucoma (obstruction of canal of Schlemm)

Conjunctivitis

Retinal vein thrombosis

Optic neuritis

Retinal artery thrombosis

Chorioretinitis

BLURRED VISION, BLINDNESS, AND SCOTOMATA

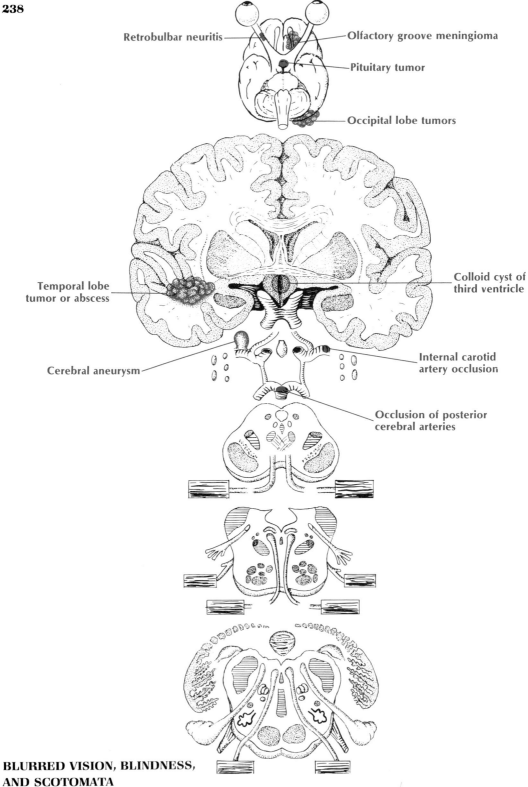

Retrobulbar neuritis

Olfactory groove meningioma

Pituitary tumor

Occipital lobe tumors

Temporal lobe
tumor or abscess

Colloid cyst of
third ventricle

Cerebral aneurysm

Internal carotid
artery occlusion

Occlusion of posterior
cerebral arteries

**BLURRED VISION, BLINDNESS,
AND SCOTOMATA**

third ventricle, aneurysms, and cavernous sinus thrombosis are possible causes. Syphilitic or tuberculosis meningitis may also involve the chiasma, as may the spread of a Schmincke tumor from the nasopharynx. Basilar skull fractures infrequently involve the chiasma.

Optic tract, optic radiations, and **occipital cortex.** Intracranial hematomas, cerebral thrombi or emboli, transient ischemic attacks (TIA), aneurysms, cerebral tumors, and abscesses all may involve these structures. Certain forms of acute and chronic encephalitis may also involve these areas, causing blurred vision and blindness. Cortical blindness may result from an occlusion of both posterior cerebral arteries at their origin from the basilar artery.

Approach to the Diagnosis

A careful eye examination with magnification and fluorescence to rule out a foreign body and ulcers is essential in the acute case of blurred vision. Ophthalmoscopic examination may demonstrate optic neuritis or a retinal vein thrombosis. Visual field examination by confrontation may reveal a field defect. If these test results are negative, ocular tension should be checked to rule out glaucoma. A history of migraine, the use of birth control, and alcohol intake must be investigated. If there is headache on the side of the lesion a sedimentation rate is done, steroids should probably be started immediately and referral to a neurologist made promptly in case temporal arteritis is possible, especially in the aged. Otherwise referral to an ophthalmologist is necessary. He will perform visual field examinations with perimetry, a slit lamp examination, and look for refractive errors. If other neurological findings are present, a CT scan, skull x-ray film, and spinal tap may be indicated. A neurological consultant can determine this.

BRADYCARDIA ■

Bradycardia (a heart rate below 60) is not infrequently found during a routine physical examination. Visualizing the conduction system of the heart recalls the sick sinus syndrome, A-V nodal rhythm, or A-V block, but unfortunately it does not help recall the many causes of these disorders. The mnemonic **VINDICATE** is the most useful aid in my experience.

V—Vascular diseases suggest myocardial infarction, especially inferior wall and anteroseptal infarctions. Arteriosclerosis may also cause focal ischemia of the conducting system.

I—Inflammatory disease suggests viral myocarditis, diphtheria, and Chagas' disease.

N—Neurological disorders, because neoplasms of the heart are infrequent. Neurological disorders include vasovagal syncope (common faint), cerebral concussion, and anything else that might cause an increased intracranial pressure (*e.g.*, subarachnoid hemorrhage and cerebral tumors).

D—Degenerative and **deficiency** disease suggests beriberi and myocardial fibroelastosis.

I—Intoxication suggests alcoholic myocardiopathy, digitalis, propranolol (Inderal), procainamide, and quinidine toxicity or effects, as well as other cardiac drugs. The hypokalemia of chlorothiazide diuretics and the hyperkalemia of uremia, triamterene (Dyrenium), and spironolactone also are suggested.

C—Congenital disorders that might cause bradycardia include many congenital heart diseases, sickle cell anemia, glycogen storage disease, and muscular dystrophy.

A—Autoimmune disorders constitute a large group of diseases that may cause bradycardia or heart block. Sarcoidosis, amyloidosis, lupus erythematosus, and rheumatic fever are some of the most important ones.

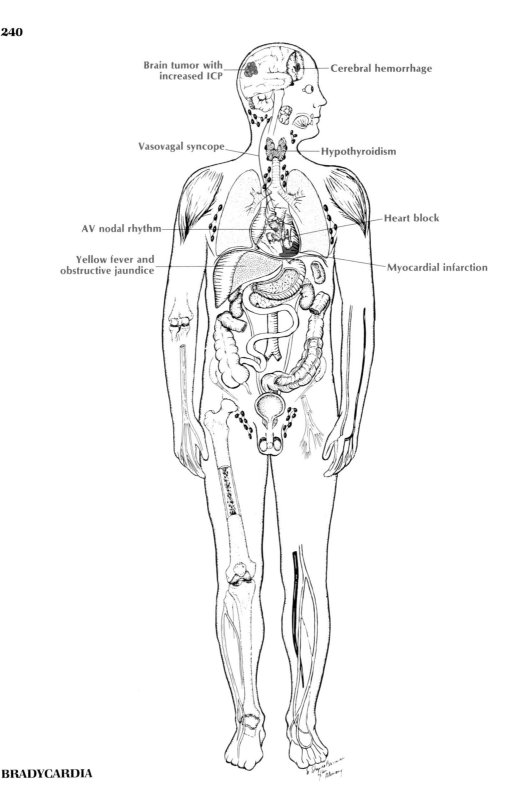

Brain tumor with increased ICP

Cerebral hemorrhage

Vasovagal syncope

Hypothyroidism

AV nodal rhythm

Heart block

Yellow fever and obstructive jaundice

Myocardial infarction

BRADYCARDIA

T—Trauma is not a significant cause; a stab wound, however, could sever the conduction system.

E—Endocrine disorders include myxedema and endocrine disorders that cause electrolyte disturbance like Addison's disease (hyperkalemia), aldosteronism (hypokalemia), and hyperparathyroidism (hypercalcemia).

Approach to the Diagnosis

The diagnosis is most frequently made by the association of other signs and symptoms. A history of ingestion of cardiac drugs and diuretics and doing blood levels for these as well as serum electrolytes will be helpful. Otherwise the diagnosis depends on ordering specific tests for the diseases mentioned above from Appendix II.

CARDIAC ARRHYTHMIAS

With few exceptions the etiologies of cardiac arrhythmias like those of bradycardia can best be recalled using the mnemonic **VINDICATE.** The exceptions are from one pathophysiological cause: **obstruction** and consequent dilatation of one or more of the chambers of the heart. Thus mitral stenosis with obstruction and dilatation of the left atrium is a prominent cause of atrial arrhythmias, especially auricular fibrillation. Hypertension and aortic stenosis may cause a number of atrial and ventricular arrhythmias. Pulmonary hypertension resulting from pulmonary emphysema, fibrosis, or pneumonia with consequent right ventricular and atrial obstruction, and dilatation causes arrhythmias, especially atrial arrhythmias.

Getting back to **VINDICATE** completes the recall of the causes of arrhythmias.

V—Vascular diseases include myocardial infarction, coronary insufficiency, and coronary artery emboli.

I—Inflammatory diseases include viral myocarditis, diphtheria, syphilis, tuberculosis, and Chagas' disease.

N—Neoplasms include atrial myxomas, but the **N** also stands for neuropsychiatric causes. Paroxysmal atrial tachycardia is especially likely to result from emotional causes.

D—Degenerative diseases include Friedreich's ataxia, myotonic dystrophy, myocardial fibroelastosis, and other myocardopathies.

I—Intoxication suggests the largest number of causes of arrhythmia: alcohol, caffeine, tobacco, digitalis, quinidine, propranolol, and procainamide are just a few. Diuretics cause electrolyte disturbances that may cause or contribute to cardiac arrhythmias.

C—Congenital disorders recall congenital heart diseases, many of which cause recurrent arrhythmias. The Wolff–Parkinson–White syndrome predisposes to atrial tachycardia. Muscular dystrophy may cause myocardopathy and arrhythmias. Von Gierke's disease and gargoylism also need to be remembered.

A—Autoimmune disorders suggest the arrhythmias of amyloidosis, sarcoidosis, scleroderma, periarteritis nodosa, and rheumatic fever,

T—Trauma suggests the arrhythmias in shock, burns, stab wounds to the heart, and head injuries. Electric shock is a cause of ventricular fibrillation.

E—Endocrinopathies should remind one of hyperthyroidism, a prominent cause of atrial fibrillation; Addison's disease; and aldosteronism, which disturb the electrolytes sufficiently to cause arrhythmias. Pheochromocytomas may cause atrial tachycardia from the tremendous output of epinephrine.

(Text continues on p. 244)

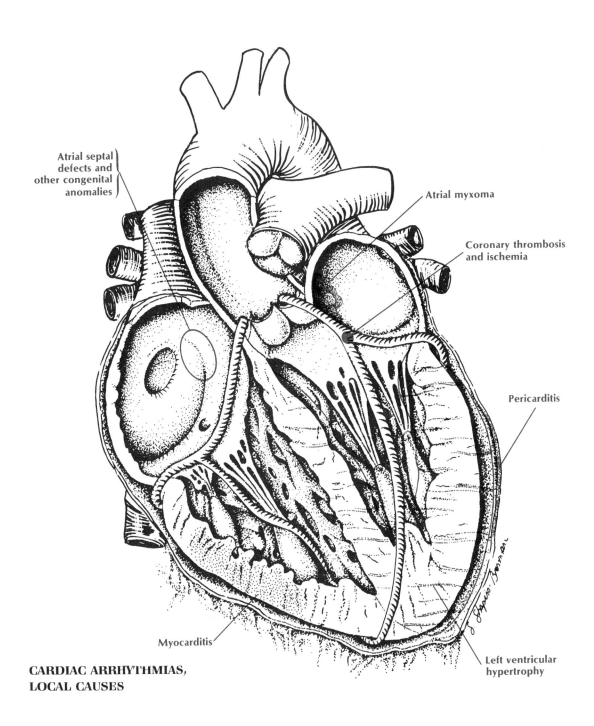

Atrial septal defects and other congenital anomalies

Atrial myxoma

Coronary thrombosis and ischemia

Pericarditis

Myocarditis

Left ventricular hypertrophy

**CARDIAC ARRHYTHMIAS,
LOCAL CAUSES**

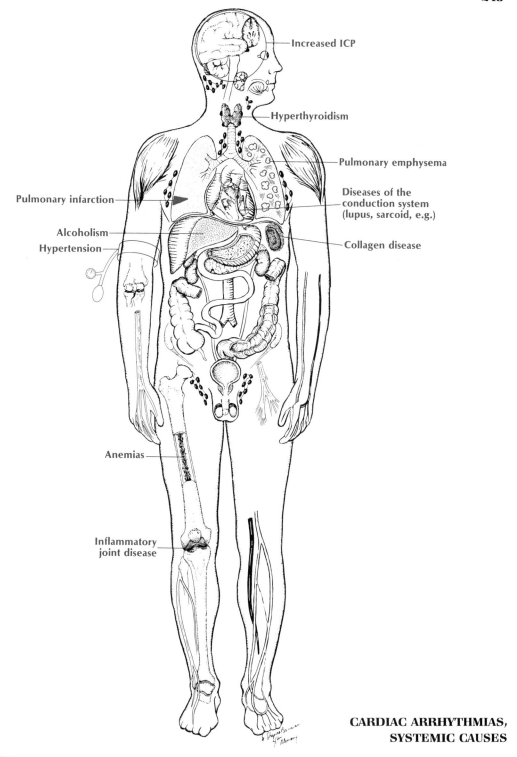

Increased ICP

Hyperthyroidism

Pulmonary emphysema

Diseases of the
conduction system
(lupus, sarcoid, e.g.)

Pulmonary infarction

Collagen disease

Alcoholism

Hypertension

Anemias

Inflammatory
joint disease

**CARDIAC ARRHYTHMIAS,
SYSTEMIC CAUSES**

Approach to the Diagnosis

The diagnosis depends a lot on the type of arrhythmia. Atrial premature contractions are usually benign and an extensive workup is unnecessary unless other physical signs indicate the need for it. Infrequent ventricular premature contractions (VPCs) in otherwise healthy individuals probably can be handled the same way. When VPCs are frequent or multifocal, an exercise tolerance test, echocardiogram, and perhaps coronary angiography are indicated. Runs of ventricular tachycardia require an extensive workup, including coronary angiography, but usually there will be other signs to indicate the need for this.

Atrial tachycardia and fibrillation require a workup of hyperthyroidism and pulmonary disease, systemic hypertension, and congestive heart failure. Atrial obstruction and dilatation should be excluded by echocardiography.

Any arrhythmia warrants an ECG and possibly repeats. The Holter monitor should be used if there is doubt about the type of arrhythmia. Other tests are listed in Appendix I.

CHILLS

A chill with chattering of the teeth and shaking followed by a fever is almost invariably due to an infectious process. Furthermore, the infection is usually bacterial, and the chill indicates that the bacteria have invaded the blood stream. The exceptions to the above are discussed later in the chapter.

Anatomy is the key to a differential diagnosis. To start with, each organ in the body can be infected by an "itis" of the parenchyma, an "itis" of the capsule, or an abscess.

1. **"Itis" of the parenchyma.** Here one should recall encephalitis, otitis media, mastoiditis, pharyngitis, pneumonitis, endocarditis, pyelonephritis, hepatitis, cholecystitis or cholangitis, gastroenteritis, appendicitis, diverticulitis, prostatitis, orchitis, endometritis, salpingitis, cellulitis, osteomyelitis, and arthritis. Since some of the above infections are frequently viral (e.g., hepatitis, gastroenteritis, and encephalitis), a chill would be unusual. Myositis is usually viral but in trichinosis a chill is not rare.

2. **"Itis" of the capsule.** In this group are meningitis, pleuritis or pleurisy, pericarditis, and peritonitis.

3. **Abscess.** This should prompt the recall of cerebral abscess, epidural or subdural abscess, dental abscess, retropharyngeal abscess, lung abscess or empyema, liver abscess, subdiaphragmatic abscess, perinephric abscess, abscessed diverticulum, appendiceal abscess, tubo-ovarian abscess, pelvic abscess, prostatic abscess, and furuncles or carbuncles. Abscesses are especially prone to cause chills.

4. **Systemic infection.** Some systemic infections are particularly likely to be associated with a chill. Malaria, relapsing fever, Weil's disease, rat-bite fever, yellow fever, smallpox, Rocky Mountain spotted fever, acute poliomyelitis, and pulmonary tuberculosis belong in this group.

5. **Venous thrombosis.** Phlebitis in various portions of the body is often associated with chills. Cavernous sinus thrombosis, lateral sinus thrombosis, pyelophlebitis, and, less frequently, thrombophlebitis of the extremities may be associated with a chill.

6. **Miscellaneous.** Chills are often associated with injection of drugs or antibiotics, intravenously, transfusions hemolytic anemia, and introduction of contaminated equipment into the body. Chills are rare in rheumatic fever.

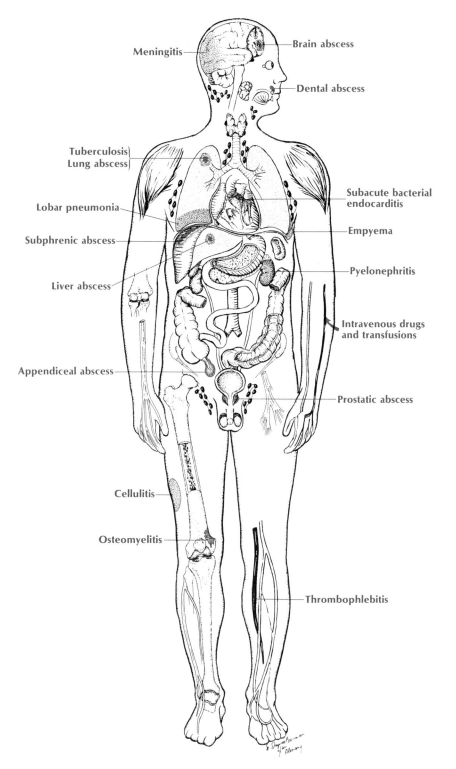

Meningitis

Brain abscess

Dental abscess

Tuberculosis
Lung abscess

Subacute bacterial
endocarditis

Lobar pneumonia

Empyema

Subphrenic abscess

Pyelonephritis

Liver abscess

Intravenous drugs
and transfusions

Appendiceal abscess

Prostatic abscess

Cellulitis

Osteomyelitis

Thrombophlebitis

CHILLS

Approach to the Diagnosis

The approach to the diagnosis of a disease with chills is similar to that of fever. Association with other signs (*e.g.,* jaundice or dysuria) will often point to the organ involved. However, when fever and chills are the only symptoms a workup like that found in Appendix I may be necessary. Careful charting of the temperature while the patient remains off aspirin or other antipyretics will be rewarding, especially in the diagnosis of malaria.

CHOREA ◾

The causes of this symptom lend themselves easily to recall. Simply remember the word **VINDICATE.** There are usually just one or two diseases for each letter.

V—**Vascular** suggests an infarct of the subthalamic nucleus, which produces hemibalism.

I—**Inflammatory** lesions suggest the various forms of viral encephalitis.

N—**Neoplasms** of the brain stem include gliomas and metastatic carcinoma.

D—**Degenerative** disease suggests Huntington's chorea.

I—**Intoxication** suggests Wilson's disease, phenothiazine, lead or manganese toxicity, and carbon monoxide poisoning.

C—**Congenital** chorea suggests the chorea of cerebral palsy.

A—**Autoimmune** disease suggests the Sydenhan's chorea of rheumatic fever.

T—**Trauma** suggests chorea from concussion, basilar skull fracture, or intracerebral hematoma.

E—**Endocrine** and **Epilepsy** suggest the possibility that the chorea is related to an epileptic focus. The hyperkinesis of hyperthyroidism sometimes stimulates chorea.

The workup of chorea is similar to the workup of tremor (see p. 396).

COMA AND SOMNOLENCE ◾

Somnolence is a deep sleep from which the patient can be aroused. Coma is an unconscious state from which the patient cannot be aroused. Since somnolence may be simply an early stage of coma, its etiologies are almost all identical with the etiologies of coma. The few exceptions are mentioned at the close of this discussion.

While in medical school, I discovered a little text, *Aids to Medical Diagnosis* by GEF Sutton. I have never forgotten the unique little mnemonic provided in the text for remembering the causes of coma, **A—E—I—O—U,** the vowels.

A—**Accidents** suggest cerebral concussion and epidural and subdural hematomas. The **A** also stands for arterial occlusions, arteriosclerosis, aneurysms, and autoimmune disorders.

E—**Endocrine** disorders such as myxedema coma, hyperparathyroidism, diabetic coma, and insulin shock are included in this category. The **E** also stands for the coma following an epileptic seizure.

I—**Inflammatory** and **Intoxication** disorders such as encephalitis, cerebral abscess, meningitis, alcoholism, and opiates or barbiturates are included in this category.

O—**Organ** failure should suggest hepatic coma, respiratory failure, and uremia.

U—**Uremia** was used by Dr. Sutton, but because it is included above in organ failure, I prefer to use the **U** to designate the "**undefined**" disorders like narcolepsy and conversion hysteria.

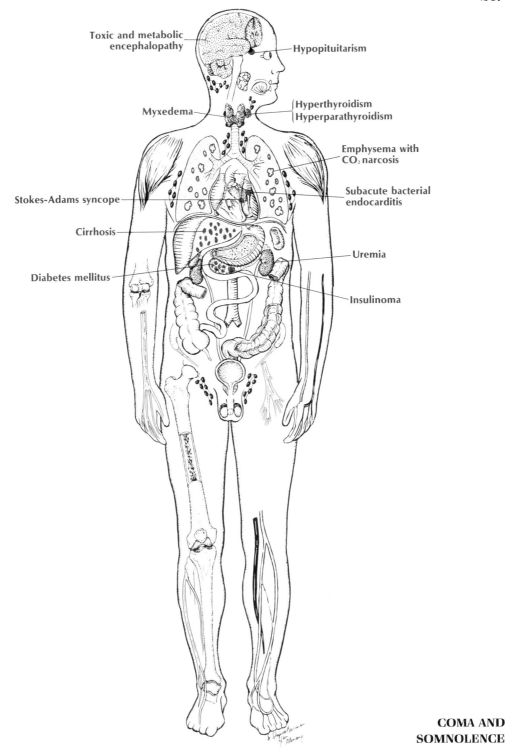

Toxic and metabolic encephalopathy

Hypopituitarism

Myxedema

Hyperthyroidism
Hyperparathyroidism

Emphysema with CO₂ narcosis

Stokes-Adams syncope

Subacute bacterial endocarditis

Cirrhosis

Diabetes mellitus

Uremia

Insulinoma

**COMA AND
SOMNOLENCE**

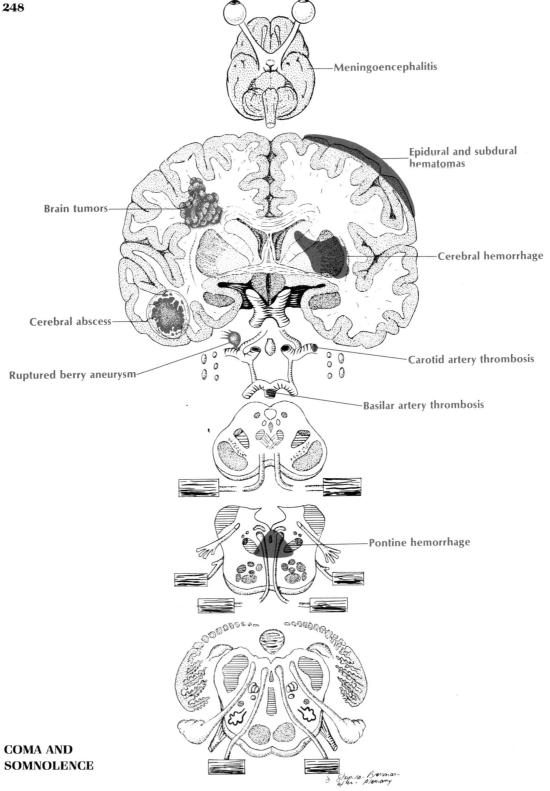

Meningoencephalitis

Epidural and subdural hematomas

Brain tumors

Cerebral hemorrhage

Cerebral abscess

Carotid artery thrombosis

Ruptured berry aneurysm

Basilar artery thrombosis

Pontine hemorrhage

**COMA AND
SOMNOLENCE**

And so with the vowels **A, E, I, O, U**, one has a useful system for recalling the causes of coma and somnolence. **VINDICATE** can be used in a similar manner, but I prefer to let the reader develop the etiologies using this mnemonic as an exercise. There are two other approaches to the differential diagnosis of coma that may be more instructive. These are the **anatomical** and **physiological** approach.

If one visualizes the **anatomy** of the head from the skull on into the ventricles and cross-indexes the various layers with the mnemonic **MINT**, one will have an excellent means of recalling the causes of coma and somnolence demonstrated in Table 5-1. The important conditions resulting from disease of each anatomical structure are reviewed here.

Thinking of the **skull** reminds one of depressed skull fractures and epidural and subdural hematomas. In visualizing the **meninges** meningitis and subarachnoid

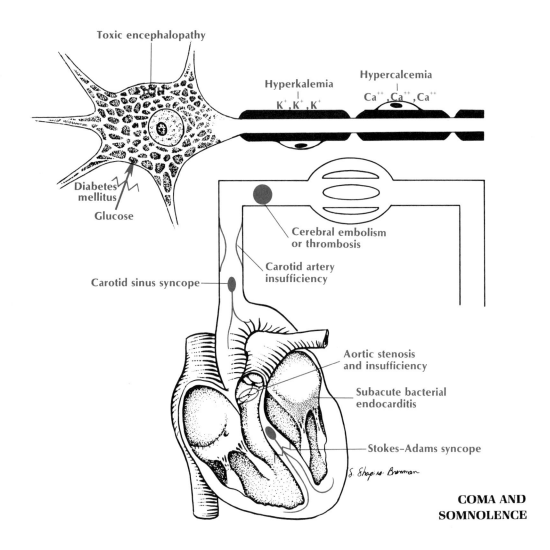

Toxic encephalopathy

Hyperkalemia
K^+, K^+, K^+

Hypercalcemia
$Ca^{++}, Ca^{++}, Ca^{++}$

Diabetes mellitus

Glucose

Cerebral embolism or thrombosis

Carotid artery insufficiency

Carotid sinus syncope

Aortic stenosis and insufficiency

Subacute bacterial endocarditis

Stokes–Adams syncope

S. Shapiro-Brennan

COMA AND SOMNOLENCE

hemorrhages are recalled. Moving deeper into the **brain** itself will suggest encephalitis, encephalopathies (*e.g.*, alcoholic), and brain tumors. Considering the **arteries** at the base of the brain, one should recall arterial occlusions, hemorrhages, and emboli. The **blood supply** prompts the recall of anoxia and other metabolic disorders that may be responsible for coma. The **veins** suggest venous sinus thrombosis as the cause of coma. Finally, the **pituitary** should help recall not only the coma of hypopituitarism but all the other endocrinopathies. This, then, is the anatomical approach to the differential diagnosis of coma and somnolence.

For the physiologic approach simply ask the question, "What does the brain cell need to "keep awake" or to continue functioning?" It needs a good supply of oxygen, glucose, and vitamins; the proper amount of insulin; an appropriate electrolyte and acid-base medium; and a proper amount of fluid in that medium. In addition, the brain cell can not afford to have any toxic substance in that medium that might block the use or action of these metabolic substances. Now one is in a

TABLE 5-1.   COMA AND SOMNOLENCE

	M **Malformations**	**I** **Inflammation**	**N** **Neoplasms**	**T** **Trauma**
Skull				Depressed skull fracture Epidural or subdural hematomas
Meninges	Subarachnoid hemorrhage (from aneurysms)	Meningitis		Subarachnoid hemorrhage
Brain and Parenchyma	Porencephalic cyst Birth trauma or anoxia Kernicterus	Encephalitis Toxic and metabolic encephalopathies Alcoholism	Brain tumors	Cerebral concussions or contusions
Arteries	Arterial occlusions Hemorrhage Embolisms	Subacute bacterial endocarditis Embolism Anoxia	Hemangiomas	Fat emboli Arterial emboli
Veins	Arteriovenous malformations	Venous sinus thrombosis		
Pituitary	Hypopituitarism and other endocrinopathies		Pituitary adenomas	Postpartum hemorrhage

position to take each category and discuss the diseases that may result in a disturbance of brain cell function.

1. **Decreased supply of oxygen.** Focal anoxia from an arterial thrombosis, embolism, or hemorrhage falls in this category. Generalized anoxia from severe anemia and pulmonary or heart disease can also be recalled here.
2. **Decreased or increased supply of glucose.** Any hypoglycemic state (*e.g.*, malabsorption syndrome, severe cirrhosis, glycogen storage disease, and hypopituitarism) may cause coma. On the other hand, coma may be caused by hyperglycemia (nonketotic hyperosmolar diabetic coma).
3. **Too much or too little insulin.** In this category one should recall excessive exogenous insulin, insulinomas, and functional hypoglycemia, as well as diabetic acidosis (too little insulin).
4. **Avitaminosis.** Wernicke's encephalopathy from thiamine deficiency, the hypocalcemia and possible tetany of rickets, and the dementia with somnolence of pellagra might be recalled here.
5. **Disturbances of electrolyte and acid-base equilibrium.** Here one should recall the coma of hyponatremia, hypokalemia, hyperkalemia (*e.g.*, Addison's disease, uremia, and diuretics), hypocalcemia (hypoparathyroidism, rickets, uremia, and malabsorption syndrome), hypercalcemia (*e.g.*, hyperparathyroidism and metastatic tumors of the bone), and hypomagnesemia. The coma of diabetic acidosis, lactic acidosis, CO_2 narcosis, and alkalosis (hyperventilation syndrome) will also be recalled here.
6. **Increased fluid in the cell medium.** This should suggest cerebral edema from brain tumors, hemorrhages, hydrocephalus, encephalitis and meningitis, and cerebral concussions.

7. **Toxic substances that block the utilization or action of metabolic substances.** In this category are extrinsic substances like lead, alcohol, lysergic acid diethylamide (LSD), opiates, and a list of other drugs. It should also include intrinsic toxins from hepatic coma, uremia, and CO_2 narcosis.

Somnolence, as suggested in the introduction, is an indication of a few conditions that are not as likely to present with frank coma: These are endogenous depression narcolepsy, cerebral arteriosclerosis, and encephalitis lethargica. The physiological approach should also suggest myxedema coma somewhere, but it is difficult to fit it into any of the aforementioned categories.

Approach to the Diagnosis

Obviously the neurological examination and a good history from a member of the family or friend are invaluable in the diagnosis of coma. However, one should not delay ordering stat. laboratory work until the examination and history are accomplished. A cbc, blood urea nitrogen (BUN), FBS, serum osmolality, electrolytes, blood gases, urinalysis, and drug screen are ordered immediately. If there is little or no history available and insulin shock is suspected, glucose or glucagon is administered before the laboratory reports are back, although this is done with more caution today for fear of aggravating a case of nonketotic, hyperosmolar diabetic coma.

It has been my experience that the neurological examination is best performed simultaneously with taking a history from a relative or friend. In this way various telltale neurological signs can be found with alacrity. A unilateral dilated pupil (suggesting a subdural hematoma or aneurysm), an acetone breath (suggesting diabetic acidosis), a contusion of the skull (suggesting cerebral concussion or hematoma), and nuchal rigidity (suggesting a subarachnoid hemorrhage in meningitis) are just a few of the signs that can help identify the cause of the coma rapidly.

Coma without focal neurological findings should suggest a metabolic or toxic cause. In that case an intensive laboratory workup as listed in Appendix I would be indicated. A spinal tap may be indicated if there is fever as well. On the other hand, coma with focal neurological signs suggests a tumor, abscess, hematoma or cerebral embolism, thrombosis, or hemorrhage. The clinician should proceed with a skull x-ray film and CT scan immediately. When these are not available, immediate referral to a large medical center is necessary. Electroencephalography and a spinal tap may identify the cause. A spinal tap should be considered with extreme caution even if there is no papilledema. Of course, a spinal tap is never done in the presence of papilledema unless a neurologist is consulted and a CT scan is negative. One indication for a spinal tap under these circumstances might be meningitis. Another might be "benign intracranial hypertension."

CONSTIPATION

The causes of constipation can be recalled on a physiological basis. Normal defecation requires feces that are of proper consistency, good muscular contraction of the walls of the large intestine, and unobstructed passage of the stool. It follows that constipation will result from insufficient intake of food and water, inhibition of muscular contraction of the bowels, or obstruction to the passage of stools. The obstruction can be high or low and intrinsic or extrinsic.

1. **Insufficient intake of food and water.** Starvation or anything that interferes with the appetite will cause constipation. Senility, anorexia nervosa, chronic tonsillitis and cardiospasm of the esophagus are examples. Lack of fluid intake will cause a hard stool and constipation.
2. **Poor bowel motility and contractability.** Neurological conditions such as poliomyelitis and tabes dorsalis may be considered in this group. In Hirschsprung's disease there is lack of the myenteric plexus, causing poor contraction of the bowel wall. Anxiety and depression may interfere with bowel motility and lead to constipation. Certain drugs (such as atropine derivatives, tranquilizers, opiates, and barbiturates) interfere with bowel motility and cause constipation. Uremia and diabetic acidosis may cause a paralytic ileus.
3. **Obstruction.**
   A. **High obstruction** includes pyloric stenosis, volvulus, intussusception, regional ileitis, adhesions, and incarcerated hernias.
   B. **Low obstruction** includes **intrinsic** lesions such as polyps, carcinomas, fecal impactions, and conditions that cause spasm of the rectal sphincter, such as proctitis, hemorrhoids, rectal fissures, rectal fistulas, and abscesses and spinal cord lesions like multiple sclerosis. **Extrinsic** conditions that cause low obstructions include pelvic inflammatory disease, a retroverted uterus, endometriosis, pregnancy, fibroids, ovarian cysts, and a large prostate or pelvic abscess.

Approach to the Diagnosis

Rectal examination for a fecal impaction and subsequent enemas if no contraindication exists are the first steps. This may disclose a

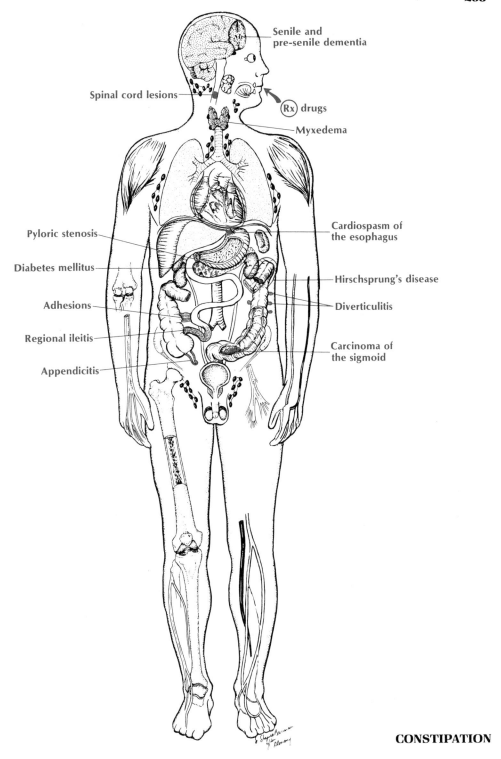

Senile and
pre-senile dementia

Spinal cord lesions

Rx drugs

Myxedema

Pyloric stenosis

Cardiospasm of
the esophagus

Diabetes mellitus

Hirschsprung's disease

Adhesions

Diverticulitis

Regional ileitis

Carcinoma of
the sigmoid

Appendicitis

CONSTIPATION

fissure, inflamed hemorrhoid, or abscess. Pelvic examination must be done in all females. If nothing is found here a proctoscopic examination and barium enema would be indicated, provided the neurological examination and a flat plate of the abdomen are normal. Careful inquiry about diet, drugs, and emotional stress should be made.

CONSTRICTED PUPILS (MIOSIS)

The best method to develop a list of the causes of a constricted pupil is to use **neuroanatomy.** One simply follows the nerve pathways from the end organ (iris) through the peripheral portion of the nerves to the central nervous system (brain stem) (Table 5-2).

1. **End organ.** Iritis, keratitis, and the cholinergic drugs may be the cause of the constricted pupil in this location. Hyperopia and presbyopia are also possible causes.
2. **Peripheral nerves.** Constriction of the pupil may occur from lesions anywhere along the sympathetic pathway as it branches around the internal carotid artery (aneurysms, thrombosis, and migraine), enters the stellate ganglion in the neck (scalenus anticus syndrome, tumors or adenopathy in the neck), and follows

TABLE 5-2. CONSTRICTED PUPILS (MIOSIS)

	V Vascular	I Inflammatory	N Neoplasm	D Degenerative
End Organ		Iritis Keratitis		Hyperopia Presbyopia
Peripheral Sympathetic Pathways	Carotid aneurysms and thrombosis Migraine Aortic aneurysms	Cervical adenitis Mediastinitis	Hodgkin's disease Mediastinal tumors Pancoast's tumor	
Brain Stem	Posterior inferior cerebellar artery occlusion Pontine hemor- rhage	Encephalitis Argyll Robertson (neurosyphilis)	Brain stem tumors	
Spinal Cord		Poliomyelitis Tuberculosis Epidural abscess Transverse myelitis	Spinal cord tumors Metastatic tumors to the spine	Syringomyelia

the preganglionic pathway into the spinal cord (aneurysm of the aorta, mediastinal tumors, spinal cord tumors, or other space-occupying lesions).

3. **Central nervous system.** Lesions involving the sympathetic pathways of the brain stem (posterior inferior cerebellar tumors, occlusion, brain stem tumors, hemorrhages, encephalitis, or toxic encephalopathy) will cause miosis. Both pupils are constricted in the Argyll Robertson pupil of neurosyphilis in which the damage is located in the pretectal nucleus of the midbrain. Morphine characteristically causes bilateral constriction of the pupils, probably based on its central nervous system effects.

Approach to the Diagnosis

In unilateral miosis the clinician must look for local conditions such as iritis and keratitis. If there is an associated ptosis and enophthalmos then Horner's syndrome is present. The lesion is undoubtedly located somewhere along the sympathetic pathway. Miosis alone, however, may be due to a sympathetic lesion. Bilateral miosis and coma should suggest narcotic intoxication or a brain stem lesion (possibly a pontine hemorrhage). Bilateral miosis in an alert individual with pupils that fail to react to light but react to accommodation is clear evidence of an Argyll Robertson pupil. Partial Argyll Robertson pupils do occur. Bilateral miosis in older individuals

(*Text continues on p. 258*)

I Intoxication	C Congenital	A Allergic and Autoimmune	T Trauma	E Endocrine
Cholinergic drugs	Hyperopia Congenital myosis Arachnodactyly	Amyloidosis		Hypoparathyroidism
	Cervical rib Klumpke's paralysis		Brachial plexus trauma	
Toxic encephalopathy (*e.g.*, morphine)				
		Multiple sclerosis	Fracture Herniated discs	

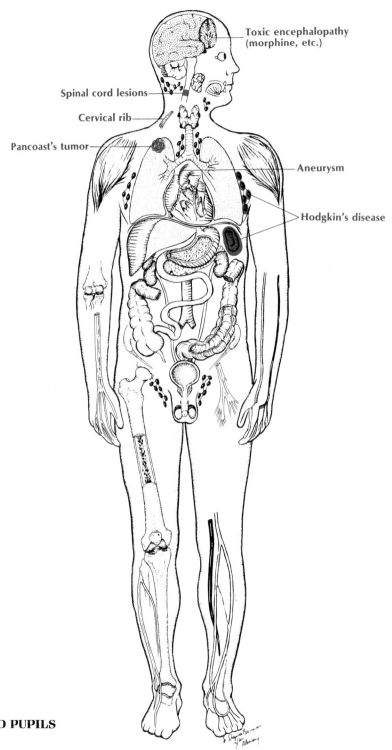

Toxic encephalopathy
(morphine, etc.)

Spinal cord lesions

Cervical rib

Pancoast's tumor

Aneurysm

Hodgkin's disease

CONSTRICTED PUPILS
(MIOSIS)

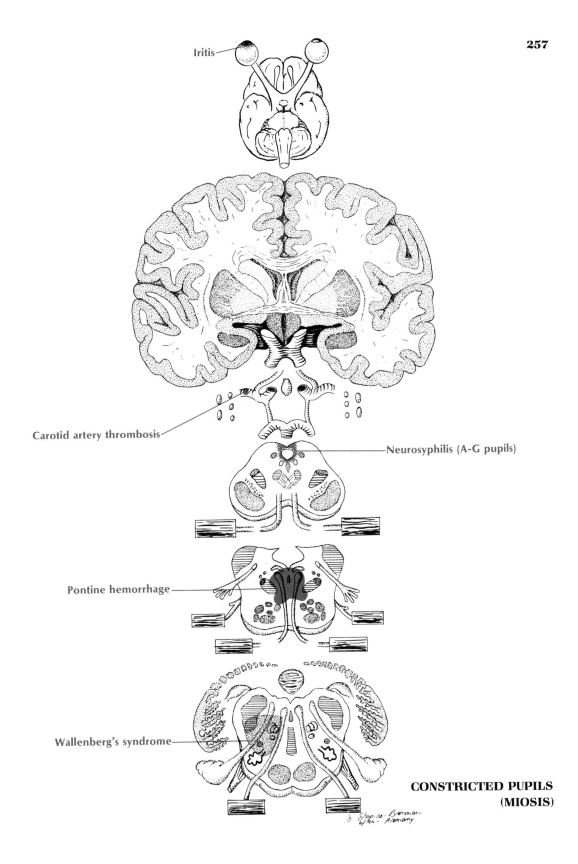

Iritis

Carotid artery thrombosis

Neurosyphilis (A-G pupils)

Pontine hemorrhage

Wallenberg's syndrome

**CONSTRICTED PUPILS
(MIOSIS)**

without loss of the light reflexes suggests hyperopia or arteriosclerosis.

The laboratory workup may include an x-ray film of the cervical spine, chest and skull roentgenogram, a CT scan, and a spinal tap or arteriograms, depending on the association of other symptoms and signs. A starch test to determine if sweating function is lost on the side of the lesion will help locate the level of the sympathetic nerve lesion.

CONVULSIONS

To formulate a differential diagnosis of convulsions, one must use both **physiology** and **anatomy.** The anatomical causes are charted in Table 5-3.

Irritability of the nerve cell is caused by the same physiological factors that lead to irritability of a muscle cell: anoxia, hypoglycemia, and electrolyte imbalances. Any condition causing anoxia may cause a seizure; thus, focal arterial spasm (TIAs) may lead to seizures. Obstruction of the artery by emboli, thrombi, or atheromatous plaques may cause focal anoxia and seizures, while diffuse cerebral anoxia is more likely to cause syncope and coma. Acute blood loss (anemic anoxia) or acute reduction in cardiac output (as in Stokes–Adams disease and various arrhythmias) are infrequent causes of seizures. Aortic stenosis and insufficiency may occasionally cause seizures by relative reduction in cardiac output compared to demand (as during exercise).

Hypoglycemia is more likely to cause a coma than a seizure. Anything that reduces the blood sugar severely (below 40 mg/dl), such as exogenous insulin overdose, islet cell adenoma, Addison's disease, and hypopituitarism, may cause a seizure.

Irritability of the nerve cell is more often caused by electrolyte alterations. The same equations that applied to muscle applies here:

$$\text{Neuronal Irritability} \times \frac{\text{NA}^+, \text{K}^+, \text{pH}}{\text{CA}^{++}, \text{Mg}^{++}, \text{H}^+}$$

Hypocalcemia may at first lead to tetany, simulating a convulsion. The causes of hypocalcemia include hypoparathyroidism, vitamin D deficiency, malabsorption syndrome, calcium losing nephropathy, and chronic nephritis. Ionizable calcium is decreased by alkalosis, respiratory or metabolic. Hypomagnesemia must be ruled out, especially in chronic alcoholics and malabsorption syndromes. Water intoxication should be considered in inappropriate antidiuretic hormone (ADH) syndrome (relative dilution of both calcium and magnesium).

Moving from the physiological causes of seizures to the anatomical analysis, the physician's main consideration is that something mechanical is irritating the nerve cell. The nerve cell may be irritated by a tumor of the supporting tissue, an abscess or a hematoma. Pressure from inflammatory lesions in the meninges (meningitis or epidural abscess) or hemorrhage into this layer (subdural or epidural hematoma and subarachnoid hemorrhages) may be the mechanical irritant. Focal accumulation of fluid in the brain substance as in encephalitis, concussions, and increased intracranial pressure from whatever causes may lead to a seizure. A depressed skull fracture is occasionally the mechanical irritant, as is a scar from an old skull injury. Infiltration of the brain by metals such as lead and copper (Wilson's disease) are worth considering in children, particularly infiltration of the brain by a foreign cell (leukemia); reticuloendotheliosis and glycogen should be considered. Turning to exogenous factors, one must consider a host of chemicals and drugs that may cause seizures, most commonly alcohol, paint thinners, lidocaine (Xylocaine),

(Text continues on p. 262)

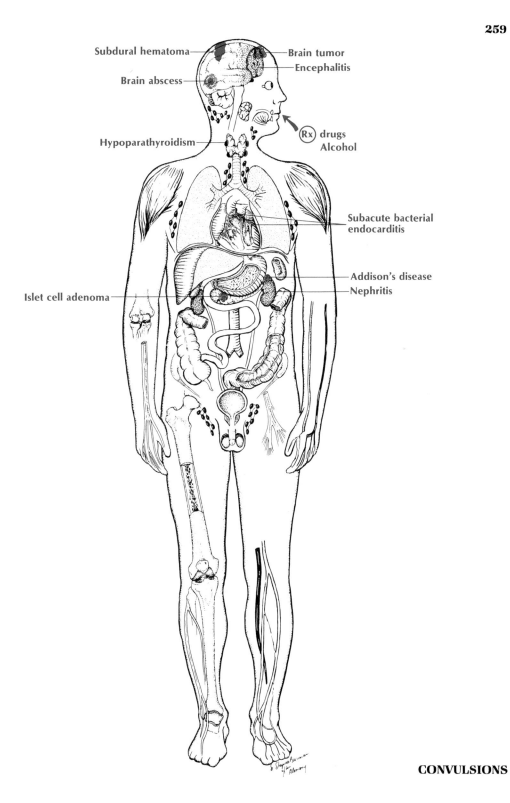

Subdural hematoma

Brain tumor

Brain abscess

Encephalitis

Hypoparathyroidism

Rx drugs
Alcohol

Subacute bacterial
endocarditis

Addison's disease

Nephritis

Islet cell adenoma

CONVULSIONS

TABLE 5-3. CONVULSIONS

	V Vascular	**I** Inflammatory	**N** Neoplasm	**D** Degenerative and Deficiency
Brain Cell and Axon	TIA Hypertensive hemorrhage	Viral encephalitis Syphilis Tetanus Rabies		Pyridoxine deficiency Cortical atrophy
Supporting Tissue		Tuberculoma Cysticercosis Other parasites	Gliomas Neurofibromas Metastasis	Tay–Sachs Histiocytosis X
Meninges	Subarachnoid hemorrhage	Meningitis Epidural abscess	Meningioma Hodgkin's disease	
Skull				
Arteries	Infarct Embolism		Hemangioma Angioma	
Veins		Venous sinus thrombosis		
Blood		Septicemia	Leukemia Polycythemia vera	Aplastic anemia
Heart	Arrhythmias Heart block Myocardial infarction	Subacute bacterial endocarditis	Atrial myxoma with embolism	

I Intoxication and Idiopathic	C Congenital	A Autoimmune Allergic	T Trauma	E Endocrine and Metabolic
Lead Wilson's disease Bromides Alcohol Kernicterus Idiopathic epilepsy Uremia Eclampsia	Schilder's disease Porencephaly Birth trauma Anoxia	Multiple sclerosis	Concussion Intracerebral hematoma	Hypoglycemia Hypopcalcemia (see physiology)
	von Gierke's disease	Cerebral urticaria		Addison's disease
Phenylketonuria (PKU)			Subdural hematoma	
			Depressed fracture Epidural hematoma	
	Aneurysms A-V anomaly	Periarteritis nodosa Lupus	A-V aneurysms	
	A-V anomaly Sturge–Weber syndrome			
Coumadin and heparin therapy		ITP		
Drug-induced arrhythmia Heart block	Aortic stenosis	Rheumatic heart disease with aortic stenosis		Hyperthyroidism with auricular fibrillation and embolism

phenothiazine drugs, and bromides. A bolus of almost any substance may occasionally cause seizures if it is large enough.

Occasionally, degenerative and demyelinating disease may present with seizures. On the other hand, lupus erythematosus and other collagen diseases may frequently present with seizures. Finally, one should not forget idiopathic epilepsy.

Approach to the Diagnosis

The clinician must first be sure that the motor disturbance was really a seizure. Tremors, dystonia, tetany, and hysteria may mimic convulsions. A careful family history from the patient or relative should be done next, making certain to ask about previous head trauma (especially at birth), anoxia, and meningitis or

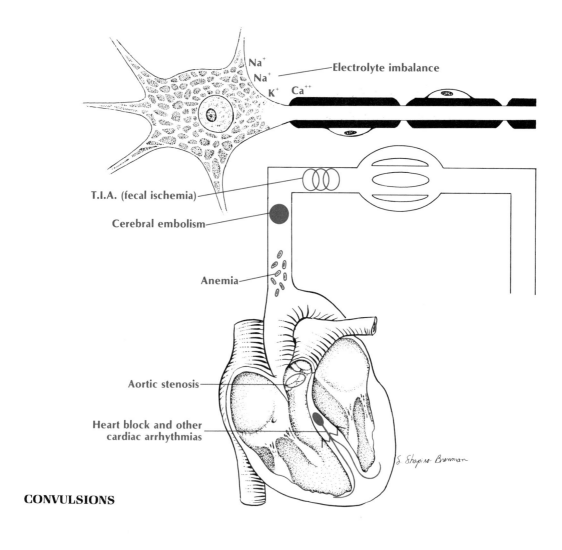

CONVULSIONS

encephalitis. A social history and drug history are essential.

Examination for focal neurological signs will help identify a tumor or other space-occupying lesions, but EEGs, CT scans, or radiocontrast studies are essential to rule these out. Laboratory studies include a blood sugar, calcium, electrolytes, and an alcohol and drug screen in many cases. Appendix I lists the most useful of these tests.

COUGH ■

The differential diagnosis of cough is best developed with the use of **anatomy.** Cough may arise from an irritative focus anywhere along the respiratory tract. The irritation may be **intrinsic,** in which case it is usually inflammatory, neoplastic, or toxic; or it may be **extrinsic,** in which case it is often neoplastic or vascular (Table 5-4).

Intrinsic Irritation. Pharyngitis, whether due to virus, streptococcus, or diphtheria, is a common cause of cough. Hypertrophied tonsils or adenoids may also initiate the cough reflex. Other pharyngeal causes are angioneurotic edema, leukemia, and agranulocytosis. The **esophagus** is an extrinsic cause of cough in most cases, but a tracheoesophageal fistula from esophageal carcinoma or reflux esophagitis with repeated aspiration of HCl may cause a chronic cough. **Diverticuli** of the esophagus may press on the trachea and cause a cough.

In the **larynx** the numerous infections of the pharynx discussed above may irritate the cough centers, but in addition laryngeal polyps, tuberculosis, and trauma from overuse are important causes. The more common causes of cough, especially a nonproductive

cough, are in the **tracheobronchial** area. Numerous viruses cause tracheobronchitis, especially influenza, but bacterial causes such as whooping cough should always be considered. Tuberculosis and carcinoma are important here, as are toxic gases such as chlorine and cigarette smoke. Bronchiectasis, whether congenital or acquired, and the associated postnasal drip from chronic sinusitis must not be forgotten. A search for asthma is important in areas with high pollen counts.

In the **alveoli,** in addition to pneumonia, tuberculosis, and carcinoma (particularly metastatic), several new etiologies are added. Thus, pulmonary embolism, parasites, fungi (such as actinomycosis), pneumoconiosis, reticuloendothelioses, and autoimmune diseases (Wegener's granuloma) should be included.

Extrinsic Irritation. The extrinsic causes are mainly from the structures of the mediastinum, especially the heart. A large heart from congestive heart failure or a single chamber enlargement (as in mitral stenosis) may compress the bronchus and recurrent laryngeal nerve and cause a cough. Pericarditis, aortic aneurysms, and rings are other cardiovascular causes. Finally, other structures in the mediastinum such as a substernal thyroid, a large lymph node from Hodgkin's disease, and occasionally a dermatoid cyst must be considered. Trauma can lead to a cough whether it hits the lung, mediastinum, or pericardium.

Approach to the Diagnosis

Clinically, exposure to dust, smoke, and various gases should be looked for in the patient presenting with a cough. An allergic history (*e.g.,* hay fever) is important. Careful exclusion of cardiovascular disease should be done, especially when sputums are negative for rou-

(Text continues on p. 266)

TABLE 5-4. COUGH

	V Vascular	I Inflammatory	N Neoplasm	D Degenerative and Deficiency

Pharynx		Bacterial or viral
		  pharyngitis,
		  (diphtheria),
		  tonsillitis
			Leukemia
			Hypertrophied tonsils
			  and adenoids	

Esophagus		Reflux esophagitis	Carcinoma	
Larynx		Laryngitis Singers' nodes Tuberculosis	Carcinoma	

Trachea		Tracheitis
		Tuberculosis
		Influenza
		Measles
			Adenoma or
			  carcinoma or
			  polyps	

Bronchi		Whooping cough
		Acute or chronic
		  bronchitis,
		Sinusitis
			Bronchogenic
			  carcinoma or
			  adenoma
				Bronchiectasis

Alveoli	Pulmonary embolism	Pneumonia
		Tuberculosis
		Parasites
		Fungi
			Metastatic carcinoma
			  or oat cell carci-
			  noma
				Emphysema bullae
				Pulmonary fibrosis

Pleura	Pulmonary embolism
	  or congestive heart
	  failure
		Tuberculosis or
		  other empyema
			Mesenthelioma	

Mediastinum	Aortic aneurysm	Mediastinitis	Hodgkin's disease Metastatic carcinoma	

Heart	Congestive heart
	  failure
		Syphilitic
		  aneurysm
		Acute pericarditis
				Dissecting aneurysm

I Intoxication	C Congenital	A Autoimmune Allergic	T Trauma	E Endocrine
Agranulocytosis with pharyngitis		Angioneurotic edema		
	Diverticulum Tracheoesophageal fistula		Traumatic rupture or fistula	
			Laryngitis from overuse	
Chlorine or smoke				
Gas, smoking, paint	Bronchiectasis Cystic fibrosis	Asthmatic bronchitis	Foreign body	
Pneumoconiosis Lipoid pneumonia	Reticuloendotheliosis Congenital cyst	Lupus Wegener's granulomatosis	Pneumothorax Contusion or hemorrhage or laceration	
			Rib fracture	
	Dermoid cyst		Stab wound Gunshot	Substernal thyroid
	Aortic ring Patent drugs	Mitral stenosis with large atrium		

tine cultures, tuberculosis, fungi, and Papanicolaou smears and chest roentgenograms, bronchoscopy and bronchography are normal. Hysterical cough should be considered, however, as well as reflux esophagitis and hiatal hernia. A sputum and nasal smear for eosinophils should be done to rule out asthma. A trial of therapy may be indicated. Other tests for the workup of cough are listed in Appendix I.

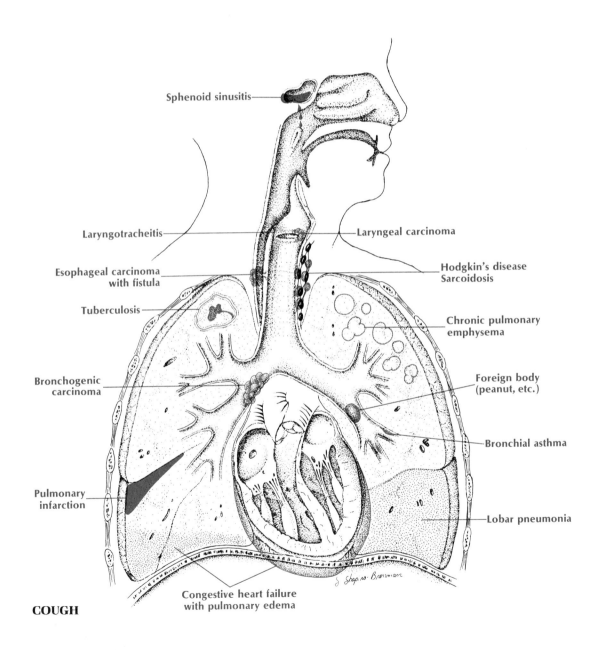

Sphenoid sinusitis

Laryngotracheitis

Laryngeal carcinoma

Esophageal carcinoma with fistula

Hodgkin's disease
Sarcoidosis

Tuberculosis

Chronic pulmonary emphysema

Bronchogenic carcinoma

Foreign body (peanut, etc.)

Bronchial asthma

Pulmonary infarction

Lobar pneumonia

Congestive heart failure with pulmonary edema

COUGH

DECREASED RESPIRATIONS, APNEA, AND CHEYNE–STOKES BREATHING ◼

Nurses frequently become distressed and summon the intern during the night about these signs. Cheyne–Stokes respirations are a frequent source of bewilderment because they may occur at times with no direct evidence of damage to the nervous system. It would be interesting to discuss the physiology of respiration at length in this section, but it will be of little help in the differential diagnosis of apnea and in slow or Cheyne–Stokes respirations except in a few instances. In all cases these are a result of an insult to the respiratory centers in the brain by some etiological agent. The causes of these signs can best be remembered by the mnemonic **VINDICATE.**

V—Vascular includes cerebral thrombosis, embolism, and especially hemorrhage of the brain stem, which may cause depressed respirations or periodic apnea. Diffuse cerebral arteriosclerosis is another cause in this category.

I—Inflammatory disorders signify encephalitis, poliomyelitis, meningitis, and brain abscesses, particularly with increased intracranial pressure.

N—Neoplasms of the brain stem (primary or metastatic) and neoplasms of the cerebrum are associated with increased intracranial pressure and may cause depression of respirations and Cheyne–Stokes breathing.

D—Degenerative diseases of the brain, including senile and presenile dementia and Schilder's disease, may cause these signs in the terminal stages.

I—Intoxication is an important category of etiologies of depressed or irregular respirations because the toxic substance may not be obvious at first. Failure of any organ system to function may lead to respiratory depression. When there is respiratory failure from emphysema or other causes, carbon dioxide builds up in the blood and CO_2 narcosis develops. In this state the important stimulus of high blood CO_2 on the respiratory centers is gradually lost and anoxia is the only stimulus left. Periodic or Cheyne–Stokes breathing frequently develops in the following manner: During respiration the blood oxygen builds up to a level at which the respiratory stimulus to anoxia is lost. Respirations cease. During apnea the blood oxygen falls to a point where there is sufficient anoxia to kick the respiratory center over again. The electrolyte disturbances and build up of toxins in uremia, the high blood ammonia and other toxins that result from hepatic failure, and the anoxia of congestive heart failure may all lead to apnea or depressed respirations.

Exogenous toxins are more commonly the cause in young people. Alcoholism, morphine, barbiturates, and a host of tranquilizers will cause respiratory depression in sufficient quantities.

C—Congenital disorders that cause these respiratory disturbances include Tay–Sachs disease, cerebral palsy, glycogen storage disease, reticuloendothelioses, epilepsy, and cerebral aneurysms with subarachnoid hemorrhage.

A—Autoimmune disorders such as lupus erythematosus and multiple sclerosis must be considered in this category.

T—Trauma is another frequent cause of apnea or Cheyne–Stokes respiration. Cerebral concussion, subdural, epidural, and intracerebral hematomas all may cause depressed respirations, especially when associated with increased intracranial pressure.

E—Endocrine disease reminds the reader that whereas diabetic coma may begin with Kussmaul's breathing, in the advanced

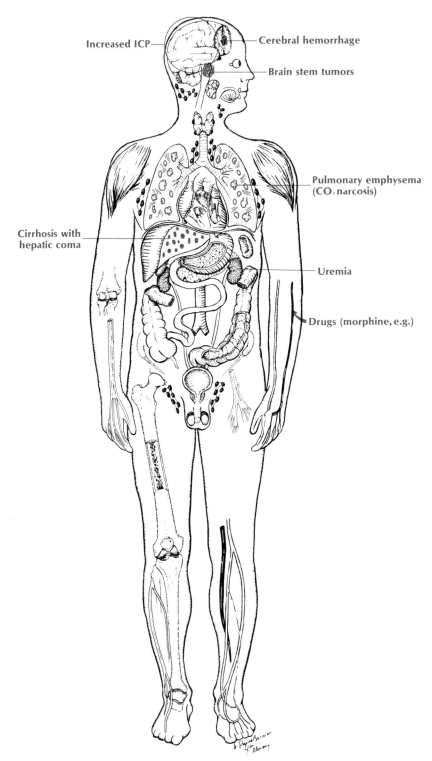

Increased ICP

Cerebral hemorrhage

Brain stem tumors

Pulmonary emphysema
(CO₂ narcosis)

Cirrhosis with
hepatic coma

Uremia

Drugs (morphine, e.g.)

**DECREASED RESPIRATIONS, APNEA,
AND CHEYNE-STOKES BREATHING**

stages bradypnea and Cheyne–Stokes respirations develop from the severe acidosis. Pituitary and suprasellar tumors may grow sufficiently to compress the brain stem and cause apnea.

Approach to the Diagnosis

Obviously, the association of other signs and symptoms will determine the workup in most cases. The most important things to do are to order a BUN, electrolytes, FBS, and arterial blood gases, a drug screen, and to check for increased intracranial pressure by examining the eye grounds. If the history or physical findings suggest increased intracranial pressure, and other metabolic studies (*e.g.*, BUN) are normal, a Mannitol or urea drip is begun while awaiting the results of other investigations such as CT scans, EEG, and echoencephalography. A neurosurgeon should be consulted without delay.

DELUSIONS ▪

A delusion is a persistent false belief. The feeling that one is being followed or watched, that one has a bad odor even after frequent and careful bathing, that one is superior to others—all are examples of delusions. Although most patients presenting with a delusion have a functional disorder, the astute clinician knows the organic disorders of the brain that may be associated with a delusion. The mnemonic **VINDICATE** forms a simple method for ready recall of these disorders.

V—Vascular disorders suggest cerebral arteriosclerosis with lacunar infarcts or cerebral emboli.

I—Inflammatory disorders suggest cerebral abscess, tuberculomas, viral encephalitis (*e.g.*, herpes simplex), and general paresis.

N—Neoplasms, both primary and metastatic, should always be considered, as these are potentially treatable.

D—Degenerative diseases include senile and presenile dementia. Huntington's chorea, diffuse sclerosis, and many other conditions.

I—Intoxication brings to mind alcoholism, bromism, chronic use of both uppers and downers, LSD, and cannabis. Uremia, CO_2 narcosis, chronic anoxia, electrolyte disorders, and early hepatic coma should also be considered.

C—Congenital diseases suggest Schilder's disease, mongolism, Wilson's disease, and many other conditions associated with mental retardation.

A—Autoimmune diseases focus on lupus erythematosus, allergic angiitis, and multiple sclerosis.

T—Trauma facilitates the recall of concussion and chronic subdural hematomas.

E—Endocrine disorders include suprasellar tumors that invade the hypothalamus, acromegaly, hypopituitarism, hyperthyroidism, Cushing's syndrome, and adrenal insufficiency. Parathyroid dysfunction can also cause delusions.

Approach to the Diagnosis

The important thing to do before referring these patients to a psychiatrist is to perform an evaluation of the mental status and a neurological examination. Memory for recent events, orientation in time and place, ability to perform serial seven's, and interpretation of proverbial phrases should all be tested for. Psychological testing may be warranted in borderline cases as well as an EEG, CT scan, skull roentgenogram, and spinal tap. A drug screen may also be indicated. Additional tests are listed in Appendix I.

(Text continues on p. 272)

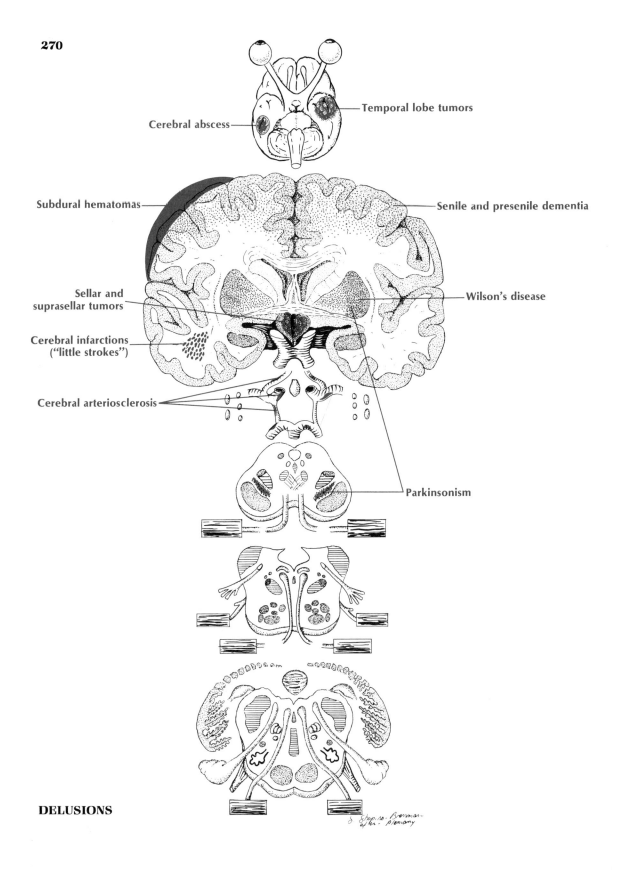

Temporal lobe tumors

Cerebral abscess

Subdural hematomas

Senile and presenile dementia

Sellar and
suprasellar tumors

Wilson's disease

Cerebral infarctions
("little strokes")

Cerebral arteriosclerosis

Parkinsonism

DELUSIONS

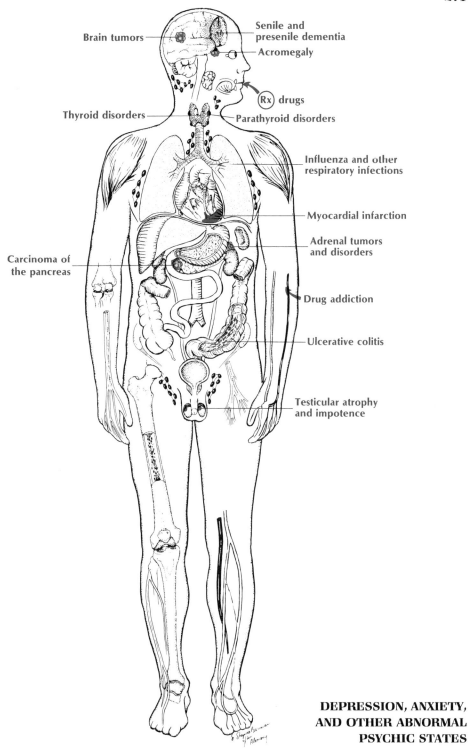

Brain tumors

Senile and
presenile dementia

Acromegaly

(Rx) drugs

Thyroid disorders

Parathyroid disorders

Influenza and other
respiratory infections

Myocardial infarction

Adrenal tumors
and disorders

Carcinoma of
the pancreas

Drug addiction

Ulcerative colitis

Testicular atrophy
and impotence

**DEPRESSION, ANXIETY,
AND OTHER ABNORMAL
PSYCHIC STATES**

DEPRESSION, ANXIETY, AND OTHER ABNORMAL PSYCHIC STATES ■

It is simple enough to administer a sedative and refer the emotionally distressed patient to a psychiatrist, but the astute diagnostician will want to rule out an organic disease first. Almost every endocrine disease is associated with emotional disturbances, all of which are potentially curable. In addition, electrolyte and other metabolic disturbances, chronic anoxia, or failure of any organ system may lead to anxiety, depression or a psychotic state. The mnemonic **VINDICATE** will help to recall this important group of disorders.

V—Vascular diseases include myocardial infarction, congestive heart failure, cerebral arteriosclerosis, and thrombosis.

I—Inflammatory diseases recall syphilis, encephalitis, tuberculosis, brain abscess, influenza, pneumonia, and any prolonged infectious state, particularly that of the hospitalized patient with tubes in every orifice.

N—Neoplasms include cerebral tumors, tumors of the endocrine glands, and any neoplasm which is metastatic or which affects the metabolism of the body by a hormone or enzyme which it secretes. Pancreatic carcinoma is frequently associated with depression.

D—Degenerative diseases and **deficiency** diseases suggest presenile and senile dementia, pellagra, Wilson's disease, and atrophy of the various endocrine glands.

I—Intoxication suggests lead poisoning, alcoholism, bromism, hypercalcemia, hypocalcemia, manganese toxicity, hypokalemia, hypovolemia, uremia, anoxia from pulmonary disease, anemias and heart diseases, and corticosteroid therapy, as well as many other drugs. Porphyria may cause depression or a psychotic state.

C—Congenital suggests the depression associated with many congenital neurological diseases: epilepsy, muscular dystrophy, Friedreich's ataxia, myotonic dystrophy, and the depression associated with congenital heart disease and congenital defects of many organ systems.

A—Autoimmune diseases include multiple sclerosis and lupus erythematosus.

T—Traumatic disorders include the now well-recognized post-traumatic neurosis or depression, neurocirculatory asthenia, and postconcussion syndrome. Compensation neurosis should be mentioned here.

E—Endocrine diseases include hypopituitarism, acromegaly, hypothyroidism, apathetic hyperthyroidism, hypoparathyroidism, hyperparathyroidism, diabetes mellitus, insulomas, hypogonadism, menopause, Cushing's syndrome, and adrenal insufficiency.

Approach to the Diagnosis

The association of other symptoms and signs is all important. A T3–T4 and free thyroxine index (T7), a urine for porphobilinogen, serum electrolytes, bromide, lead level, 24-hour urine, 17-ketosteroids, and 17-hydroxycorticoids should be done on anyone suspected of endogenous depression. (Possibly all depressed patients should get this screen.) Skull x-ray film, EEG, CT scan and even a spinal tap (to rule out MS and lues) may be worthwhile when other neurological signs are present.

DIARRHEA ■

The differential diagnosis of diarrhea may be approached from either an anatomic or a physiological basis. The **anatomical** approach is used in Table 5-5. In the **stomach** and **duodenum** pernicious anemia and

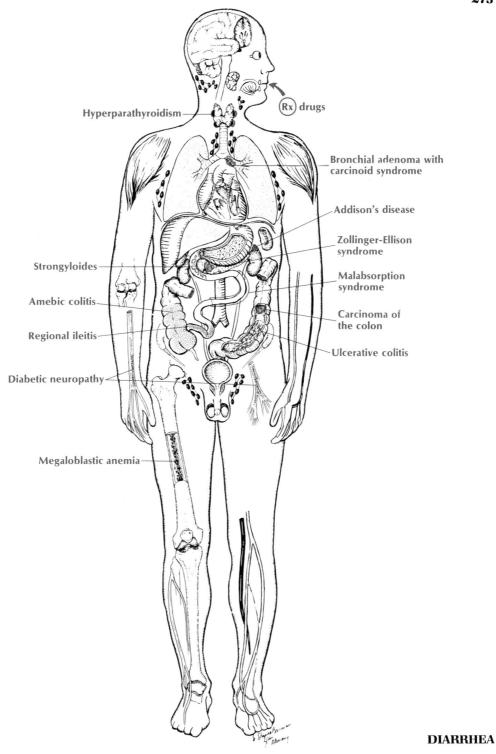

Hyperparathyroidism

Rx) drugs

Bronchial adenoma with carcinoid syndrome

Addison's disease

Zollinger-Ellison syndrome

Malabsorption syndrome

Strongyloides

Amebic colitis

Carcinoma of the colon

Regional ileitis

Ulcerative colitis

Diabetic neuropathy

Megaloblastic anemia

DIARRHEA

Zollinger–Ellison syndrome are prominent causes. A carcinoma may form a fistula with the transverse colon and cause diarrhea. Viral gastroenteritis, and *Giardia* may also be prominent causes.

Liver and biliary tract diseases of all types may cause diarrhea (steatorrhea) by decreasing the secretion of bile. Ampullary carcinoma and cirrhosis are illustrated here, but one should not forget the diarrhea of chronic cholecystitis. The **pancreas** is the source of important digestive enzymes; as a result chronic pancreatitis and pancreatic carcinomas may

be associated with diarrhea (steatorrhea) in adults, whereas cystic fibrosis should be considered in children. The pancreatic islet cell tumors may secrete gastrin or vasoactive intestinal peptide, causing diarrhea.

Most of the lesions causing diarrhea are in the **small intestine.** Thus, cholera, salmonella, staphylococcus, typhoid, and tuberculosis attack here. The carcinoid syndrome, various polyps, (especially Peutz–Jeghers), and regional ileitis are also important causes. Toxins and drugs (Table 5-5) are common causes acting here, as are pellagra and other

TABLE 5-5. DIARRHEA—ANATOMICAL CLASSIFICATION

	V Vascular	I Inflammatory	N Neoplasm	D Degenerative and Deficiency
Stomach and Duodenum		Viral gastroenteritis Parasites	Carcinoma with fistula into intestines	Pernicious anemia Iron deficiency
Liver and Biliary Tract		Chronic cholecystitis and lithiasis	Neoplasms obstructing bile ducts	Cirrhosis
Pancreas		Chronic pancreatitis	Pancreatic carcinoma Islet cell adenoma	
Small Intestine	Mesenteric artery insufficiency	Cholera Botulism Staphylococcus Salmonella *E. coli* Parasites Tuberculosis	Carcinoid Polyps Sarcomas Lymphoma	Pellagra Pyridoxine deficiency
Large Intestine	Mesenteric artery insufficiency	Shigella Amebiasis Other parasites	Polyps Carcinomas and other neoplasms	

vitamin deficiencies, as well as food allergies. Systemic autoimmune diseases such as scleroderma and Whipple's disease are also important. Mesentery artery insufficiency or obstruction should be considered both here and in the colon.

A wide variety of etiological agents cause diarrhea by their action on the **colon.**

V—Vascular diseases include ischemic colitis.

I—Infectious agents such as bacillary dysentery (shigella), *E. coli,* camphylobacter, yersinia, and amebiasis may ulcerate or inflame the colon.

N—Neoplasms such as carcinomas and polyps cause chronic irritation and exudates from the colon with hypermotility and diarrhea.

D—Degenerative lesions of the muscularis that cause diverticulosis and allow overgrowth of bacteria and chronic inflammation may lead to diarrhea, but this may be classified under the idiopathic category as well.

I—Intoxicating substances, osmotic cathar-

I Intoxication and Idiopathic	C Congenital	A Autoimmune Allergic	T Trauma	E Endocrine
Uremia Antacids			Surgery (*e.g.* blind loop)	Zollinger–Ellison syndrome
Cirrhosis				
Radiation	Cystic fibrosis			Pancreatic cholera
Sprue Cathartics Mercurials Reserpine Antibiotics Alcohol Other drugs	Peutz–Jehger's diverticuli (Meckel's)	Regional ileitis Whipple's disease Scleroderma	Fistulas	Hypoparathyroidism Hyperthyroidism Addison's disease
Mucus colitis Diverticulosis Antibiotics Hypervitaminosis Uremia	Familial polyposis	Ulcerative colitis Granulomatous colitis Food allergy		

tics, and antibiotics (by allowing overgrowth of bacteria and fungi) may involve the colon (*e.g.,* pseudomembranous colitis). Mucous colitis or irritable bowel syndrome may best be classified as idiopathic.

C—Congenital lesions of the colon include the solitary diverticulum of the cecum, malrotation (more frequently associated with intestinal obstruction), and familial polyposis.

TABLE 5-6.   DIARRHEA—PHYSIOLOGICAL CLASSIFICATION

	Hyposecretion	Hypersecretion	Hypomobility	Hypermobility	Primary Malabsorption	Exudative
Gastric	Pernicious anemia Iron deficiency Gastric resection	Zollinger–Ellison syndrome		Dumping syndrome		
Duodenal	Lactase deficiency Sucrase deficiency		Blind loop syndrome	Secretion induced		
Biliary	Liver disease Obstructive jaundice			Cholecystokinin induced	Cholecystokinin induced Regional ileitis	
Pancreatic	Cystic fibrosis Chronic pancreatitis	"Pancreatic cholera" (islet cell adenoma with vasoactive intestinal peptide)		Gastrin Vasoactive intestinal peptide		
Small Intestine		Cholera (*e.g., E. coli*)	Diabetic diarrhea Drugs	Coffee Serotonin induced Cathartics Parasympatho-mimetics	Celiac sprue Tropical sprue Whipple's disease Intestinal lymphoma Extensive resection	Regional ileitis Salmonellosis
Large Intestine		Protein-losing enteropathy (*e.g.,* villous adenoma)				Shigella Ulcerative colitis Amebiasis

A—Autoimmune disease of the colon is common and includes both ulcerative colitis and granulomatous colitis.

T—Trauma is not a common cause of diarrhea anywhere in the intestinal tract, but certainly surgically induced fistulas may occur in the colon or anywhere else.

E—Endocrine disorders do not usually affect the colon directly.

Having considered the local causes of diarrhea, do not forget reflex diarrhea from diseases of other organs, such as pyelonephritis, salpingo-oophoritis, and central nervous system diseases.

Using Table 5-6 the reader can develop the differential diagnosis of diarrhea with **physiology.** Diarrhea may result from **increased intake** of fluids or bulk foods; **hyposecretion** of enzymes necessary for digestion of food; **hypersecretion** of gastrointestinal fluids and enzymes; **malabsorption** of various substances, particularly protein and fat; **exudations** of pus induced by granulomatous or ulcerative colitis and salmonella or shigella infections; **hypermobility** from stimulation by cathartics, various hormones (*e.g.,* vasoactive intestinal peptides and gastrin), and **hypomobility** from autonomic dysfunction as occurs in diabetic neuropathy.

Approach to the Diagnosis

Whichever method is applied (anatomical or physiological) most causes of diarrhea can be recalled before interviewing the patient. Then one can proceed to ask the right questions to eliminate each suspected cause. Combinations of symptoms and signs will assist greatly in narrowing the differential diagnosis. For example, chronic diarrhea and copious mucous without blood suggests irritable bowel syndrome. Chronic diarrhea with mucous and blood suggests ulcerative colitis.

Physical examination is often unrewarding but it may disclose a hepatic, rectal, or pelvic source for the diarrhea; it may also indicate that the diarrhea is a sign of a systemic disease (*e.g.,* scleroderma or hyperthyroidism). Rectal examination may reveal a fecal impaction. A warm stool examination for pus, pH (acid stool suggests lactase deficiency), fat and meat fibers, blood, ova, and parasites is most essential. A stool culture is done. Proctoscopy (immediately if there is blood) followed by colonoscopy, barium enema, and upper GI series is usually necessary in all cases. Appendix I gives additional tests to be ordered in the elusive case.

DIFFICULTY SWALLOWING (DYSPHAGIA)

Swallowing is the function of the pharynx, larynx and esophagus. This function may be impaired by two mechanisms: mechanical obstruction (*e.g.,* carcinoma of the esophagus) and physiological obstruction (*e.g.,* pseudobulbar palsy).

Mechanical obstruction may result from intrinsic disease of the pharynx, larynx, and esophagus or extrinsic disease of the organs around the esophagus.

The mnemonic **VINDICATE** is useful in recalling the causes of mechanical obstruction as follows:

V—Vascular indicates aortic aneurysms and cardiomegaly.

I—Inflammatory should suggest pharyngitis, tonsillitis, esophagitis, and mediastinitis.

N—Neoplasm should bring to mind esophageal and bronchogenic carcinoma, and dermoid cysts of the mediastinum.

D—Degenerative and **deficiency** disease should suggest Plummer–Vinson syndrome of iron deficiency anemia.

I—Intoxication immediately indicates lye strictures.

C—Congenital and acquired anomalies should suggest esophageal atresia and diverticuli.

A—Autoimmune disease suggests scleroderma.

T—Trauma would prompt the recall of ruptured esophagus, pulsion diverticulum, and foreign bodies that obstruct or injure the wall of the esophagus.

E—Endocrine disorders suggest the enlarged thyroid of endemic goiter and Graves' disease.

Physiological obstruction results from neuromuscular disorders at the end organ, myoneural junction, lower and upper motor neurons.

1. **End organ.** This should suggest myotonic dystrophy, dermatomyositis, achalasia, and diffuse esophageal spasm.
2. **Myoneural junction.** This brings to mind myasthenia gravis.
3. **Lower motor neuron.** In this category one would recall poliomyelitis, diphtheritic polyneuritis, and brain stem tumors or infarcts.
4. **Upper motor neuron.** This structure prompts the recall of pseudobulbar palsy from cerebral thrombosis, embolism, or hemorrhage, multiple sclerosis, presenile dementia, and diffuse cerebral arteriosclerosis. It should also bring to mind Parkinson's disease and other extrapyramidal disorders.

Approach to the Diagnosis

The age of onset is significant since carcinoma of the esophagus is rare before age 50, whereas achalasia and reflux esophagitis are more common in young and middle-aged adults. The onset is gradual in carcinoma and aortic aneurysms but more acute in reflux esophagitis and foreign bodies. Patients with achalasia have trouble swallowing both food and water, but those with carcinoma suffer the most, and often the only difficulty is swallowing food.

Association of other symptoms and signs is important. Neurological findings will focus on the diagnosis of bulbar and pseudobulbar palsy whereas hematemesis and heartburn will suggest esophageal carcinoma or reflux esophagitis.

The barium swallow is still the most useful initial study to order. However, esophagoscopy and biopsy will lead to a definitive diagnosis in most cases of mechanical obstruction. If esophagoscopy is negative one may resort to a Mecholyl test to diagnose achalasia, a Tensilon test to exclude myasthenia gravis, and esophageal manometry to diagnose reflux esophagitis, scleroderma, and diffuse esophageal spasm. Additional useful tests for the workup are listed in Appendix I.

DILATED PUPILS (MYDRIASIS) ■

Like that of myosis, the differential diagnosis of dilated pupils or mydriasis can best be developed by applying **neuroanatomy** (Table 5-7). "Knowing where the lesion is, tells us what the lesion is." One simply follows the nerve pathway from the end organ up the third nerve to the termination in the brain stem. A dilated pupil, however, may also signify a lesion of the optic nerve and its pathways.

1. Lesions of the third nerve and pathways:
   A. End organ. Lesions of the eye that cause dilated pupils include glaucoma,

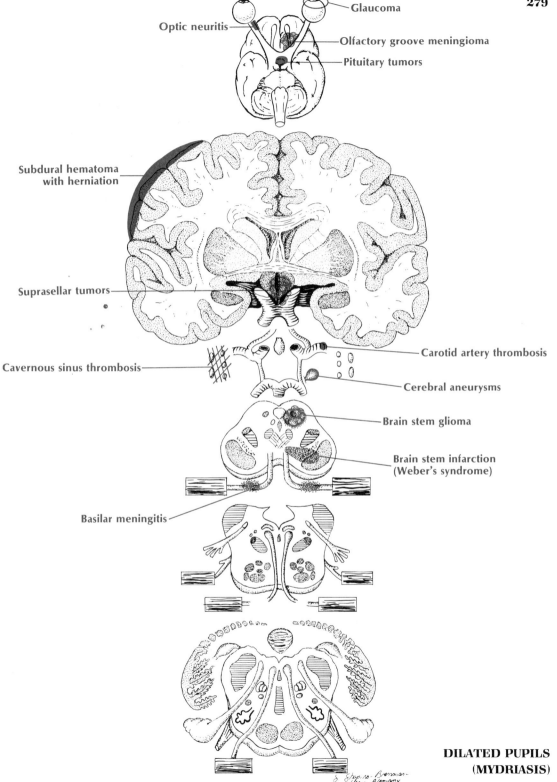

Glaucoma

Optic neuritis

Olfactory groove meningioma

Pituitary tumors

Subdural hematoma
with herniation

Suprasellar tumors

Carotid artery thrombosis

Cavernous sinus thrombosis

Cerebral aneurysms

Brain stem glioma

Brain stem infarction
(Weber's syndrome)

Basilar meningitis

**DILATED PUPILS
(MYDRIASIS)**

high myopia, anticholinergic drugs (*e.g.*, atropine), and sympathomimetric drugs (such as neosynephrine).

B. Peripheral portion of the oculomotor nerve. Important lesions here include aneurysms of the internal carotid artery and its branches, herniation of the brain in brain tumors, subdural hematomas and other space-occupying lesions, cavernous sinus thrombosis, sellar and suprasellar tumors, tuberculosis and syphilitic meningitis, and sphenoid ridge meningiomas. Diabetic neuropathy of

the third cranial nerve does not usually cause mydriasis. Most of these lesions are associated with ptosis and paralysis of the other extraocular muscles supplied by the third nerve.

C. Brain stem. Lesions here include multiple sclerosis, syphilis, encephalitis, Wernicke's encephalopathy, brain stem gliomas, and Weber's syndrome. Barbiturates and other drugs may cause dilated pupils by their central nervous system effects.

2. Optic nerve and pathways.

TABLE 5-7. DILATED PUPILS (MYDRIASIS)

	V Vascular	I Inflammatory	N Neoplasm	D Degenerative and Deficiency
3rd Nerve				
End Organ		Orbital cellulitis		
Peripheral portion of the oculomotor nerve	Aneurysm Sinus thrombosis	Tuberculosis Syphilis Cerebral abscess	Pituitary and brain tumors	
Brain stem	Weber's syndrome	Syphilis Encephalitis	Brain stem gliomas	Wernicke's encepha- lopathy
Optic Nerve				
End organ	Occlusion of oph- thalmic artery Occlusion of in- ternal carotid	Keratitis Retinitis	Retinoblastoma	Cataracts Retinitis pigmentosa
Peripheral portion	Cerebral aneurysm	Optic neuritis Basilar arachnoiditis	Pituitary and brain tumors Optic nerve glio- mas	Weber's optic atro- phy
Brain stem	Aneurysm Sinus thrombosis	Tuberculosis Syphilis	Pituitary and brain tumors	

A. End organ. Keratitis, cataracts, retinitis, and occlusion of the opthalmic artery are included here.

B. Peripheral portion of the optic nerve. Aneurysms, optic neuritis, sellar and suprasellar tumors, optic nerve gliomas, primary optic atrophy from lues and other conditions, orbital fractures, exophthalmos, and cavernous sinus thrombosis are recalled in this category.

C. Brain stem. The lesions involving the optic tract here are similar to those that involve the oculomotor nerve discussed above. The optic cortex (calcerine fissure) lesions may cause blindness, but there is no mydriasis.

Approach to the Diagnosis

The association of other signs and symptoms will pinpoint many causes in the differential. Laboratory tests useful in narrowing the diagnosis further are listed in Appendix I.

I Intoxication	C Congenital	A Allergic and Autoimmune	T Trauma	E Endocrine
Anticholinergic drug Neosynephrine	Glaucoma Myopia		Trauma to the globe Hematomas Orbital fracture	Pheochromocytoma Pituitary tumors (advanced)
Barbiturate		Multiple sclerosis		
	Cataracts	Temporal arteritis		Cataracts
Methyl alcohol Tobacco		Multiple sclerosis	Orbital fracture	Exophthalmos
		Multiple sclerosis	Hematomas	Cranial concussions

DIZZINESS

Dizziness may mean true vertigo, which is a hallucination of movement of the patient or his environment, or light-headedness, which is a feeling that one is going to faint (and sometimes does). The causes of light-headedness are developed under Syncope, page 382.

The diagnostic approach to dizziness or true vertigo uses **anatomy,** on page 208, beginning with the external ear and working inwards towards the middle ear, labyrinth, auditory artery and nerve, and vesticular nuclei in the brain stem. Impacted wax or other foreign bodies in the **external ear** may cause

vertigo. Otitis media, especially when it invades the mastoid or petrous bone, is the most important cause of vertigo in the middle ear. One should not forget serous otitis media from allergies or upper respiratory infections (URI). If the **drum** is perforated, however, or if there is a perforation into the perilymph system, vertigo will occur, especially when water enters the ear.

The **inner ear** is the site of two important causes of vertigo, acute labyrinthitis and Meniere's disease. Acute labyrinthitis is more often toxic than infectious (viral) in nature. Drugs such as streptomycin and gentomycin are common causes, but aspirin and quinidine should be considered with a host of

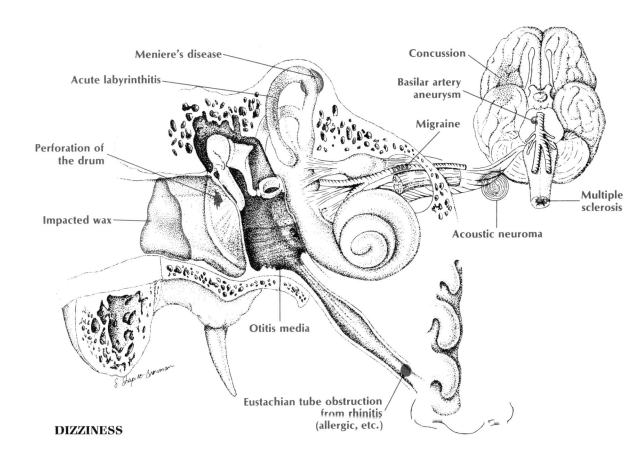

Meniere's disease
Acute labyrinthitis
Perforation of the drum
Impacted wax
Otitis media
Concussion
Basilar artery aneurysm
Migraine
Acoustic neuroma
Multiple sclerosis
Eustachian tube obstruction from rhinitis (allergic, etc.)

DIZZINESS

other drugs. This can be determined by a good history without looking up the long list of drugs. Perhaps more common and more important from a legal standpoint is traumatic labyrinthitis from head injuries. The cause of Meniere's disease is not known, but swelling of the endolymphatic ducts is probably the major pathophysiological mechanism. If the **internal auditory artery** is obstructed by spasm, as occurs in migraine, basilar artery insufficiency, or thrombosis, vertigo will result. Rarely, an aneurysm of this artery or the basilar artery at its branching may compress or hemorrhage into the vestibular nerve and cause vertigo.

Additional neurological causes of vertigo are acoustic neuromas and other brain stem tumors, petrositis, and vestibular neuronitis, which may involve the vestibular nerve or nucleus. Finally, central vertigo may result from multiple sclerosis, concussion, epilepsy, and cerebral tumors.

Approach to the Diagnosis

Clinically, the approach to the patient with vertigo is as follows:

1. Make sure it is true vertigo and not light-headedness, ataxia, or diplopia.
2. Get a list of diagnostic possibilities fixed in mind.
3. Eliminate possibilities by the presence or absence of combinations of other symptoms and signs established by the history and physical. For example, vertigo with tinnitus, deafness, and fullness in the ear points to Meniere's disease, especially when there have been previous episodes. Vertigo with a history of head injury suggests traumatic labyrinthitis or postconcussion syndrome. Vertigo with focal neurological signs suggests a brain-stem lesion (MS, vascular occlusion, or tumor).
4. Laboratory, roentgenogram, and special

diagnostic procedures (Appendix I) provide additional means of establishing the diagnosis and are necessary in most cases.

DOUBLE VISION ■

Most physicians know that double vision is a neurological condition and may refer these cases immediately to a neurologist: but what about the cases of double vision with one eye closed? Surprisingly enough, this condition really does exist. Monocular diplopia results from dislocation of the lens (*e.g.*, from injury and Marfan's syndrome), from the incipient stage of cataracts, corneal opacities, double pupils (from surgery or trauma), or from hysteria. Fortunately for us but unfortunately for the patient, double vision is usually binocular and due to paralysis of the extraocular muscles. The causes can be recalled best by anatomically grouping them into those that involve the muscles themselves, those that involve the myoneural junction, those that involve the peripheral portion of the cranial nerve, and those that involve the nucleus of the cranial nerve in the brain stem and supranuclear causes.

1. **Extraocular muscle.** Using the mnemonic **MINT** the following differential can be developed:

    M—Malformations such as myotonic dystrophy and congenital opthalmoplegia belong here.

    I—Inflammatory conditions such as dermatomyositis and orbital cellulitis are considered here.

    N—Neoplasms of the orbit and exophthalmic goiter are classified here.

    T—Trauma suggests orbital fractures and contusions or lacerations of the muscles.

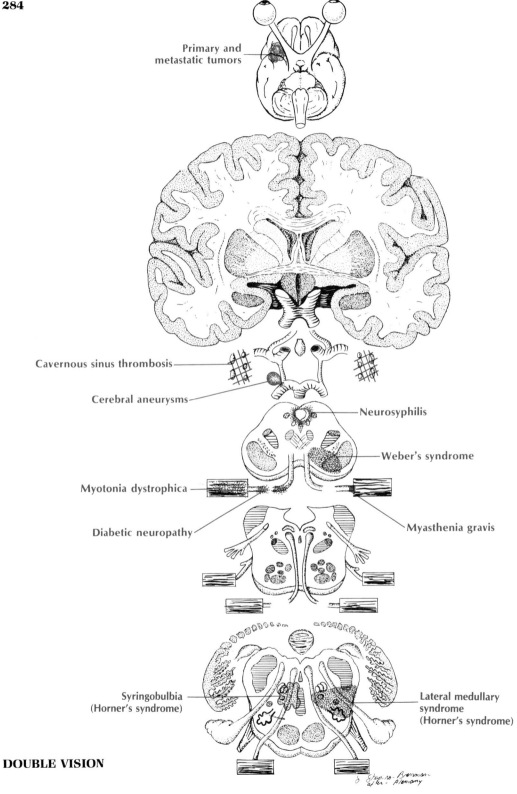

Primary and
metastatic tumors

Cavernous sinus thrombosis

Cerebral aneurysms

Neurosyphilis

Weber's syndrome

Myotonia dystrophica

Diabetic neuropathy

Myasthenia gravis

Syringobulbia
(Horner's syndrome)

Lateral medullary
syndrome
(Horner's syndrome)

DOUBLE VISION

2. **Myoneural junction.** This suggests the important condition myasthenia gravis.
3. **Peripheral portion of the cranial nerve.** Recall of these conditions is assisted by the mnemonic **VINCE.**

 V—Venous sinus thrombosis (cavernous sinus in this case) is suggested.

 I—Inflammatory conditions remind one of syphilis and tuberculous meningitis, postdiphtheritic neuritis, sphenoid sinusitis, and petrositis, as well as increased intracranial pressure.

 N—Neoplasms suggest pituitary tumors, suprasellar tumors, nasopharyngeal carcinomas, chordomas, and sphenoid ridge meningiomas.

 C—Congenital lesions suggest aneurysms.

 E—Endocrine disorders suggest diabetic neuropathy, a common cause of sudden extraocular muscle palsy.
4. **Brain stem.** Recall of these conditions is best undertaken with the mnemonic **VINDICATE.**

 V—Vascular lesions include basilar artery thrombosis, hemorrhages, emboli, and aneurysms. Migraine perhaps belongs here too.

 I—Inflammatory lesions include syphilis, tuberculosis, and viral encephalitis.

 N—Neoplasms include brain stem gliomas, metastatic carcinomas, and Hodgkin's disease.

 D—Deficiency diseases suggest Wernicke's encephalopathy.

 I—Intoxication suggests botulism, bromide, and iodide poisoning.

 C—Congenital conditions suggest hydrocephalus and Arnold–Chiari malformation.

 A—Autoimmune disease suggests multiple sclerosis, postinfectious encephalitis, and lupus.

 T—Traumatic condition suggests subdural hematomas, and basilar skull fractures and pontine hematomas.

 E—Endocrine reminds one of the increased incidence of basilar artery thrombosis in diabetes.
5. **Supranuclear causes (including cortical).** These recall a pineal tumor, the conjugate palsy of cerebral thrombosis or hemorrhage, the conjugate gaze in focal cortical epilepsy, and the dilated pupil in early herniation through the tentorium.

Approach to the Diagnosis

This is similar to that for all neurological disorders. It depends on the association of other signs. Isolated palsies of the third or sixth nerve without pupillary changes suggest diabetic neuropathy, so a glucose tolerance test would be done. As isolated palsy of the third nerve with pupillary changes (mydriasis) suggests an aneurysm and angiography is indicated. Roentgenograms of the skull and orbits, a spinal tap, and CT scans would all be useful under certain circumstances, but a neurologist is in a better position to determine this. A cavernous sinus thrombosis is possible if the patient is febrile and has more than one cranial nerve palsy along with loss of the corneal reflex, chemosis and ecchymosis, and distended retinal veins. Treatment should be started immediately.

DWARFISM

A list of possible causes of dwarfism may be developed anatomically or physiologically and biochemically. Visualizing the many organs of the body is an excellent way to recall the causes. Beginning with the **pituitary** one thinks of hypopituitarism and Lawrence–Moon–Biedl syndrome. The **thyroid** suggests cretinism. The **heart** suggests the many congenital anomalies there (*e.g.,* tetralogy of Fal-

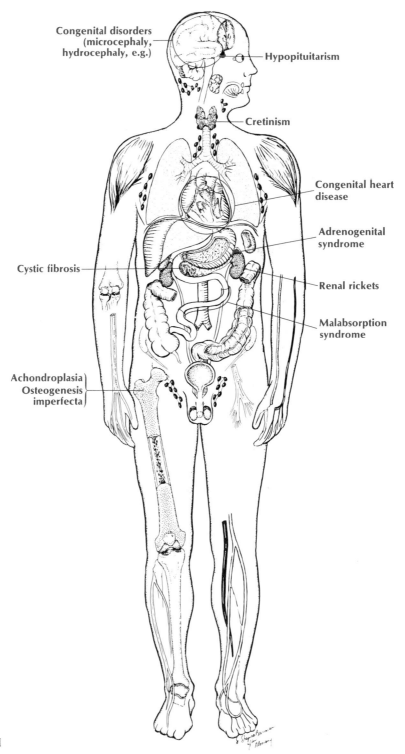

Congenital disorders
(microcephaly,
hydrocephaly, e.g.)

Hypopituitarism

Cretinism

Congenital heart
disease

Adrenogenital
syndrome

Cystic fibrosis

Renal rickets

Malabsorption
syndrome

Achondroplasia
Osteogenesis
imperfecta

DWARFISM

lot) that are associated with dwarfism. The **gastrointestinal tract** suggests the malabsorption syndrome and its many causes. The **pancreas** suggests cystic fibrosis. The **kidney** suggests chronic nephritis with renal rickets. The **bone** suggests rickets and achondroplasia. The **brain** suggests microcephaly and all the other causes of mental retardation (such as mongolism) that are associated with stunted growth. The **ovary** suggests Turner's syndrome. (This method will not help recall the primordial dwarf and some of the other genetic dwarfs but it is a good start.)

Applying physiology and biochemistry, one must consider the intake of food and oxygen, its absorption and transport, and its uptake by the cells and excretion of waste products. For the regulations and promotion of this metabolic process, adequate vitamins and hormones are essential. With these processes in mind, one can recall the diseases that interfere with each.

Intake. Starvation and malnutrition cause dwarfism and various vitamin deficiency states, rickets being the most significant.

Absorption. Malabsorption syndromes may create dwarfism by preventing food and vitamins from getting into the body.

Transport. Congenital anomalies of the heart prevent distribution of oxygen and glucose to the cells.

Cell uptake. Impaired cell uptake of glucose in diabetes may cause a short stature; the bulging of the cells with glycogen in glycogen storage disease may do the same. Galactosemia is a possible cause. Reticuloendotheliosis and gargoylism may be recalled under this heading.

Excretion of waste products. This heading should help recall renal rickets.

Regulation. This heading helps recall the hormonal deficiency states: cretinism-deficiency of thyroxine, Turner's syndrome-deficiency of estrogen and progesterone, and hypopituitarism-deficiency of growth hormone. Poor function of all of the above would suggest progeria. The adrenal carcinomas may cause precocious puberty and premature closure of the epiphysis. The above method fails to include most of the genetic causes of dwarfism so perhaps this group can be remembered by its exclusion.

Approach to the Diagnosis

The workup of dwarfism should probably be done by an endocrinologist. Many of the causes are genetic and untreatable, but it would be a shame to miss cretinism, hypopituitarism, or a Turner's syndrome. All of these have associated findings that should help differentiate them, but hypopituitarism may be very subtle. Cystic fibrosis can be diagnosed by a sweat test. Mongolism, Turner's syndrome, and certain other genetic causes can be determined by a chromosomal analysis.

DYSARTHRIA AND SPEECH DISORDERS

Besides dysarthria three other types of speech disorders should be considered here: dysphasia, cerebellar speech, and extrapyramidal speech. In each case the anatomical location in the nervous system is fairly specific.

Dysarthria. This may be due to a lesion at the end organ (muscles of the mouth and tongue), the myoneural junction, the peripheral branches of the fifth and twelfth cranial nerves, the brain stem, or the cerebrum.

1. End organ. Hypertrophy of the tongue from myxedema, carcinoma of the tongue, and painful lesions of the mouth and tongue may cause speech difficulty. Inabil-

288

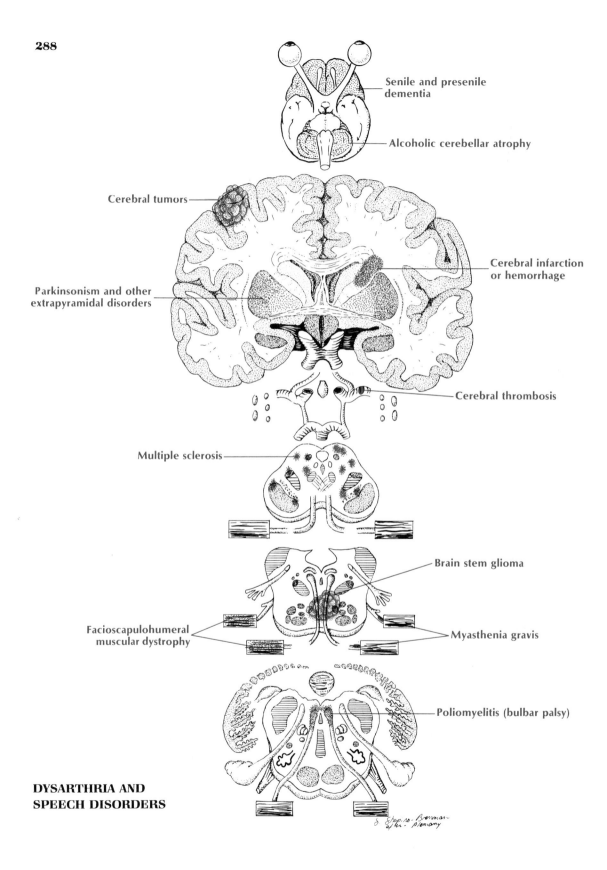

Senile and presenile dementia

Alcoholic cerebellar atrophy

Cerebral tumors

Cerebral infarction or hemorrhage

Parkinsonism and other extrapyramidal disorders

Cerebral thrombosis

Multiple sclerosis

Brain stem glioma

Facioscapulohumeral muscular dystrophy

Myasthenia gravis

Poliomyelitis (bulbar palsy)

DYSARTHRIA AND SPEECH DISORDERS

ity to swallow may leave saliva and food in the mouth and interfere with speech. The facioscapulohumeral form of muscular dystrophy may cause dysarthria.

2. **Myoneural junction.** Myasthenia gravis, a treatable form of dysarthria, should always be ruled out.
3. **Peripheral nerve.** Hypoglossal nerve damage from trauma and severing of the motor portion of the trigeminal nerve in trauma and surgery are the principal lesions here.
4. **Brain stem.** Poliomyelitis, Guillain–Barré syndrome, disseminated encephalomyelitis, brain stem gliomas, and basilar artery occlusions are the most important lesions to recall in this category.
5. **Cerebrum.** Any disorder that may cause hemiplegia from cerebral involvement may cause dysarthria and pseudobulbar palsy. Cerebral thrombi, emboli, or hemorrhages are perhaps the most significant of these. Frontal lobe tumors or abscesses may be the cause here. Diffuse cerebral diseases such as alcoholism, Huntington's chorea, and general paresis may cause dysarthria, but they are more likely to cause other speech disorders.

Cerebellar Speech.   This may be scanning or staccato (clipped). Multiple sclerosis is often the first condition to consider, but the hereditary cerebellar ataxias (*e.g.*, Marie's ataxia), alcoholic cerebellar atrophy, syphilis, and cerebellar tumors may also be the etiology.

Dysphasia.   In this condition words cannot be pronounced properly (motor dysphasia), there is difficulty naming objects (nominal aphasia), or the words cannot be placed properly in a sentence (syntactic aphasia). In determining the etiology, it is not important to know the exact location of the lesion in the cerebrum because any disease of the cerebrum may cause aphasia or dysphasia. Cere-

bral hemorrhages, thrombi, emboli, and tumors or other space-occupying lesions are the most important ones to remember. The others are listed on page 349 (memory loss).

Extrapyramidal Speech.   This is the monotone, rapid, dysarthric speech of paralysis agitans, but it may be found in cerebral palsy, Wilson's disease, or Huntington's chorea. The last two conditions may also have a jerky speech or dysarthria.

Approach to the Diagnosis

Dysarthria without other symptoms or signs requires that myasthenia gravis be ruled out with a Tensilon test and psychometrics be done to rule out hysteria. In the presence of other neurological signs, speech disorders require a thorough neurological workup with an EEG, skull x-ray film, CT scan, and even a spinal tap or arteriography may be indicated. The clinician should remember that dysarthria may be only the first sign of a serious neurological disease such as multiple sclerosis, Wilson's disease, lupus erythematosus, or chronic alcoholism so that close follow-up is important.

DYSPNEA, TACHYPNEA, AND ORTHOPNEA   ■

Dyspnea is the subjective feeling of rapid or difficult breathing. The patient will often say, "I can't get my breath!" **Tachypnea** is the objective finding of a rapid respiratory rate and may or may not be associated with the feeling of not being able to breathe properly. One is a symptom and the other is a sign, but the mechanisms for producing them are the same: inadequate oxygen for body needs or inability to excrete carbon dioxide. A few other mechanisms that produce hyperventilation and tachypnea will be discussed later on in this chapter. The best basic science for developing a list of the causes of dyspnea and tachypnea is **pathophysiology.** Difficulty breathing or rapid breathing will develop when there is decreased intake of oxygen, impaired absorption of oxygen, inadequate perfusion of the lungs with blood, inability of the body to transport enough oxygen to the tissues, increased demand of the tissues for oxy-

gen, and inability of the body to excrete carbon dioxide and other waste products of body metabolism. These are tabulated in Table 5-8.

Disorders of Oxygen Intake. In this category are the conditions that may block the respiratory passages such as laryngitis, foreign bodies, an aortic aneurysm or mediastinal tumor pressing on the trachea or bronchi, bronchial asthma, acute infectious bronchitis, and pulmonary emphysema. Also considered in this category are conditions

TABLE 5-8.   DYSPNEA, TACHYPNEA, AND ORTHOPNEA

	V Vascular	I Inflammatory	N Neoplasm	D Degenerative
Disorders of Oxygen Intake		Laryngitis Bronchitis	Bronchogenic carcinoma	Pulmonary emphysema
Disorders of Oxygen Absorption	Pulmonary edema	Pneumonia Tuberculosis Lung abscess	Alveolar carcinoma Metastatic carcinoma	Pulmonary emphysema and fibrosis
Disorders of Perfusion	Pulmonary embolism		Hemangioma	Pulmonary fibrosis Pulmonary emphysema
Disorders of Transport	Congestive heart failure	Septicemia with shock		Aplastic anemia
Disorders of Increased Oxygen Demands	Polycythemia	Fever	Leukemia Hodgkin's disease Metastatic carcinoma	
Disorders of Excretion of Carbon Dioxide and Other Wastes of Body Metabolism		Septicemia with lactic acidosis	Pulmonary emphysema	

that interfere with the "respiratory pump" (thoracic cage, thoracic and diaphragmatic muscles, and respiratory centers in the brain) such as kyphoscoliosis, Pickwickian syndrome, myasthenia gravis, peritonitis, encephalitis, and brain tumors.

Disorders of Oxygen Absorption. Lobar pneumonia, sarcoidosis, silicosis and various causes of pulmonary fibrosis, and pulmonary edema are considered here. Oxygen diffusion across the alveolocapillary membrane is af-

fected in all of these. Alveolar proteinosis, shock lung, and the adult respiratory distress syndrome must also be considered here.

Disorders of Perfusion of the Pulmonary Capillaries. Pulmonary emboli, hemangiomas of the lungs, and congenital heart increases such as tetralogy of Fallot belong in this category. In all of these conditions unoxygenated blood bypasses the alveoli. Also included in this category are diseases with a ventilation–perfusion defect. In other words

I Intoxication	C Congenital	A Allergic and Autoimmune	T Trauma	E Endocrine
Pneumoconiosis	Kyphoscoliosis Bronchiectasis	Bronchial asthma	Foreign body Injury to ribs	
Lipoid pneumonia Toxic pneumonitis Shock lung	Atelectasis	Periarteritis nodosa Wegener's granuloma Sarcoidosis Scleroderma	Pneumothorax	
	Congenital heart disease			
Methemoglobinemia Shock from drugs and toxins	Sickle cell anemia Congenital heart disease	Shock	Hemorrhagic shock	Waterhouse– Friderichsen syndrome
				Hyperthyroidism
Uremia Lactic acidosis				Diabetic acidosis

some alveoli are being ventilated but not perfused with blood, while at the same time some alveoli are being perfused but not ventilated. Pulmonary emphysema and the various

conditions associated with pulmonary fibrosis (*e.g.*, pneumoconiosis) cause dyspnea on this basis, as well as other physiological reasons mentioned above.

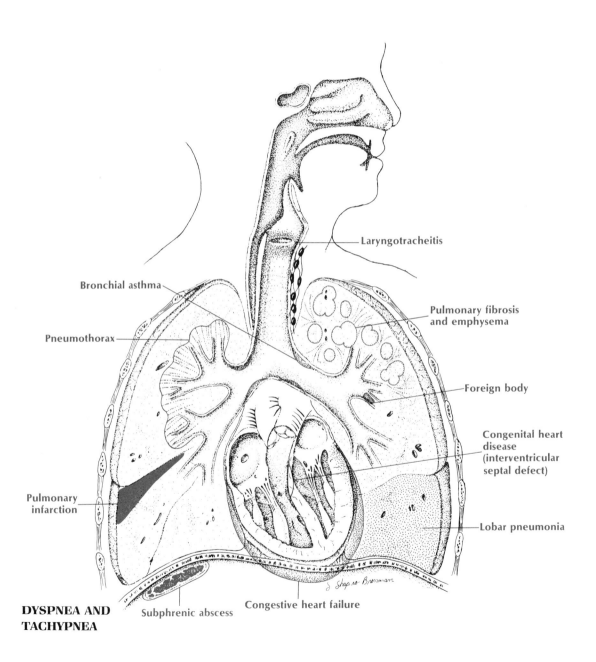

DYSPNEA AND TACHYPNEA

Disorders of Oxygen Transport. The tissues will not get oxygen if there is not enough blood to transport it, as in anemia and hemorrhagic shock; or if there is not enough blood pressure to perfuse the tissues, as in vasomotor and cardiogenic shock; or if the heart pump fails, as in congestive heart failure from many causes. In methemoglobinemia and sulfhemoglobinemia there may be enough blood but it is unable to carry the oxygen.

Increased Tissue Oxygen Demand. During exercise and nervous stress, and in febrile states, leukemia and other malignancies, and hyperthyroidism there is an increase in tissue metabolism and consequently tachypnea may develop to increase the supply.

Inadequate Excretion of Carbon Dioxide and Other Wastes of Tissue Metabolism. Inability to excrete carbon dioxide may occur without anoxia in pulmonary emphysema and other chronic obstructive lung diseases and initiate dyspnea, especially on exertion. Other wastes of tissue metabolism may cause an acidosis and stimulate the respiratory centers in this fashion. Lactic acidosis, diabetic acidosis, and uremia may cause dyspnea on this basis.

From the above discussion it should be evident that the clinician can develop an excellent list of the causes of dyspnea and tachypnea with an understanding of the pathophysiology involved. A few conditions cannot be recalled with this method: hyperventilation syndrome, ingestion of acids (e.g., methyl alcohol poisoning) and drugs that stimulate the respiratory centers (such as amphetamines), and atmospheric reduction in oxygen tension.

Approach to the Diagnosis

The history and physical examination will almost invariably disclose the cause of dyspnea. To confirm pulmonary disease one will order pulmonary function studies, a chest roentgenogram and arterial blood gases. If routine pulmonary function studies are normal, more sophisticated studies such as the nitrogen washout test and perfusion and ventilatory scans may be necessary. To diagnose cardiac conditions, an ECG and venous pressure and circulation times may be necessary.

Any patient with dyspnea and normal physical findings deserves a circulation time at least to rule out early congestive heart failure. A hemogram will diagnose anemias but it will not diagnose methemoglobinemia. A determination of the erythrocytes methemoglobin, arterial oxygen saturation, and diaphorase I must be done. Other tests to work up dyspnea and tachypnea are listed in Appendix I.

DYSTOCIA

Both **physiology** and **anatomy** must be applied to develop the differential diagnosis of dystocia. An abnormally long labor may result from inadequate abdominal muscle or uterine muscle contractions, obstruction of the birth canal, abnormalities of the fetus or placenta, and unusual positions of the fetus in the abdomen and pelvis.

1. **Inadequate abdominal muscle contractions.** This may be due to diastasis recti, ventral hernias, and obesity.
2. **Inadequate uterine muscle contractions.** This may result from malformations of the uterus, such as bicornuate uterus; from multiple fibroids and other neoplasms of the uterus; from drugs that inhibit uterine contractions, such as morphine and other sedatives; and from primary uterine inertia.
3. **Obstruction of the birth canal.** Look for

ovarian cysts, uterine fibroids, cervical stenosis, deformities of the pelvis, impacted feces and an enlarged bladder in this category.

4. **Abnormalities of the fetus.** This category includes large babies, polyhydramnios due to diabetes mellitus, hydrocephalus, abdominal neoplasms or ascites in the fetus, and twins or additional multiple births.

5. **Abnormal position of the fetus.** Breech presentation, transverse lie, face or brow presentation, and occipital-posterior presentations are included in this category.

Approach to the Diagnosis

Thorough examinations, ultrasonic scans, roentgenograms of the abdomen for fetal size and position, and amniocentesis are all useful procedures to assist in the diagnosis.

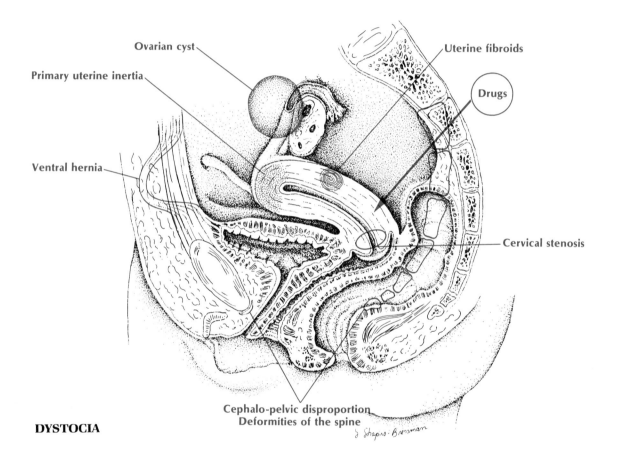

Ovarian cyst

Primary uterine inertia

Ventral hernia

Uterine fibroids

Drugs

Cervical stenosis

Cephalo-pelvic disproportion
Deformities of the spine

DYSTOCIA

ENURESIS (BEDWETTING)

By following the innervation of the bladder from its termination to the spinal cord, brain, and "supratentorium," one can develop an extensive list of possibilities for this mischievous condition. Thus **anatomy** is the key and the mnemonic **MINT** is the door.

Termination.   The bladder and entire urinary tract should be suspect for pathology in any case of enuresis beyond the age of six.

M—Malformations include phimosis, small urinary meatus, and vesicoureteral reflux.

I—Inflammatory conditions form the largest group and include balanitis, urethritis, cystitis and pyelonephritis. If a child develops chronic nephritis at an early age his bladder simply may be too small to retain the polyuria during sleep.

N—Neoplasms are an unlikely cause in children but they occur in adults.

T—Trauma from a vesical calculus or other foreign bodies inserted into the bladder must also be considered. Postprostatectomy enuresis should be considered here in the adult.

Spinal Cord.   The following are included in this group:

M—Malformations such as spina bifida

I—Inflammatory conditions such as poliomyelitis and transverse myelitis

N—Neoplasms such as spinal cord tumors

T—Traumatic conditions such as fracture, hematomyelia, and herniated discs

Brain.   This is an important group of conditions to consider if only briefly, for if the patient has a form of epilepsy a cure may be easily obtained. Other neurological conditions include mental retardation, multiple sclerosis, general paresis, brain tumors, and chronic encephalidites.

Supratentorium.   A child may react violently to the pressure of toilet training by deliberately wetting the bed; his bed-wetting may also be a way of getting back at generally strict parents or a way of getting their attention. Recent studies show that a child should not be considered to be a bed-wetter until after the age of six. Parents who put that label on a child too early may assure that his enuresis will continue for emotional reasons. Labeling the child as a bed-wetter at any age is not a solution but an aggravation of the problem.

Approach to the Diagnosis

From the above discussion it should be obvious that simple bed-wetting prior to age six may not require a workup at all. After that age a careful examination of the urine, including smear and culture for bacteria, should be done. An intravenous pyelogram and voiding cystogram are usually necessary. If these suggest a congenital lesion or are negative, cystoscopy may need to be done. An x-ray film for spina bifida and a sleep EEG are probably worthwhile if urological investigation is negative.

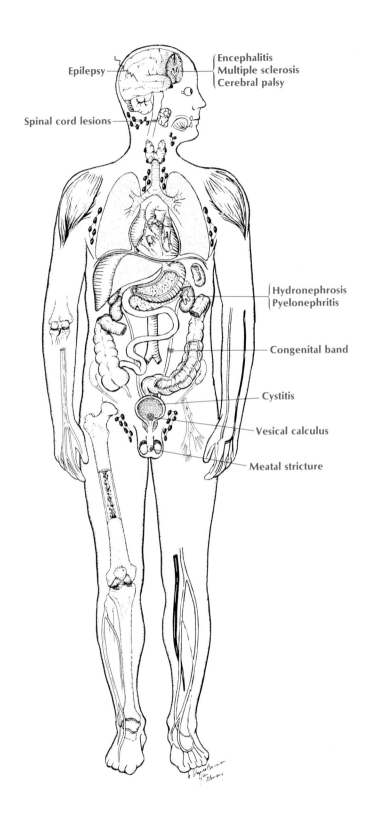

Epilepsy

Encephalitis
Multiple sclerosis
Cerebral palsy

Spinal cord lesions

Hydronephrosis
Pyelonephritis

Congenital band

Cystitis

Vesical calculus

Meatal stricture

**ENURESIS
(BED WETTING)**

EXCESSIVE SWEATING ◼

It is uncommon for patients to present with the chief complaint of excessive sweating (diaphoresis, hyperhidrosis); when they do it is often hyperhidrosis of the hands and feet due to caffeine or nervous tension. Obese patients may complain of excessive sweating, especially under the armpits. What are the pathological causes of sweating and how can they be recalled?

Physiology is the basic science most useful in developing a differential diagnosis. The sweat glands are under the control of the sympathetic nervous system; consequently, they respond to anything that increases the level of adrenalin in the body. Shock from any cause causes a reflex stimulation of the sympathetic nervous system and adrenal gland and an outpouring of adrenalin. Thus diaphoresis may be found in mycardial infarctions and congestive heart failure (cardiogenic shock), in pulmonary embolism, renal embolism, and peripheral embolism (vasomotor shock), and in bleeding peptic ulcer, pyloric obstruction with vomiting, cholera, intestinal obstruction, and other forms of shock due to a drop in blood volume. Acute labryrinthitis or seasickness causes sweating by neurogenic shock pathways.

The adrenalin level may also be increased in the body in hypoglycemic states. Thus a diabetic in insulin shock will sweat while a diabetic in acidosis will not. Islet cell adenomas cause diaphoresis during the hypoglycemic attacks. Hepatic hypoglycemia, glycogen storage disease, and hypopituitarism may all be associated with excessive sweating on the same basis. Excessive adrenalin output is the cause of diaphoresis in pheochromocytomas. It may well be the cause in hyperthyroidism also, although another mechanism discussed below is undoubtedly involved.

Hypermetabolism causes excessive sweating by hypothalamic stimulation of the sweating center to assist in the cooling of the body. Thus any cause of fever is associated with sweating. The sweating induces a drop in temperature. Most notable of these are rheumatic fever, pulmonary tuberculosis, and septicemia. An abscess large enough to cause fever will probably cause sweating. Hypermetabolism in hyperthyroidism is largely responsible for the continuous sweating, although excessive adrenalin is involved too. Neoplasms, especially leukemia and metastatic carcinoma, are associated with sweating on the same basis.

A miscellaneous group of conditions associated with diaphoresis that are also due to physiological mechanisms include neurocirculatory asthenia, chronic anxiety neurosis, menopause; and various drugs, including camphor, morphine, and ipecac.

Approach to the Diagnosis

Pinpointing the diagnosis involves a search for other symptoms and signs of the above conditions. A chest x-ray film to rule out pulmonary tuberculosis is especially important in a patient presenting with night sweats. Accurate charting of the temperature will indicate those cases due to fever. Urine vanillylmandelic acid (VMA) levels and a thyroid workup will spot pheochromacytomas and hyperthyroidism. A 36- to 48-hour fast with frequent glucose determinations will help diagnose insulinomas and other hypoglycemic states. Since this is not usually the major presenting symptom the workup will usually center around another symptom. Asking about coffee ingestion will often spot the cause without expensive laboratory testing.

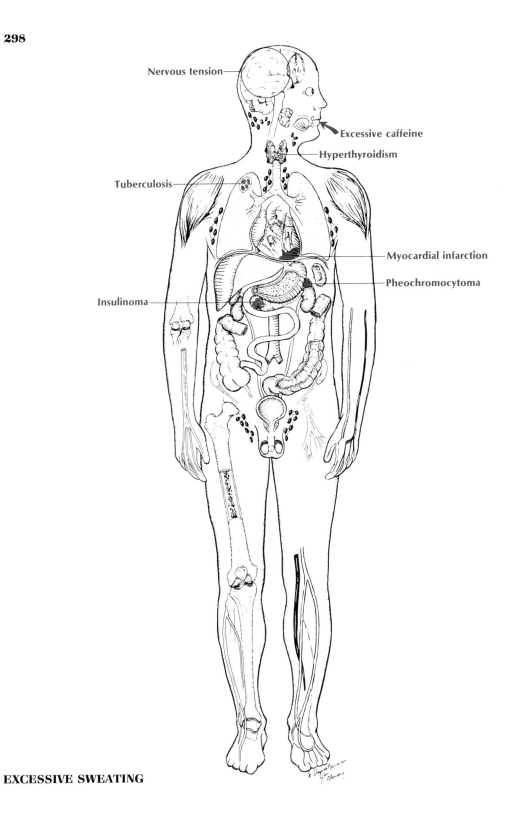

Nervous tension

Excessive caffeine

Hyperthyroidism

Tuberculosis

Myocardial infarction

Pheochromocytoma

Insulinoma

EXCESSIVE SWEATING

FACIAL PARALYSIS ■

A facial palsy is usually considered to be Bell's palsy and it frequently is. Nevertheless, the clinician who begins treatment without ruling out other possibilities will eventually get burned. **Anatomy** is the key to recalling these possibilities before the patient leaves the office. Follow the facial nerve from its origin along its pathway to its termination and all the causes should come to mind.

Origin. Diseases of the brain and brain stem are considered here. They are usually distinguished from a Bell's palsy by the presence of other neurological findings. The mnemonic **ANITA** will help recall them in an organized fashion.

A—**Arterial** diseases include aneurysms, emboli, thrombosis, and hemorrhage. Occlusion of the posterior-inferior cerebellar artery will cause a peripheral facial palsy, but it can easily be distinguished from a Bell's

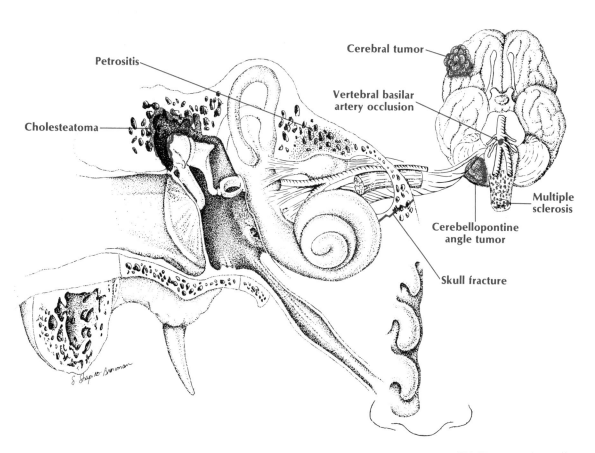

Petrositis

Cholesteatoma

Cerebral tumor

Vertebral basilar
artery occlusion

Multiple
sclerosis

Cerebellopontine
angle tumor

Skull fracture

FACIAL PARALYSIS

palsy by the presence of a Horner's syndrome, hoarseness, ataxia, and crossed hemianalgesia.

N—Neoplasms include gliomas and the cerebellopontine angle tumor or acoustic neuroma.

I—Inflammation suggest neurosyphilis, tuberculosis, brain abscess, and encephalitis.

T—Trauma helps recall skull fractures and epidural and subdural hematomas.

A—Autoimmune disease suggests multiple sclerosis, the collagen diseases, and early Guillain–Barré syndrome.

Pathway. The facial nerve has a long pathway and along that path it can be destroyed by the following:

A—Arterial aneurysms

N—Neoplasms such as acoustic neuromas and parotid gland tumors

I—Inflammatory conditions like herpes zoster, petrositis, mastoiditis, and cholesteatomas

T—Trauma such as basilar skull fractures and otological surgery

A—Autoimmune disease such as Bell's palsy, or uveoparotid fever

Termination. The site of termination of the facial nerve should suggest myasthenia gravis, muscular dystrophy, and facial hemiatrophy. These rarely present with an isolated facial palsy.

Approach to the Diagnosis

What tests can be done to determine the exact cause of a facial palsy? First of all, it must be decided whether the lesion is peripheral or central. In a peripheral lesion the patient cannot close his eye or wrinkle his brow; when he smiles there is little or no movement of the involved side. Lacrimation may also be lost. In central lesions, there is almost always an as-

sociated hemiplegia or monoplegia. Electromyography is useful in difficult cases. If it is determined that the lesion is peripheral, roentgenograms of the skull, mastoids, and petrous bones need to be done, and possibly an audiogram to rule out an acoustic neuroma. A Tensilon test may be helpful. If the lesion is central, the workup of hemiplegia (see p. 410) may be appropriate.

FASCICULATIONS

This sign is generally considered pathognomonic for anterior horn cell or root disease. It may occur, however, in certain cases of peripheral neuropathy, in electrolyte disturbances, and in myasthenia gravis, especially under treatment. It is also found in healthy states, most commonly in the twitching of the orbicularis oculi muscle from nervous tension or eyestrain. Fasciculations must be distinguished from fibrillations which are not visible, are detected only with EMG, and are caused by muscle disease. The causes can easily be recalled by visualizing the anterior horn cells and nerves and applying the mnemonic **VINDICATE** to this area.

V—Vascular conditions include anterior spinal artery occlusion and intermittent claudication from peripheral vascular disease.

I—Inflammatory diseases include poliomyelitis, viral encephalomyelitis, tetanus, syphilis, and diphtheria.

N—Neoplasm suggests intramedullary tumors of the cord such as ependymomas and extramedullary tumors such as meningiomas, Hodgkin's disease, metastatic carcinomas, and multiple myeloma must be considered.

D—Degenerative diseases are the most important causes of fasciculations. They include progressive spinal muscular atrophy, amyotrophic lateral sclerosis, Werdnig–Hoffmann disease, and syringomyelia.

I—Intoxication includes lead poisoning and alcoholism.

C—Congenital disorders suggest Werdnig–Hoffmann, spondylolisthesis, and other anomalies of the spinal cord that may compress the anterior horn and roots.

A—Autoimmune disorders recall transverse myelitis, myasthenia gravis (under treatment), periarteritis nodosa, and Guillain–Barre syndrome.

T—Trauma suggests herniated discs and fractures that compress the anterior horn or roots.

E—Endocrine and metabolic diseases include hypoparathyroidism and other causes of tetany, magnesium deficiency and other electrolyte disturbances, and diabetic myelopathy and hypothyroid myopathy (more commonly the cause of fibrillations which can only be detected by electromyography).

Approach to the Diagnosis

Deciding on the cause of fasciculations will usually be based on other neurological symptoms and signs. Muscular atrophy without sensory changes suggests progressive muscular atrophy, whereas atrophy and fasciculations with sensory changes suggest syringomyelia, peripheral neuropathy, and root compression (e.g., a herniated disc). Treatable neurological disorders should be considered first. Thus, roentgenograms of the spine, spinal fluid analysis, and myelography should be performed to rule out a space-occupying lesion. Electromyography is useful in detecting which level is involved as well as in following the progress of the disease. Serum electrolytes, calcium, phosphorus, and magnesium are useful in selected disorders.

FEVER ▪

The differential diagnosis of fever is best developed using **physiology** first and **anatomy** second.

Physiology. Increased heat in the body is caused by increased production or decreased elimination of dysfunction of the thermoregulatory system in the brain. Increased production of heat occurs in conditions with increased metabolic rate such as hyperthyroidism, pheochromocytomas, and malignant neoplasms. Poor eliminations of heat may occur in congestive heart failure (poor circulation through the skin) and conditions where the sweat glands are absent (congenital) or poorly functioning (heat stroke). Most cases of fever are caused by the effect of toxins on the thermoregulatory centers in the brain. These toxins may be exogenous from drugs, bacteria (endotoxins), parasites, fungi, rickettsiae and virus particles, or they may be endogenous from tissue injury (trauma) and breakdown (carcinomas, leukemia, infarctions, and autoimmune disease).

Anatomy. With the etiologies suggested by the mnemonic **VINDICATE,** one can apply anatomy and the various organ systems and make a useful chart (see p. 304). The infections should be divided into the **systemic diseases** that affect more than one organ, such as typhoid, brucellosis, tuberculosis, syphilis, leptospirosis, and bacterial endocarditis, and the **localized diseases** that usually affect the same specific organ, such as infectious hepatitis, subacute thyroiditis, pneumococcal pneumonia, and cholera. It is wise to divide the localized infectious diseases into the **"itises"** (e.g., pneumonitis, hepatitis, and prostatitis), and the **abscesses** (dental abscesses, empyema, perinephric abscess, liver abscess, and subdiaphragmatic abscess).

(Text continues on p. 304)

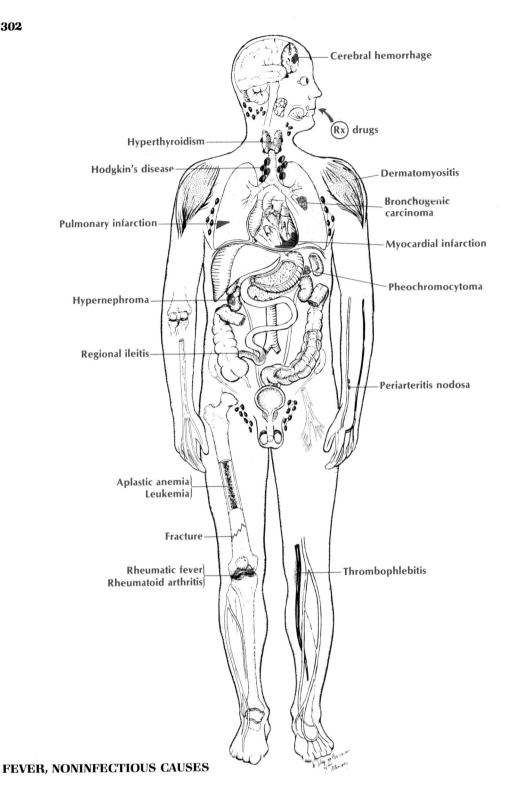

Cerebral hemorrhage

Rx drugs

Hyperthyroidism

Hodgkin's disease

Dermatomyositis

Bronchogenic carcinoma

Pulmonary infarction

Myocardial infarction

Pheochromocytoma

Hypernephroma

Regional ileitis

Periarteritis nodosa

Aplastic anemia
Leukemia

Fracture

Rheumatic fever
Rheumatoid arthritis

Thrombophlebitis

FEVER, NONINFECTIOUS CAUSES

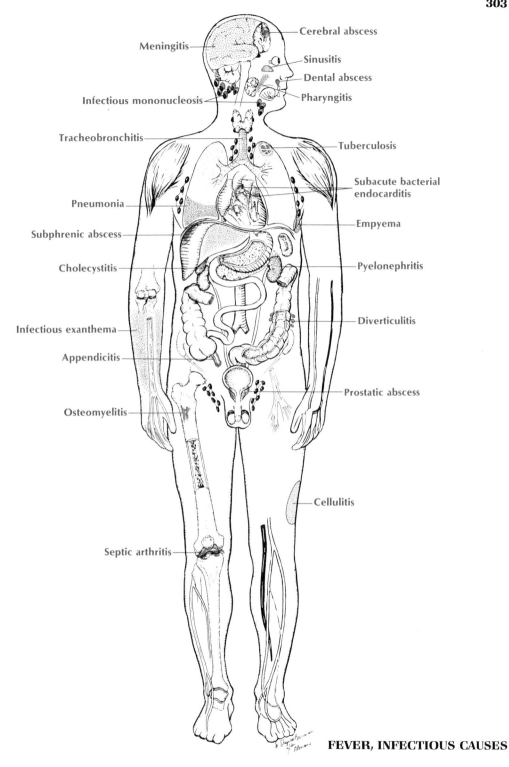

Meningitis

Cerebral abscess

Sinusitis

Dental abscess

Infectious mononucleosis

Pharyngitis

Tracheobronchitis

Tuberculosis

Subacute bacterial endocarditis

Pneumonia

Empyema

Subphrenic abscess

Cholecystitis

Pyelonephritis

Infectious exanthema

Diverticulitis

Appendicitis

Prostatic abscess

Osteomyelitis

Cellulitis

Septic arthritis

FEVER, INFECTIOUS CAUSES

Also, when the physician attempts to recall the specific infections, he can group them into six categories beginning with the smallest organism and working onto the largest as follows: viruses, rickettsiae, bacteria, spirochetes, fungi, and parasites. Endogenous toxins released by infarctions of various organs form another convenient group. Finally, the most common neoplasms to cause fever (by tissue breakdown) are illustrated on page 302.

Approach to the Diagnosis

There are certain things to remember when a patient with fever is approached. First, a mild elevation up to 100.5° rectally may be normal in some people. Second, one should rule out malingering by the patient or incorrect recording by hospital personnel. Finally, psychogenic disorders must be ruled out.

The duration and severity of the fever are

TABLE 5-9.   FEVER

	V Vascular	I Inflammatory	N Neoplasm	D Degenerative
Brain	Occlusions Infarctions Hemorrhage	Meningitis Encephalitis Abscess Epidural abscess	Glioma Metastasis	
Ear, Nose, and Throat		Otitis media Mastoiditis Petrositis Dental abscess		
Lungs	Pulmonary infarction	Pneumonia Lung abscess Empyema Tuberculosis	Carcinoma	
Heart	Myocardial infarction	Myocarditis Subacute bacterial endocarditis		
Liver and Biliary Tract	Budd–Chiari syndrome Pyelophlebitis	Hepatitis Amoebic abscess Cholangitis Cholecystitis Diaphragmatic abscess	Hematoma Metastasis Hodgkin's disease	
Pancreas		Pancreatitis Pancreatic cyst	Carcinoma	

important. If possible, a careful chart of the fever should be made with the patient off all drugs (especially aspirin and steroids). Conditions with intermittent or relapsing fever such as brucellosis, malaria and Mediterranean fever will be elucidated in this fashion (Table 5-9).

The association with other symptoms is important. Fever, right upper quadrant pain, and jaundice suggest cholecystitis or cholangitis, whereas fever when right flank pain suggest pyelonephritis. After taking a few moments to jot down the differential before launching into the history and physical examination, one can question and examine the patient more appropriately. The differential diagnosis will also lead to more appropriate use of the laboratory. Appendix I shows the most useful tests to include in a workup of fever.

(*Text continues on p. 308*)

I Intoxication	C Congenital	A Autoimmune Allergic	T Trauma	E Endocrine Metabolic
Pyrogens Endotoxins Heat stroke	Ruptured aneurysm	Collagen diseases	Epidural and subdural hematoma Cerebral contusion	Pituitary tumors
	Bronchiectasis	Wegener's granulomatosis Periarteritis nodosa Lupus erythematosus	Contusion Hemorrhage	
		Collagen diseases	Hemopericardium and contusion	
Alcoholic cirrhosis Toxic hepatitis Calculi		Collagen diseases	Contusion Lacerations	
				Diabetes mellitus

TABLE 5-9. (*continued*)

	V Vascular	I Inflammatory	N Neoplasm	D Degenerative
GI Tract	Mesenteric thrombosis	Tuberculosis Typoid Abscess of appendix or diverticuli	Carcinomas Sarcomas	
Urinary Tract	Embolism Renal vein throm- bosis Infarct	Perinephric abscess Pyelonephritis cysti- tis	Hypernephroma	
Reproductive Organs	Torsion of testicle	Orchitis Epidydimitis Prostatis Endometritis	Seminoma Carcinomas Endometrial carci- noma	
Bones	Infarction Aseptic bone necrosis	Osteomyelitis Bone abscess	Sarcoma Metastasis	
Skin		Rocky Mountain spotted fever Syphilis Abscess Cellulitis	Pemphigus	
Blood and Blood- Forming Organs		Malaria Oroya fever Kala-azar	Leukemia	
Lymphatics		Tuberculosis Mononucleosis Many specific infec- tions	Hodgkin's disease Lymphosarcoma	
Endocrine Glands		Subacute thyroiditis Orchitis	Graves' disease Carcinoma	
Eye	Retinal vein or arterial occlusions	Scleritis Uveitis Retinitis Orbital abscess	Retinoblastoma	
Muscle		Trichinosis Epidemic myalgia		

I Intoxication	C Congenital	A Autoimmune Allergic	T Trauma	E Endocrine Metabolic
Ulcers with hemorrhage or perforation	Meckel's diverticulum	Ulcerative colitis Regional enteritis	Perforated viscus	
Calculi	Anomalies (*e.g.,*polycystic kidney)	Glomerulonephritis Collagen disease	Contusion Hemorrhage	Calculi
Progesterone	Torsion of testicle			Pregnancy
			Fracture	
Exfoliative dermatitis	Diffuse atopic dermatitis		Multiple contusions	
Agranulocytosis		Hemolytic anemia Blood transfusion	Hemolysis from valve prosthesis	
Radiation				
		Uveitis	Orbital fractures	
		Dermatomyositis	Crush syndrome	

FLASHES OF LIGHT

Flashes of light usually result from involvement of the retina, optic nerve, optic cortex, or the arterial circulation to these areas.

1. **Retina.** Conditions of the retina to be considered in this symptom are exudative choroiditis, retinal detachment, venous thrombosis, and embolism.
2. **Optic nerve.** Optic neuritis at the onset may cause flashes of light. Multiple sclerosis is prone to present this way.
3. **Optic cortex.** Transient ischemic attacks in the posterior cerebral circulation and epileptic auras may cause this symptom.
4. **Arterial circulation to the eye and brain.** Migraine, cerebral thrombosis, and emboli present with this symptom.

Approach to the Diagnosis

This is similar to the workup of blurred vision (see p. 236).

FLATULENCE AND BORBORYGMI

Flatulence is increased output of gas by mouth or rectum. Borborygmi are audible sounds of hyperperistalsis of gas. Both are caused by similar physiological mechanisms.

The increase of gas in the intestinal tract depends on three physiological mechanisms:

1. Increased intake of air
2. Increased production of gas in the intestinal tract
3. Decreased absorption of gas

Increased Intake

This is probably one of the most frequent causes of flatulence and borborygmi. Aerophagia in neurosis is a well-known psychogenic cause. However, compulsive eating, compulsive drinking, excessive smoking, or excessive talking may produce the same effect. All of us take in a certain amount of air when we swallow food or liquids. When we overeat, however, or when we drink too much, the amount of gas taken in may exceed our ability to absorb it. Salesmen and public speakers have an additional problem because talking increases salivation and swallowing, and frequently air is swallowed between sentences.

Some people have a particular beverage they are fond of, such as cola, coffee, or alcohol. Excessive drinking of these beverages entails the swallowing of excess air. In addition, some of these beverages release gas after ingestion (carbonated beverages especially), which causes flatulence. Reflux esophagitis is a frequent cause.

Increased Production of Gas in the Intestinal Tract

In acute bacterial gastroenteritis (*e.g.,* salmonella and shigella) gas-producing organisms multiply and produce excess gas. The diarrhea or vomiting associated with these disorders usually makes the diagnosis easy. A more obscure cause of increased production of gas is chronic mild intestinal obstruction leading to excessive bacterial overgrowth. Adhesions, intestinal polyps, regional ileitis, and all the various causes of paralytic ileus (*e.g.,* anticholinergic drugs, tranquilizers, uremia, and chronic anoxia) cause increased gas production by this mechanism. Gas production is also increased when bacteria are allowed to accumulate in large numbers in chronic in-

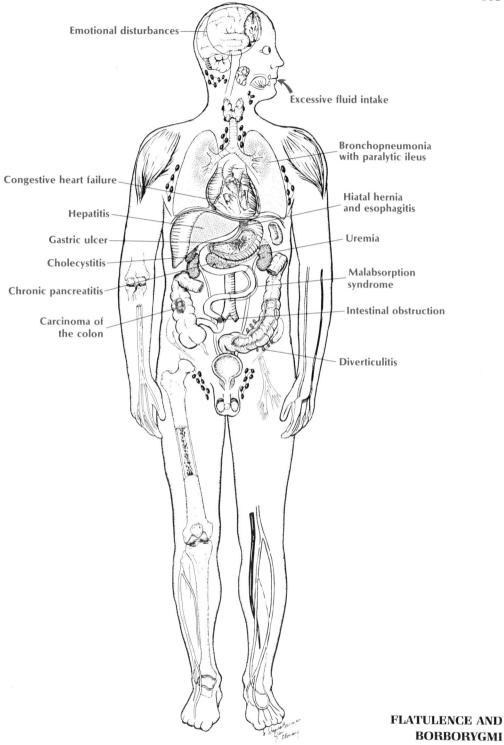

Emotional disturbances

Excessive fluid intake

Bronchopneumonia with paralytic ileus

Congestive heart failure

Hiatal hernia and esophagitis

Hepatitis

Uremia

Gastric ulcer

Cholecystitis

Malabsorption syndrome

Chronic pancreatitis

Intestinal obstruction

Carcinoma of the colon

Diverticulitis

FLATULENCE AND BORBORYGMI

testinal disorders. The blind loop syndrome, diverticulitis, and Meckel's diverticulum fall in this category. Certain cases of irritation in the intestinal tract cause a mild paralytic ileus and allow bacteria to multiply and ferment. Esophagitis and hiatal hernia, chronic gastritis, ulcers, regional ileitis, and ulcerative and mucus colitis may cause mild paralytic ileus on this basis.

When the amount of digestive juices is insufficient to digest the food, more food is available for bacterial fermentation. Thus in chronic atrophic gastritis the reduced HCl leaves undigested food for bacterial action. In cholecystitis and partial bile duct obstruction or liver disease, there are insufficient bile acids for digestion and more food is left for bacterial fermentation. In chronic pancreatitis the reduction in pancreatic enzymes causes the same problem. Lactase deficiency leaves food for fermentation.

Decreased Absorption of Gas

Malabsorption syndromes cause this condition. In acute gastroenteritis the swollen inflamed intestines cannot absorb the gas. Intestinal motility may be so rapid that there is not enough time for absorption. In celiac disease, the atrophied villi cannot pick up food and gas and it is passed on through. Intestinal parasites may pre-empt food from absorption and produce excessive gas in their own digestive processes.

Approach to the Diagnosis

If excessive food, beverages, or air swallowing from nervous tension or talking can be excluded, reflux esophagitis and diverticulitis must be considered. Upper GI series, esophagram, small bowel series, and sigmoidoscopy with a barium enema should be done. A gallbladder series is also ordered. If these are questionable, more definitive diagnosis may

be made with endoscopy. Stools for ova, parasites, and blood, and cultures should be done. When the outcome is still uncertain, evaluation of the adequacy of the intestinal digestive secretions is worthwhile. Gastric analysis with histalogue, duodenal analysis for bicarbonate, bile, and pancreatic enzymes are done. A lactose tolerance test should be done. If the digestive secretions are adequate, a small bowel biopsy may be necessary to exclude a malabsorption syndrome. Xylose absorption is a good screening test for this. Other tests are listed in Appendix I.

FREQUENCY AND URGENCY OF URINATION

Frequency of urination may be due to polyuria (increased output of urine), obstruction to the output of urine requiring frequent voiding to get the urine out because the net capacity of the bladder is reduced, or an irritative lesions in or nearby the urinary tract.

1. **Polyuria.** Increased output of urine is discussed on page 374 but, in summary, it may be caused by pituitary diabetes insipidus, nephritis, diabetes mellitus, hyperthyroidism, hyperparathyroidism, and nephrogenic diabetes insipidus.
2. **Obstruction of the bladder.** This may be mechanical, as occurs in bladder neck obstruction due to prostatic hypertrophy, prostatitis, median bar hypertrophy, urethral stricture, and bladder calculi; or it may be due to a neurogenic bladder, as occurs in poliomyelitis, parasympatholytic drugs, tabes dorsalis, multiple sclerosis, other spinal cord lesions, and diabetic neuropathy.
3. **Irritative lesions of the urinary tract.** Infection, calculus, or neoplasm of the bladder, kidney, ureters, or urethra may do

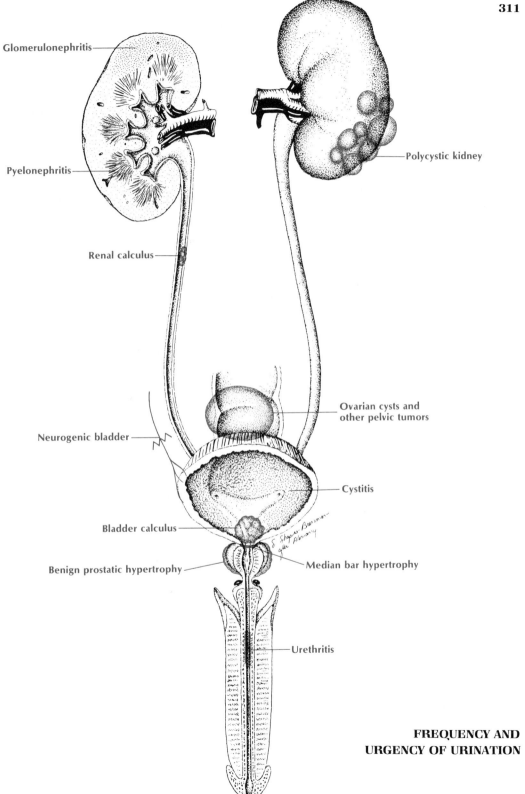

Glomerulonephritis

Pyelonephritis

Renal calculus

Polycystic kidney

Neurogenic bladder

Ovarian cysts and
other pelvic tumors

Cystitis

Bladder calculus

Benign prostatic hypertrophy

Median bar hypertrophy

Urethritis

**FREQUENCY AND
URGENCY OF URINATION**

this. Chronic or acute prostatitis is sometimes the culprit. Inflammation anywhere in the pelvis (vaginitis, hemorrhoids, diverticulitis, appendicitis, or salpingitis) may also cause this.

Approach to the Diagnosis

This is no problem. Examine a drop of unspun urine under the microscope. More than 1 or 2 motile bacteria per HPF is diagnostic of urinary tract infection (UTI). Then culture the urine; catheterize for residual urine; and do an IVP and voiding cystogram. A cystoscopy may be necessary. If these are negative it is a good idea to collect a 24-hour specimen and check the response to pitressin if this exceeds 5 liters in amount. Special cultures for chlamydia should be done if all else fails. The workup of polyuria (see p. 374) can be followed further if necessary.

FRIGIDITY ▪

Frigidity may be due to an organic cause, in which case the differential diagnosis is similar to dyspareunia (see p. 35), or it may be functional. The **organic** causes can be recalled with the mneumonic **MINT.**

M—Malformations include a hood clitoris or imperforate hymen, vaginal stenosis, hermaphroditism, retroverted uterus, and Turner's syndrome.

I—Inflammation suggests vaginitis, Bartholinitis, endometritis, or salpingitis.

N—Neoplasms recall neoplasms of the vagina, cervix, uterus, and ovary and endome-triosis, as well as neurological conditions such as multiple sclerosis or peripheral neuropathy (diabetes).

T—Trauma includes introduction of a large male organ, masturbation, or previous rape, in addition to the emotional trauma discussed below. Unfortunately, this does not include the numerous hormonal causes of frigidity (e.g., menopause, hypopituitarism, Stein–Leventhal syndrome, and adrenal tumors). Obesity would seem to be another "organic" cause of frigidity, but this may simply be another sign of a functional disorder.

Functional or psychogenic causes of frigidity include all the neuroses and psychoses, especially schizophrenia and endogenous depression, as well as specific feelings of fear or hostility related to intercourse. These may be grouped into conscious or unconscious feelings. **Conscious fears** include a fear of pregnancy or, if pregnant, fear of damage to the fetus. It would also include fear of not being able to consummate the marriage and have a child. Another important conscious fear that many women have is that they will not be able to satisfy the husband or that they themselves will not reach a climax. Conscious hostility may be based on a disgust for male superiority or anger at the husband for the way he treats her parents or her other relatives or for his lack of respect for her. She may be disgusted because his lack of technique or premature ejaculation prevents her from reaching orgasm.

Unconscious fears include repressed anxiety from previously being raped in childhood, repressed anxiety from previous incest, and repressed guilt that sex is dirty. Unconscious hostility may come from a castration complex or a reluctance to identify with the feminine role.

Approach to the Diagnosis

The approach to the diagnosis here is to examine the patient and husband for organic causes and perhaps even do FSH, estradiol, and other hormone blood levels. Estrogen replacement therapy may be indicated in menopause. If no organic cause can be found, referral to a psychiatrist or sex therapist is indicated. A reassuring, personable, and interested physician, however, may be quite capable of getting at the psychological cause, especially if it is in the conscious mind.

GAIT DISTURBANCES ■

The anatomical location of the lesion in a gait disturbance depends on the type of disturbance.

1. **Spastic gait.** In this type of lesion, both feet shuffle along the floor in short steps and the legs are close together moving in a scissors-like fashion. It is due to lesions of both pyramidal tracts anywhere from the lower spinal cord to the brain stem and brain. The principal disorders are the following:
    A. In the cord. Multiple sclerosis, amyotrophic lateral sclerosis, spinal cord tumors, syringomyelia, and cervical trauma or spondylosis.
    B. In the brain stem. Tumors, basilar artery thrombosis, multiple sclerosis, platybasia, and progressive lenticular degeneration.
    C. In the brain. Cerebral arteriosclerosis, cerebral palsy, general paresis, and senile and presenile dementia.
2. **Hemiplegic gait.** One foot is dragged above the floor, swinging out in a semicircular fashion. This is due to involvement of only one pyramidal tract, usually in the brain. Cerebral hemorrhage, thrombosis, emboli, and space-occupying lesions may be the culprits. Multiple sclerosis, early cervical cord tumor, or disc may do the same.
3. **Steppage gait.** Because of the weakness of dorsiflexion of both feet the patient has to lift the foot high to avoid tripping. The lesion is a diffuse peripheral neuropathy which may be from lead intoxication, alcoholism, diabetes, porphyria, perineal muscular atrophy, or a cauda equina tumor. There are many other causes of peripheral neuropathy discussed on page 406.
4. **Limping gait.** Pain in one lower extremity due to bone disease, sciatica, hip disease, knee joint disease, and ankle and foot disorders of all types may cause favoring of the painful limb and quickening of the stride on that side so the victim can get back on his healthy limb. Osteoarthritis of the hip or knee, a herniated disc, an osteoarthritic spur of the heel, a sprained ankle, and fracture of any of the bones of the limb are typical conditions causing this type of gait.
5. **Ataxic gait.** The gait is wide-based, clumsy, and staggering. An ataxic gait may be sensory or cerebellar. Sensory ataxia is due to a lesion of the dorsal columns, such as tabes dorsalis, pernicious anemia, or a spinal cord tumor. In sensory ataxia the patient walks carefully with his eyes fixed on the ground. Cerebellar ataxia is due to involvement of the spinocerebellar tracts and cerebellum. This occurs in hereditary cerebellar ataxia, Friedreich's ataxia, cerebellar tumors, multiple sclerosis, and alcoholic cerebellar atrophy. In a cerebellar ataxia the patient reels about as he walks and it is not much more difficult to walk with his eyes closed. Multiple sclerosis

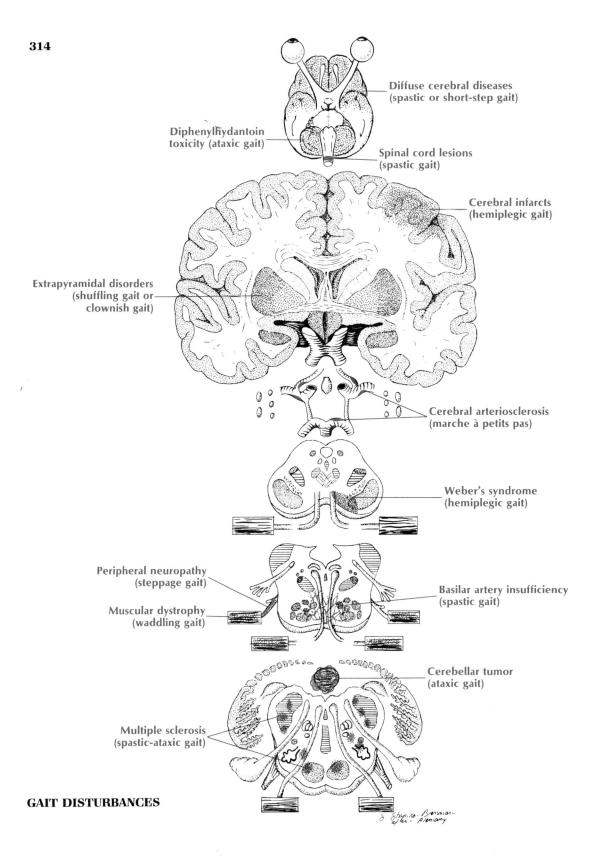

Diffuse cerebral diseases
(spastic or short-step gait)

Diphenylhydantoin
toxicity (ataxic gait)

Spinal cord lesions
(spastic gait)

Cerebral infarcts
(hemiplegic gait)

Extrapyramidal disorders
(shuffling gait or
clownish gait)

Cerebral arteriosclerosis
(marche à petits pas)

Weber's syndrome
(hemiplegic gait)

Peripheral neuropathy
(steppage gait)

Muscular dystrophy
(waddling gait)

Basilar artery insufficiency
(spastic gait)

Cerebellar tumor
(ataxic gait)

Multiple sclerosis
(spastic-ataxic gait)

GAIT DISTURBANCES

and syringomyelia may involve both the dorsal columns, pyramidal and spinocerebellar tracts, or cerebellum, producing a mixed spastic-ataxic gait.

6. **Muscular dystrophy gait.** This is wide-based with a pelvic tilt forward as if the patient is trying to "show-off," but the feet are lifted from the ground with difficulty and there is waddling or rolling from side to side.

7. **Extrapyramidal disease gait.** The gait is short-stepped, spastic, and the feet shuffle along the ground. The patient may tilt forward with trunk and head bent toward the ground, causing acceleration (propulsion). At time the reverse may occur (retropulsion). In Huntington's chorea the gait is clownish and grotesque, as if the patient were drunk but playing games.

Approach to the Diagnosis

The workup depends on the presence or absence of other neurological signs. If a peripheral nerve lesion is suspected a workup for diabetes and a careful history for alcoholism and porphyria are expected. A suspected spinal cord lesion requires x-rays of the spinal column, spinal tap, Schilling's test, and possibly a myelogram. When the lesion is believed to be in the brain or brain stem an EEG and CT scan are almost axiomatic before a spinal tap or other radiocontrast studies are considered. Other tests are listed in Appendix I. A neurologist or neurosurgeon can best decide how the workup should be conducted.

GIGANTISM ■

The differential of this symptom can be developed physiologically by overactivity or underactivity of an endocrine gland. Thus overactivity of the pituitary gland (as in eosinophilic adenomas of the pituitary) causes gigantism from too much growth hormone, whereas underactivity of the testicles (as in Klinefelter's syndrome) produces a tall individual because the inadequate secretion of testosterone delays closure of the epiphysis. Tumors of the adrenal cortex, testicle and pineal gland may produce macrogenitosomia or prepubertal gigantism by stimulation of overgrowth by androgens and estrogens only to lead to ultimate dwarfism by premature closure of the epiphysis.

Primary gigantism is like the gigantism of plants and flowers; genetic arachnodactyly is also a genetic form of gigantism, although it is a true disease and is associated with dislocation of the lens.

Approach to the Diagnosis

The approach to the diagnosis of these conditions is simple Radioimmunoassay (RIA) studies of the hormone levels are now readily available and roentgenograms of the skull with CT scans and tomography will allow a diagnosis. Referral to an endocrinologist may be wise from the start, especially because potentially tall girls may want endocrine therapy to close the epiphysis early.

316

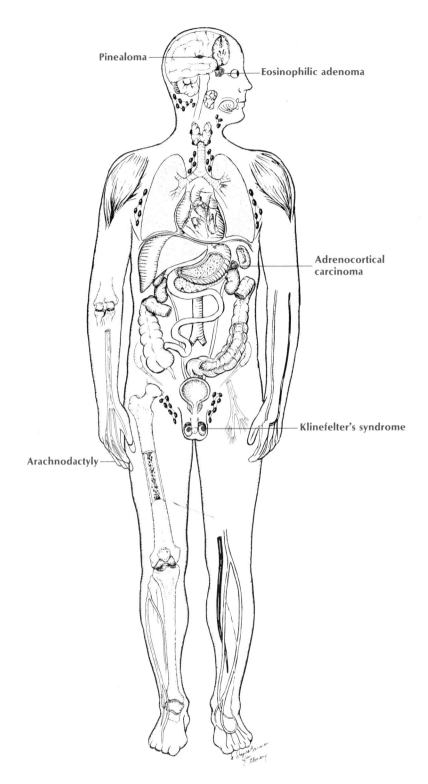

Pinealoma

Eosinophilic adenoma

Adrenocortical carcinoma

Klinefelter's syndrome

Arachnodactyly

GIGANTISM

HALLUCINATIONS ◼

A hallucination is seeing, hearing, touching, smelling, or tasting something that is not there. Auditory hallucinations without evidence of mental deterioration usually indicate schizophrenia, but epilepsy, drug toxicity, and brain tumors must be excluded. Visual hallucinations are often the sign of drug or alcohol intoxication but occasionally they occur in schizophrenia. Hallucinations with mental deterioration should prompt the recall of the differential diagnosis for memory loss (see p. 349).

When faced with a hallucinating patient, think of the mnemonic **MINT** and a list of possibilities can be recalled easily.

M—Mental disease brings to mind schizophrenia, manic-depressive psychosis, and paranoid states.

I—Intoxication and **inflammation** suggest alcoholism, cannabis, LSD, bromism, various other drugs, and encephalitis, cerebral abscess (temporal lobe especially), and syphilis. The "**I**" should also suggest **Idiopathic** disorders such as epilepsy, presenile dementia, and arteriosclerosis.

N—Neoplasm would suggest brain tumors. A tumor of the occipital lobe may present with visual hallucinations, whereas a tumor of the temporal lobe causes auditory hallucinations or uncinate fits (*i.e.*, bad smells). A tumor of the parietal lobe may present with tingling or other paresthesias of the body.

T—Trauma should suggest concussions, epidural or subdural hematomas, and depressed skull fractures.

Approach to Diagnosis

In the workup of hallucinations, it is essential to get a drug history from a relative or friend if not from the patient. Ask about a family his-

tory of epilepsy or head trauma. A drug screen should be ordered. If there is no mental deterioration, referral to a psychiatrist may be done but an electroencephalogram may still be indicated. With mental deterioration, a neurologist should be consulted. When there is doubt about mental deterioration, psychological testing may be done. CT scans, EEGs, skull x-ray films, echoencephalography, and arteriograms may be necessary in selected cases.

HICCOUGHS ◼

A list of causes of this fairly common symptom is best developed by considering the **anatomy** of the structures associated with the phrenic nerve at its origin, along its pathway, and at its termination. Applying the mnemonic **MINT** to these structures allows one to arrive at a fairly complete list of possibilities.

Origin. Impulses transmitted along the phrenic nerve originate in the brain stem and spinal cord so diseases of these structures must be considered.

M—Malformations to be considered are hydrocephalus and kernicterus.

I—Inflammatory and intoxicating conditions that are possible causes are encephalitis, toxic encephalopathy (*e.g.*, alcohol, bromides, drugs, and uremia), and, in the spinal cord particularly, tabes dorsalis. Meningitis may be associated with persistent hiccoughs. Epidemic hiccoughs is probably a form of encephalitis.

N—Neoplasms of the brain may cause hiccoughs, especially when they are associated with increased intracranial pressure.

T—Traumatic lesions (*e.g.*, concussions and

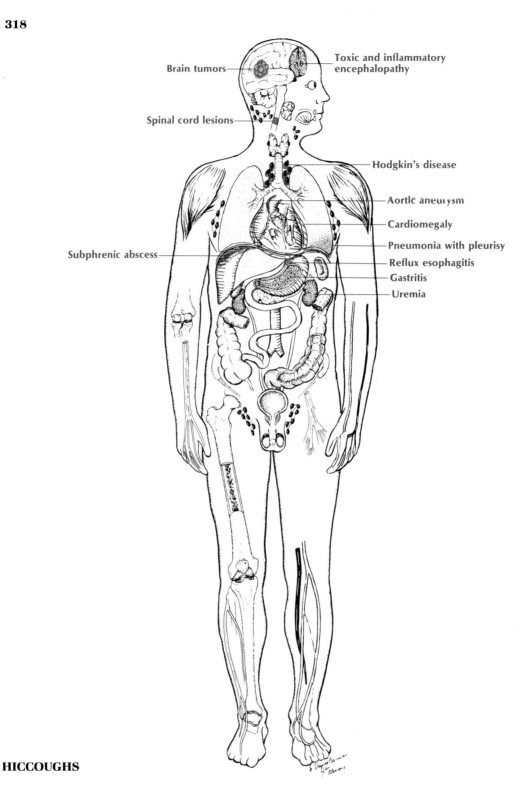

Brain tumors

Toxic and inflammatory encephalopathy

Spinal cord lesions

Hodgkin's disease

Aortic aneurysm

Cardiomegaly

Pneumonia with pleurisy

Reflux esophagitis

Gastritis

Uremia

Subphrenic abscess

HICCOUGHS

hematomas). Supratentorial conditions (such as neurosis) may be associated with hiccough, but this is present only during the waking hours and the patient eats surprisingly well.

Pathway. Along the pathway of the phrenic nerve mediastinal and chest conditions are important.

M—Malformations such as aortic aneurysm, dermoid cyst, and enlarged heart from whatever cause should be considered.
I—Inflammatory lesions such as pericarditis, mediastinitis, pneumonia, and pleurisy are equally important.
N—Neoplasm here, particularly Hodgkin's disease and bronchogenic carcinoma, may cause hiccoughs.
T—Trauma, particularly penetrating wounds of the chest causing pneumothorax and hemopneumothorax, are often associated with hiccoughs.

Termination. The most common causes of hiccoughs are found in the diaphragm.

M—Malformations include hiatal hernia, pyloric obstruction, and Barrett's esophagitis.
I—Inflammation suggests reflux or bile esophagitis, gastritis, hepatitis, cholecystitis, peritonitis, and subphrenic abscess.
N—Neoplasms include esophageal carcinoma, carcinoma of the stomach, and retroperitoneal Hodgkin's disease and sarcoma.
T—Trauma includes hemoperitoneum from ruptured spleen or liver, ruptured viscus, or ruptured ectopic pregnancy. One other group of causes is the reflex stimulation of the phrenic nerve from organs far beneath the diaphragm. For example, carcinoma of the uterus or colon without metastasis may occasionally cause hiccoughs.

Approach to the Diagnosis

The usual reaction to a patient with hiccough, is "they'll get over them regardless of what we do so why worry about them." If, however, one puts himself in the position of the patient, it behooves him to be certain a grave condition such as uremia or subdiaphragmatic abscess is not present. In the otherwise healthy patient, esophagoscopy and gastroscopy often reveal a reflux esophagitis or gastritis. Cholecystograms, liver and pancreatic function studies, spinal tap, and brain and total body scan have their place in individual cases. The laboratory workup may be found under Vomiting, page 358 (Appendix I).

HOARSENESS ■

Neuroanatomy provides the most useful basic science in developing a list of causes for hoarseness. Hoarseness may occur from involvement of the larynx, myoneural junction of the vocal cord muscles, vagus nerve, of the brain stem. When these structures are cross-indexed with the many etiologies suggested by the mnemonic **VINDICATE,** a chart like Table 5-10 can be prepared.

The **larynx** may be involved with acute infections like diphtheria and influenza and with chronic infections like tuberculosis and syphilis. It may also be involved with allergy, neoplasms, and chronic trauma from overuse of the voice. Smoking and alcohol are common causes of hoarseness. Hypothyroidism may present with hoarseness.

The **myoneural junctions** prompt the recall of myasthenia gravis, whereas the peripheral portion of the vagus nerve prompts the recall of the greatest number of disorders; thyroid tumors and surgery to the thyroid, mediastinal tumors, and aortic aneurysms are only a few. Lead and diphtheria may cause a neuritis to this nerve. The **intracranial portions of the vagus** may be involved by basilar artery aneurysms, basilar meningitis, platybasia, and foramen magnum tumors.

In the **brain stem,** the nucleus ambiguus is involved in poliomyelitis, ependymomas, Wal-

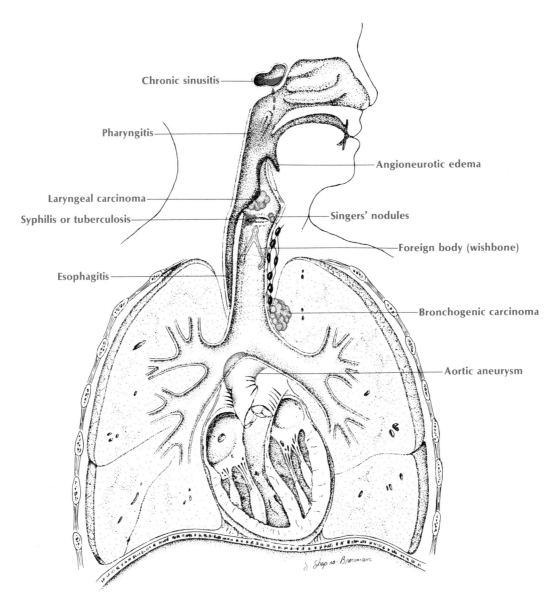

- Chronic sinusitis
- Pharyngitis
- Laryngeal carcinoma
- Syphilis or tuberculosis
- Esophagitis
- Angioneurotic edema
- Singers' nodules
- Foreign body (wishbone)
- Bronchogenic carcinoma
- Aortic aneurysm

HOARSENESS

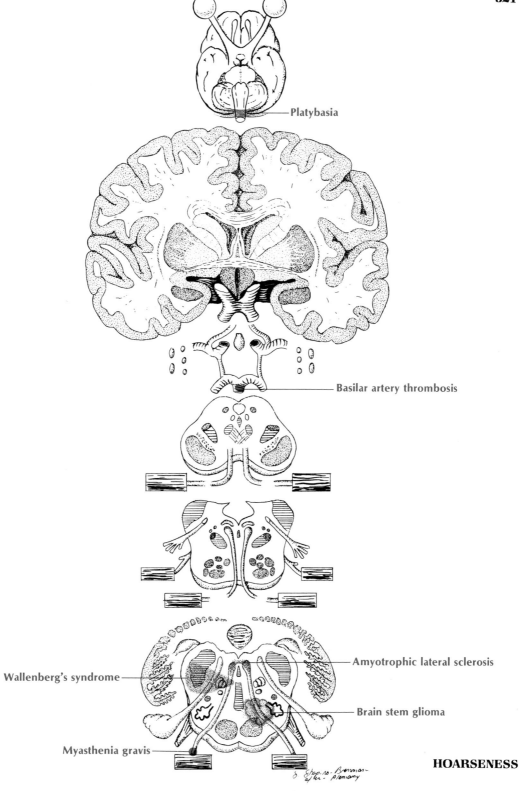

Platybasia

Basilar artery thrombosis

Wallenberg's syndrome

Myasthenia gravis

Amyotrophic lateral sclerosis

Brain stem glioma

HOARSENESS

TABLE 5-10.   HOARSENESS

	V Vascular	I Inflammatory	N Neoplasm	D Degenerative and Deficiency
Larynx		Viral upper respiratory infection Diphtheria Syphilis Tuberculosis Sinusitis Epiglottitis	Singers' nodes Polyps Carcinoma	
Myoneural Junction				
Vagus Nerve: Extracranial Portion	Aortic aneurysms Mitral stenosis	Mediastinitis Tuberculosis Sarcoid Diphtheria	Hodgkin's disease Bronchogenic carcinoma Esophageal carcinoma	
Vagus: Intracranial Portion	Aneurysms Jugular vein thrombosis	Syphilis Tuberculosis Meningitis	Tumor of ganglion Foramen magnum tumor	
Brain Stem	Wallenberg's syndrome Basilar artery insufficiency	Encephalitis Poliomyelitis Syringobulbia Syphilis	Brain stem glioma Metastasis	Amyotrophic lateral sclerosis

lenberg's syndrome, syringomyelia, and amyotrophic lateral sclerosis. Multiple sclerosis and gliomas may involve the roots of the ambiguus nucleus as they pass through the brain stem white matter.

Approach to the Diagnosis

A careful examination of the larynx with a laryngoscope or the fiberoptic bronchoscope is essential. The indirect laryngeal mirror is difficult to use and probably should be discarded by those unfamiliar with its use. If no local disease is found, evidence of vagal nerve palsy will be noted by the cord paralysis. A chest x-ray film, thyroid function tests, blood lead level, and Tensilon test may be necessary to diagnose recurrent laryngeal involvement. Intracranial lesions will demonstrate other neurological signs. A skull roentgenogram, CT scan, and spinal tap will probably give valuable clues to their cause. X-ray films of the cervical spine, a rheumatoid-arthritis (R-A) test, arteriography, and other tests that may be necessary are listed in Appendix I.

I Intoxication and Idiopathic	C Congenital	A Autoimmune Allergic	T Trauma	E Endocrine
Smoking Alcohol Gout	Laryngeal web	Angioneurotic edema Cricothyroid arthritis	Overuse of voice Foreign body Fracture	Hypothyroidism Acromegaly
Anectine Cholinergic drugs		Myasthenia gravis		
Idiopathic paralysis Lead neuropathy			Thyroid surgery	Thyroid carcinoma Reidel's struma
	Platybasia			
		Multiple sclerosis		

HYPERMENORRHEA

The causes of hypermenorrhea or excessive menstrual bleeding can be easily recalled by simply applying the mnemonic **MINTS.**

M—Malformations include bicornate uterus, congenital ovarian cysts, endometriosis, ectopic pregnancies, and retained placenta.

I—Inflammation recalls cervicitis, endometritis, and pelvic inflammatory disease.

N—Neoplasms include fibroids, carcinoma, and polyps of the cervix and endometrium. One should also not forget choriocarcinoma, hydatidiform moles, and hormone-producing tumors of the ovary.

T—Trauma includes perforation of the uterus, excessive intercourse during the menses, and introduction of foreign bodies into the uterus.

S—Systemic diseases include anemia and the coagulation disorders like hemophilia, idiopathic thrombocytopenic purpura, and scurvy. Also in this category are lupus ery-

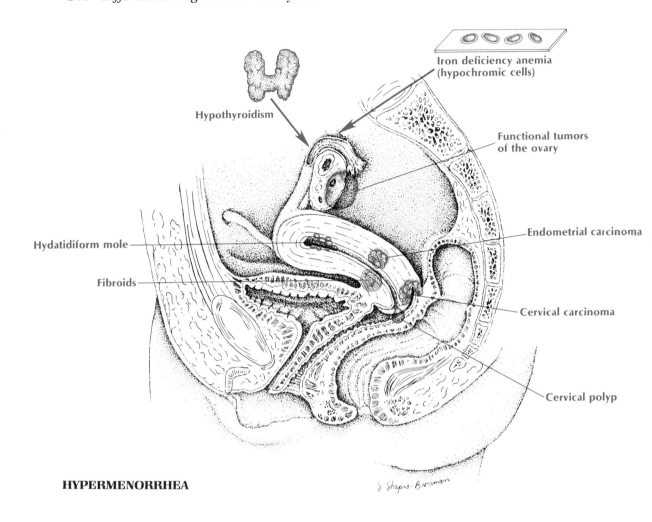

Hypothyroidism

Iron deficiency anemia
(hypochromic cells)

Functional tumors
of the ovary

Endometrial carcinoma

Hydatidiform mole

Fibroids

Cervical carcinoma

Cervical polyp

J. Shapiro-Brennan

HYPERMENORRHEA

thematosus and endocrine disorders, especially hypothyroidism and dysfunctional uterine bleeding from disproportion in the output of estrogen and progesterone by the ovary.

Approach to the Diagnosis

The diagnosis includes a thorough pelvic examination, a cbc and coagulation studies, thyroid function, and perhaps other endocrine tests. Ultrasonography is ordered next. If all these are normal, a trial of estrogen or progesterone supplementation or a D & C may be

indicated. Culdoscopy, peritoneoscopy, and a hysterosalpingogram may be necessary before performing an exploratory laparotomy and, if necessary, a hysterectomy.

HYPERTENSION ■

With the emphasis placed on the diagnosis and treatment of hypertension in the past 20 years, every physician has a fairly good knowledge of the causes of hypertension. His list

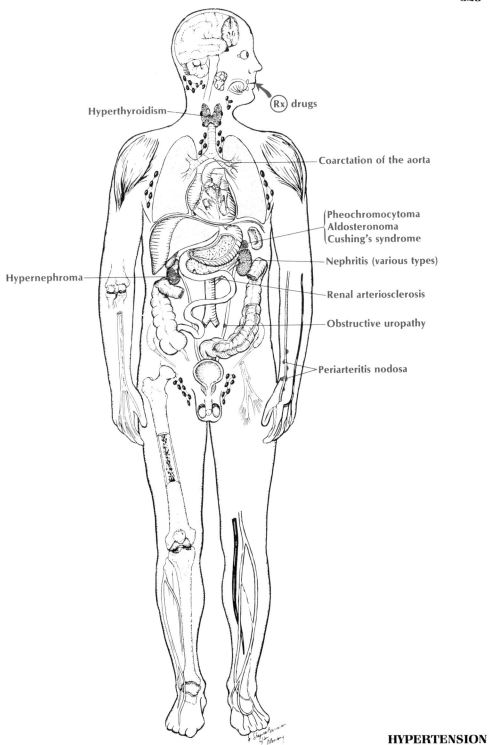

Hyperthyroidism

Rx drugs

Coarctation of the aorta

Pheochromocytoma
Aldosteronoma
Cushing's syndrome

Nephritis (various types)

Hypernephroma

Renal arteriosclerosis

Obstructive uropathy

Periarteritis nodosa

HYPERTENSION

TABLE 5-11. HYPERTENSION

	V Vascular	I Inflammatory	N Neoplasm	D Degenerative
Cardiovascular System		Aortic insufficiency	Polycythemia vera Intracranial tumors	Atherosclerosis Medionecrosis
Adrenal Gland			Pheochromocytomas Cushing's disease Primary aldosteronism	
Kidney	Atherosclerotic plague of renal artery (stenosis)	Pyelonephritis Renal tuberculosis	Hypernephroma Multiple myeloma	

nevertheless, may be incomplete. If consideration is to be given only to the treatable disorders, then one simply needs remember the cardiovascular system, adrenal gland, and kidney and apply the mnemonic **VINDICATE** to develop a list of the causes (Table 5-11). It is more instructive, however, to apply physiology in developing a differential.

Since blood pressure is maintained by an adequate blood volume, an adequate cardiac output, and appropriate vasomotor tone, it follows that hypertension may result from an increase in any one or more of these three factors.

1. **Increased blood volume.** This results in most cases from an increase in sodium chloride in the blood from primary aldosteronism (adrenal tumors) or from secondary aldosteronism (renovascular hypertension from glomerulonephritis and other primary renal diseases or obstruc-

tion of the renal arteries by atherosclerotic plagues or fibromuscular hyperplasia). Administration of corticosteroid drugs may cause hypertension by the same mechanism. Polycythemia vera is often associated with moderate hypertension because of increased red cell mass.

2. **Increased cardiac output.** This mechanism accounts for the systolic hypertension in hyperthyroidism, aortic insufficiency, patent ductus arteriosus, arteriovenous shunts, and Paget's disease.

3. **Increased vasomotor tone.** Increased output of epinephrine and norepinephrine as occurs in pheochromocytomas is one example of this type of hypertension. Administration of sympathomimetic drugs is another. Essential hypertension is probably based on this mechanism, but increased total body sodium leading to an increased blood volume is also probably a pathophysiological mechanism is essential

I Intoxication	C Congenital	A Allergic and Autoimmune	T Trauma	E Endocrine

Sympathomimetics
Exogenous corti-
  costeroids
Porphyria
	Coarctation of the aorta
	Patent ductus
	Essential hypertension
		Polyarteritis nodosa	A-V fistula
			Intracranial
			  hemorrhage
				Hyperthyroidism
				Acromegaly

				Adrenocortical hyperplasia

Toxic nephritis
Toxemia of preg-
  nancy
	Polycystic kidney
	Hydronephrosis
	Other anomalies
		Glomerulonephritis
		Vasculitis
				Kimmelstiel–
				  Wilson syndrome

hypertension. Unfortunately, this ap-proach omits dissecting aneurysm and coarctation of the aorta, two important causes of hypertension.

Approach to the Diagnosis

Take the blood pressure yourself to be sure the hypertension is real; 24-hour blood pressure monitoring is now available. The workup of hypertension includes a family his-tory, serial electrolytes, urinalysis and urine culture, and possibly "hypertensive" IVP and 24-hour urine VMA to rule out treatable causes of hypertension. A complete hyperten-sive workup is not usually performed today unless there is no family history of hyperten-sion; the hypertension does not respond to treatment; there are other symptoms suggest-ing a surgical lesion (*e.g.*, paroxysmal head-aches); or there is sudden onset of hyperten-sion in a known normotensive individual.

Appendix I gives all the tests that may be nec-essary in individual cases.

HYPOMENORRHEA AND AMENORRHEA ■

Combining the **anatomy** of the female genital tract with the **endocrine system** will key in on the major sources of absent or diminished menstrual flow. It is perhaps best to begin at the bottom and work upward to the head.

1. **Female genital tract.** Such congenital anomalies as an imperforate hymen, im-perforated vagina, cervical stenosis, double uterus, or the complete absence of any one or more of these organs would obviously cause amenorrhea. Radiation therapy may destroy the endometrium so that it cannot

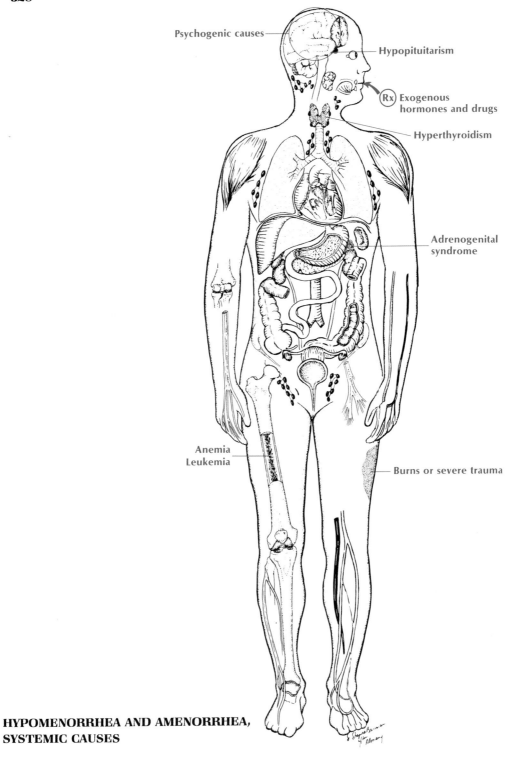

Psychogenic causes

Hypopituitarism

Rx Exogenous hormones and drugs

Hyperthyroidism

Adrenogenital syndrome

Anemia
Leukemia

Burns or severe trauma

**HYPOMENORRHEA AND AMENORRHEA,
SYSTEMIC CAUSES**

respond to female hormones. Pregnancy is the most common cause of amenorrhea, and it must be considered the cause of sudden onset of amenorrhea in an apparently normal female until proven otherwise. Excessive blood levels of endogenous or exogenous estrogen or progesterone will cause amenorrhea. The tubes should immediately suggest an ectopic pregnancy as the cause, although spotting and metrorrhagia are frequent in these cases.

2. **Ovary.** The mnemonic **MINTS** serves well in subdividing the causes here.

M—Malformations of the ovary include Turner's syndrome (where the ovaries are reduced to a fibrotic peasized nodule), Stein–Leventhal syndrome, and other congenital cysts. Acquired malformations suggest the atrophy of menopause, which may occur as early as the late 1920s.

I—Intoxication includes the ovarian dys-

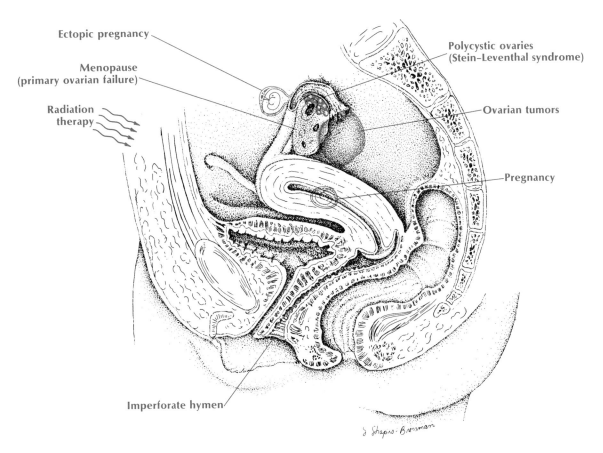

Ectopic pregnancy

Menopause (primary ovarian failure)

Radiation therapy

Polycystic ovaries (Stein–Leventhal syndrome)

Ovarian tumors

Pregnancy

Imperforate hymen

J. Shapiro-Brennman

HYPOMENORRHEA AND AMENORRHEA, LOCAL CAUSES

function of exogenous hormones, irradiation, chronic alcoholism, or drug addiction.

N—Neoplasms of the ovary frequently cause amenorrhea, especially if they secrete hormones or are bilateral. The arrhenoblastomas, granulosa cell and theca cell tumors, and cystadenocarcinomas must be considered in this category.

T—Trauma as a cause of amenorrhea is well known, but this is generally due to general body trauma like an auto accident, severe burns, or extensive surgery. Direct trauma to the ovary merely reminds one that oophorectomy can cause amenorrhea. Emotional trauma is probably a more common cause of amenorrhea than any of the above.

S—Systemic disease suggests the amenorrhea of leukemia, Hodgkin's disease, chronic nephritis, fever, and severe malnutrition.

3. **Thyroid.** It is well known that hyperthyroidism causes hypomenorrhea or amenorrhea whereas hypothyroidism causes hypermenorrhea; however, the exact reverse may occur.

4. **Adrenal gland.** Visualizing this organ should stimulate the recall of amenorrhea in the adrenogenital syndrome of adrenal hyperplasia or carcinomas and in Addison's disease.

5. **Pituitary gland. MINT** is a useful mnemonic here also.

M—Malformations here are Fröhlich's syndrome and Chiari–Frommel syndrome, but perhaps more important is the reduced output of pituitary hormone in many states of congenital mental retardation and brain damage.

I—Inflammation suggests the hypopituitarism of sarcoid and tuberculosis.

N—Neoplasm suggests the largest group of causes of hypopituitarism, including chromophobe adenomas and basophilic adenomas.

T—Trauma recalls the hypopituitarism of postpartum hemorrhage and amniotic fluid emboli or Sheehan's syndrome.

Approach to the Diagnosis

Obviously the first thing to do is rule out pregnancy both by examination and a pregnancy test, preferably the serum β subunit HCG. One must keep an ectopic pregnancy in mind even if the examination is normal and plan follow-up examinations. Altered secondary sex characteristics should be noted. If the examination fails to show evidence of pregnancy, congenital anomalies, and tumors of the ovaries, the physician should order thyroid function studies, a Wassermann test, cbc, and sedimentation rate. If these are normal a gynecologist should be consulted. He will probably give a test dose of IM progesterone to prove that the endometrium functions well. He may do a D & C first. Then serum or urine FSH, LH, and prolactin levels are done; if the FSH level is high, the ovary is probably the site of the trouble. If the levels are low, even after gonadotropin releasing factor (GRF) is administered, the pituitary is responsible. Roentgenograms of the skull, CT scans, culdoscopy, and exploratory laparotomy all share their place in the workup (Appendix I).

HYPOTENSION AND SHOCK ■

Many patients are told they have a low blood pressure and are even treated for it when that blood pressure may be entirely normal for them. Asymptomatic hypotension may not be pathological at all. At any rate, an expensive investigation for the causes of "hypotension"

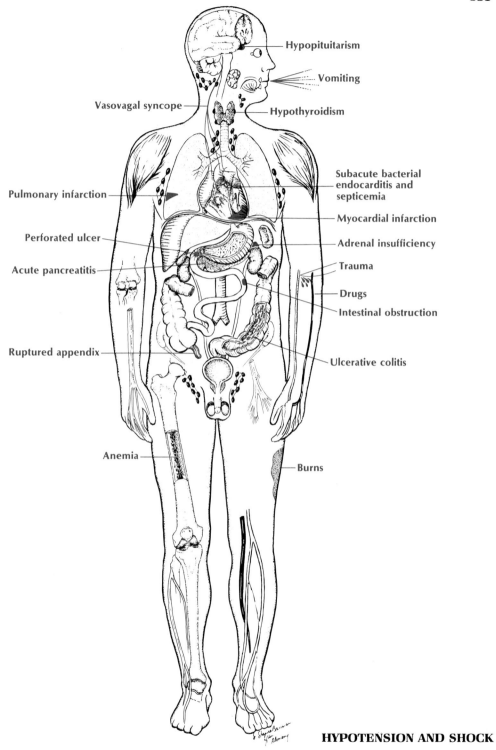

Hypopituitarism

Vomiting

Vasovagal syncope

Hypothyroidism

Pulmonary infarction

Subacute bacterial endocarditis and septicemia

Myocardial infarction

Perforated ulcer

Adrenal insufficiency

Acute pancreatitis

Trauma

Drugs

Intestinal obstruction

Ruptured appendix

Ulcerative colitis

Anemia

Burns

HYPOTENSION AND SHOCK

would seem unnecessary if the systolic pressure is above 80 mm, especially when the patient is asymptomatic.

The differential diagnosis of both hypotension and shock is best developed using **physiology**. There are three things that are necessary to sustain the blood pressure at the normal level: adequate blood volume, adequate cardiac output, and adequate tone in the arteries and arterioles. Alteration of any of these may produce hypotension.

Low blood volume may result from any of the following conditions:

1. Hemorrhagic shock such as acute upper GI bleeding
2. Chronic blood loss (*e.g.*, peptic ulcer) or anemia of decreased production (such as aplastic anemia) or increased destruction (hemolytic anemias)
3. Dehydration
4. Decreased NaCl in blood from pituitary and adrenal insufficiency, diuretics, diarrhea or vomiting, chronic nephritis, or severe diaphoresis
5. Decreased albumin in the blood from nephrosis, cirrhosis, and malnutrition or malabsorption syndrome. Any one of the conditions listed above may be associated with hypotension.

Decreased cardiac output usually results from congestive heart failure of many causes and myocardial infarction. Many valvular lesions (*e.g.*, mitral stenosis) may manifest hypotension without overt heart failure. Cor pulmonale may lead to hypotension from a decreased cardiac output.

Decreased arterial tone (*e.g.*, vasomotor shock) occurs in the following conditions:

1. When the sympathetic nerves are blocked by antihypertensive drugs (*e.g.*, alpha methyldopa, guanethidine, and pentoli-

nium tartrate), diabetic neuropathy, or after a sympathectomy
2. When there is increased vagal stimulation, as in neurogenic shock (common faint) and late stages of increased intracranial pressure
3. When toxins are introduced into the bloodstream from necrotic tissue, bacteria, or drugs that act directly on the arterioles. Examples of the last type of hypotension are pulmonary infarction (necrotic tissue), toxins, septicemia (bacterial toxins), and hydralazine therapy.

Approach to the Diagnosis

The workup of shock must be vigorous with stat cbc, blood cultures, blood gases, ECG, electrolytes, BUN, and type and cross-match of blood at the same time vigorous antishock measures are applied. Checking the GI tract for blood loss with a rectal and nasogastric tube can be both diagnostic and therapeutic.

To workup chronic hypotension, one should not forget venous pressure and circulation times (to diagnose decreased cardiac output and congestive heart failure), serial electrolytes and cortisol levels (to rule out adrenal insufficiency), and sedimentation rate and cultures of various body fluids to exclude a chronic infectious disease (*e.g.*, tuberculosis).

HYPOTHERMIA

Subnormal temperature is not usually a presenting finding, but when it is found in a case of coma, hypothyroidism (myxedema coma) is the first thing to rule out. Understanding the cause of this sign is best approached from a **physiological** standpoint. There are three basic reasons why a temperature drops: absolute decrease in metabolic rate, decreased cir-

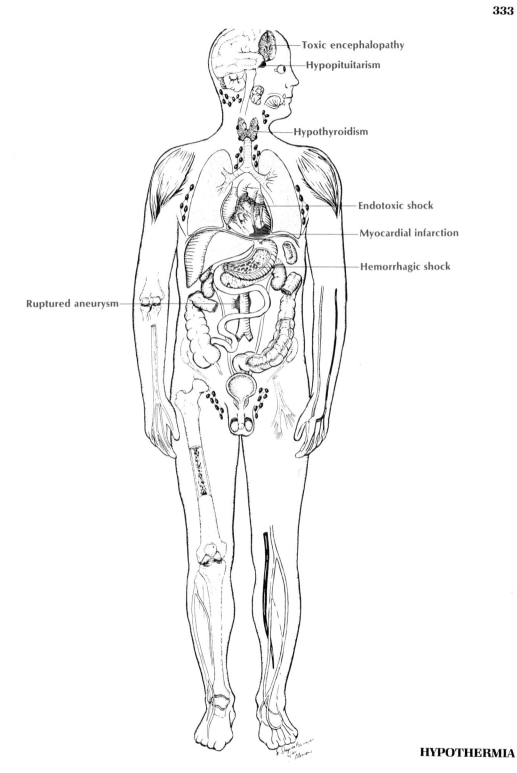

Toxic encephalopathy

Hypopituitarism

Hypothyroidism

Endotoxic shock

Myocardial infarction

Hemorrhagic shock

Ruptured aneurysm

HYPOTHERMIA

culation to the area where the temperature is being recorded, and disorders of the thermoregulatory center in the brain.

1. **Decreased metabolic rate.** Hypothyroidism and hypopituitarism are the principal conditions that fall in this category. Senility, starvation, and chronic inanition may cause hypothermia on the same basis. Diabetes mellitus may cause hypothermia because of poor cellular absorption of glucose.

2. **Poor circulation.** Shock from any cause (hypovolemia, cardiogenic, or neurogenic) falls into this category. Hemorrhagic shock, dehydration, congestive heart failure, and adrenal insufficiency are all probably based on this mechanism. With poor circulation there is tissue anoxia and a reduced metabolism in the skin and mucosa where the temperature is taken.

3. **Disorders of the thermoregulatory center.** Cerebral thrombosis and hemorrhage, certain pituitary tumors, toxic suppression of this center by barbiturates, alcohol, opiates, and general anesthesia all fit into this category. Any case of prolonged coma may cause hypothermia on this basis.

Approach to the Diagnosis

Establishing a definitive diagnosis of hypothermia depends heavily on the interpretation of other symptoms and signs. A good history is invaluable as well as laboratory studies including FBS, thyroid functions, electrolytes, BUN and drug screens; in selected cases, a spinal tap may be useful.

IMPOTENCE ■

Impotence may be due to local end-organ disease, dysfunction of the peripheral nerve pathways, disease of the spinal cord or brain, pituitary and other endocrine disorders, and "supratentorial" disorders. Thus recall of the various causes is based on both **anatomy** and **physiology.**

1. **End-organ disorders.** These include phimosis, paraphimosis, prostatitis and prostatic carcinoma, and Peyronie's disease.

2. **Peripheral nerve disorders.** Diabetic neuropathy is a common cause in this category, but alcoholic neuropathy and other neuropathies may occasionally cause impotence.

3. **Spinal cord disorders.** Transverse myelitis, poliomyelitis, compression fractures, spinal cord tumors, multiple sclerosis, and tabes dorsalis are important disorders to be considered here.

4. **Disorders of the brain.** In addition to general paresis, brain tumors, vascular occlusions, and arteriosclerosis, the degenerative diseases such as Alzheimer's disease, senile dementia, and Schilder's disease will cause impotence.

5. **Pituitary and other endocrine disorders.** Impotence is found in pituitary tumors, acromegaly, testicular atrophy from hemochromatosis, mumps, Klinefelter's syndrome and other causes, and even in Cushing's disease and hypothyroidism.

6. **Supratentorial disorders.** This is the cause of perhaps 90% of the cases of impotence. There are several reasons for this. After years of marriage and intercourse with the same sexual partner, one's libido may decline considerably. The first time the male has trouble reaching an erection he begins to believe he is "over the hill." If he should happen to acquire a young mistress he may find convincing proof that his impotence is psychological

Sometimes, in search of variety in his sexual life, a married man may decide to find a new sexual partner. When the moment of truth arrives he may be unable to get an erection be-

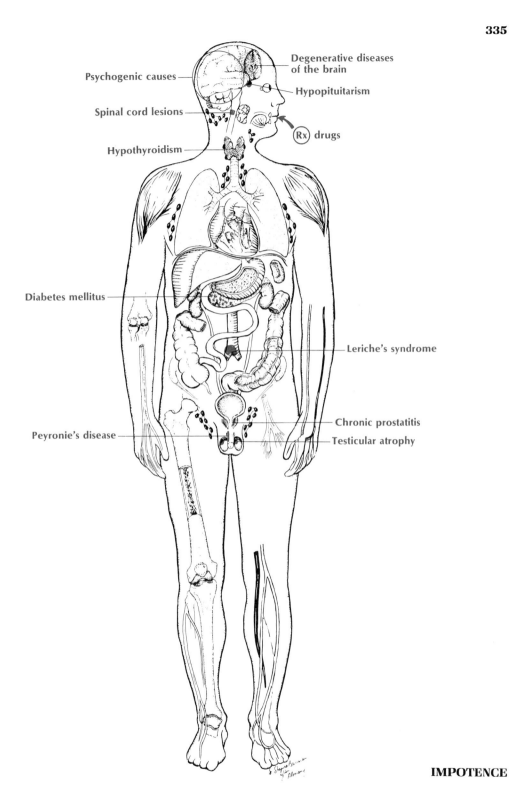

Psychogenic causes

Degenerative diseases
of the brain

Hypopituitarism

Spinal cord lesions

Rx drugs

Hypothyroidism

Diabetes mellitus

Leriche's syndrome

Chronic prostatitis

Peyronie's disease

Testicular atrophy

IMPOTENCE

cause of the associated guilt involved. Premature ejaculation is common under these circumstances also. After his first failure the fear of a repeat performance may make him impotent not only in extramarital relations, but also in marital relations.

Young men, whether married or unmarried, may "fall into impotence" quite by accident because of alcoholic intoxication. As Shakespeare correctly surmised, "alcohol provokes the desire, but it takes away the performance." Under the influence of alcohol the inspired lover may fail miserably. When sober once more, he may begin a pattern of failure to get an erection simply because of the fear that it will happen again and he will be embarrassed beyond belief.

Some other "supratentorial" causes of impotence are endogenous: depression, schizophrenia, latent homosexuality, repressed hostility toward the partner, and fear of pregnancy. It is important to note that all of the above psychological causes may occur in the female as well as the male. There are many more causes too numerous to mention in a book of this scope.

Approach to the Diagnosis

A careful examination of the external genitalia, the prostate, and secondary sex characteristics is essential. The laboratory workup may include a glucose tolerance test, blood testosterone and cortisol levels, thyroid function studies, a spinal tap, a skull roentgenogram, and a chromosomal analysis. A nocturnal penile tumescence study is performed to rule out organic causes. If the physical examination is normal it may be wise to administer psychometric tests or refer the patient to a psychiatrist before doing an extensive endocrine and neurological workup. A sympathetic physician may be able to find the "supratentorial" cause and cure it with a few long discussions with the patient. A women physi-

cian may have more success in this area than a man.

INCONTINENCE, URINARY

Incontinence may be due to loss of voluntary control of urination, in which case neurological disorders are usually the cause, or it may result from overflow of a distended bladder (overflow incontinence), in which case the causes may be bladder neck obstruction or a flaccid neurogenic bladder.

1. **Loss of voluntary control.** The neurological causes include multiple sclerosis, neurosyphilis, syringomyelia, encephalitis, cerebral arteriosclerosis, frontal lobe tumors and abscesses, senile dementia, and transverse myelitis from trauma or infection. The local causes are a cystocele (often following a hysterectomy) and a damaged urethral sphincter from prostatectomy.
2. **Bladder neck obstruction.** Benign prostatic hypertrophy, chronic prostatitis, prostatic carcinoma, median bar hypertrophy, vesical calculus, and urethral stricture are important mechanical causes of obstruction.
3. **Flaccid neurogenic bladder.** Drugs such as atropine, tranquilizers, and anesthetics and diseases of the cauda equina and nervi erigentes such as diabetic neuropathy, poliomyelitis, tabes dorsalis, and cauda equina tumors will cause a flaccid neurogenic bladder with overflow incontinence.

Approach to the Diagnosis

First, exclude stress incontinence with a pad test. Perineal pads are weighed before and after walking and stress for 30 minutes. An increase in weight identifies urine loss. Cathe-

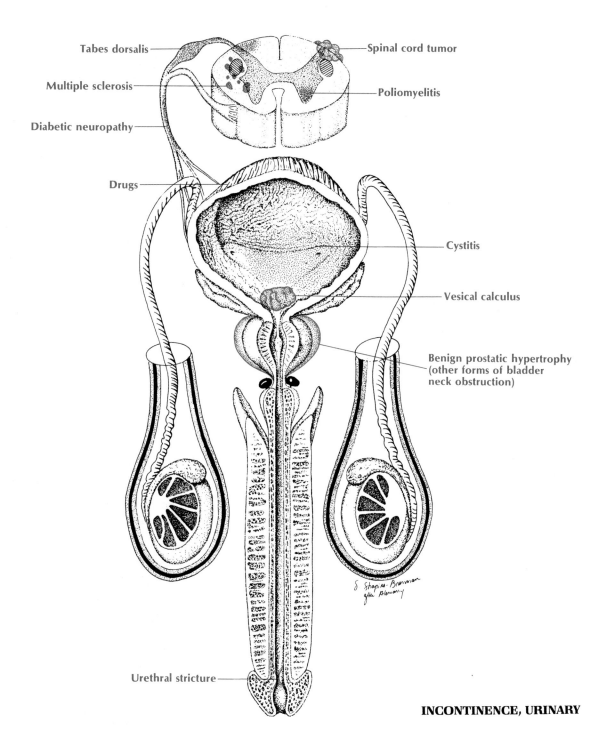

Tabes dorsalis

Multiple sclerosis

Diabetic neuropathy

Drugs

Spinal cord tumor

Poliomyelitis

Cystitis

Vesical calculus

Benign prostatic hypertrophy
(other forms of bladder
neck obstruction)

Urethral stricture

INCONTINENCE, URINARY

terization and examination, smear, and culture of the urine are essential at the outset. Cystoscopy and cystometric studies are often needed. Surgical repair of a cystocele or a parasympathomimetic drug in cases of a flaccid neurogenic bladder and probanthine (parasympatholytic drug) for spastic neurogenic bladders may be all that is necessary. A neurologist and urologist often need to cooperate in the diagnosis and treatment of these unfortunate individuals.

INDIGESTION

This is a vague term, and if the patient is put on the spot he will usually describe his problem as heartburn, regurgitation of water brash, fullness in the stomach, or frequent belching following meals. Usually the patient's appetite is not affected nor is there any weight loss.

The causes are easy to arrive at by merely asking the question, "Why would food cause these symptoms?" Obviously the food or drink ingested may be the source of irritation: spicy foods, coffee, alcohol, excessive fried food (which actually suppresses the secretion of gastric juice and slows gastric emptying), and insufficiently masticated food. The patient may sometimes be allergic to a particular food.

The upper GI tract may be already irritated with reflux esophagitis from a hiatal hernia, gastritis, gastric ulcer or duodenal ulcer; or it may be partially obstructed by a carcinoma of the esophagus or stomach or a pyloric ulcer. Chronic appendicitis and regional ileitis may cause partial obstruction or paralytic ileus. There may be diminished secretion of GI juices in pernicious anemia, cholecystitis and cholelithiasis, hepatitis, chronic pancreatitis or pancreatic carcinoma, or in patients with previous gastrectomies.

There may be a systemic illness that is associated with GI irritation or paralytic ileus. In this category one must consider congestive heart failure, electrolyte disturbances such as hypokalemia (diuretics) or hyperkalemia (Addison's disease) and abdominal angina, migraine, or epilepsy. Anemia and diabetic acidosis may produce similar symptoms.

Is there another way of recalling these conditions that may be simpler? Yes, the application of the "target" method to the anatomy of the internal organs. In the "bull's eye" one would think of the esophagus and stomach (esophagitis, esophageal carcinoma, gastritis, gastric ulcer, and gastric carcinoma); in the next circle one would consider gallbladder, pancreatic, liver, and heart disease; and, in the final circle, kidney, central nervous system, hormonal alterations, and other systemic diseases.

A third approach is simply to apply the mnemonic **MINT** to the organs of the upper abdomen. It is recommended that the reader apply this method as an exercise. Table 5-12 applies the mnemonic **VINDICATE** to the same organs.

Approach to the Diagnosis

The association of other symptoms and signs is important. If there is relief by antacids, then esophagitis, gastritis, or an ulcer may be present. If there is blood in the stool, one should suspect an ulcer or carcinoma. Roentgenographic studies in the form of an upper GI series and esophagram, a cholecystogram, and a barium enema are usually indicated. A gastric analysis, esophagoscopy, and gastroscopy often need to be done. Awareness that a systemic disease such as an electrolyte disturbance or uremia may be the cause will suggest the need for other studies, especially if there are systemic symptoms, fever, or shortness of breath. These may be found in Appendix I.

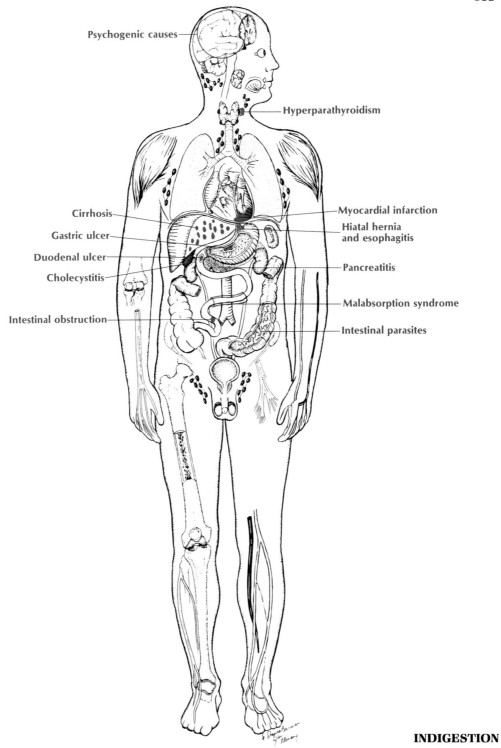

Psychogenic causes

Hyperparathyroidism

Cirrhosis

Myocardial infarction

Gastric ulcer

Hiatal hernia
and esophagitis

Duodenal ulcer

Cholecystitis

Pancreatitis

Malabsorption syndrome

Intestinal obstruction

Intestinal parasites

INDIGESTION

TABLE 5-12. INDIGESTION

	V Vascular	I Inflammatory	N Neoplasm	D Degenerative
Esophagus	Varices	Esophagitis	Esophageal carcinoma	Plummer–Vinson syndrome
Stomach		Gastritis Ulcer	Carcinoma	Atrophic gastritis Pernicious anemia
Duodenum and Small Intestines	Abdominal angina	Duodenitis Ulcer	Polyps	
Gallbladder		Cholecystitis	Cholangiocarcinoma	
Liver	Congestive heart failure	Infectious hepatitis	Hepatoma metastatic carcinoma	Cirrhosis
Pancreas		Pancreatitis	Pancreatic carcinoma	
Kidney		Pyelonephritis		

INFERTILITY ■

Fertility depends on a healthy sperm reaching a freshly laid egg and impregnating it, and the fertilized egg's digging into a healthy endometrium and being maintained in a healthy state until term. By visualizing the path the sperm must follow to reach the egg one can come up with many important causes of infertility. Male fertility, however, depends on a healthy pituitary gland and testicles, and female fertility depends on a healthy ovary and pituitary.

Thus, in the male, hypopituitarism, testicular atrophy (as in mumps), vas deferens obstruction (due to gonorrhea or tuberculosis), prostatitis and other prostatic disease, hypospadius, and other abnormalities of the urethra may cause infertility. Failure of copulation may cause infertility; the causes of this disorder are discussed under Frigidity and Impotence (see pp. 312 and 336).

In the female genital tract the sperm may encounter antibodies, vaginitis, vaginal deformities, cervicitis, cervical carcinoma, endometritis or carcinoma of the endometrium, a

I Intoxication Idiopathic	C Congenital	A Autoimmune Allergic	T Trauma	E Endocrine
Lye stricture	Hiatal hernia Diverticulitis Barrett's esopha- gitis	Scleroderma		
Aspirin Steroids Reserpine Alcohol Coffee	Cascade stomach		Gastrectomy	Zollinger–Ellison syndrome
	Diverticuli	Scleroderma	Gastrectomy with afferent loop obstruction	Zollinger–Ellison syndrome Uremic ulcer
	Stones from sickle cell anemia		Calculi	
Alcoholic cirrhosis				
	Fibrocystic dis- ease			Hyperparathyroidism
Uremia			Calculi	

retroverted uterus and other deformities, and obstruction of the tubes by a tubo-ovarian abscess or endometriosis. The ovary may not be able to develop an egg because of hypopituitarism or ovarian diseases, such as Stein–Leventhal polycystic ovaries, ovarian cysts, and tumors (especially hormone-secreting tumors of the ovary that prevent the variation in estrogen–progesterone concentration necessary during the cycle that allows maturation of the egg). There may be no ovaries present from birth (Turner's syndrome) or there may be acquired ovarian failure (surgical removal or early menopause). Thyroid disorders (hyper- and hypothyroidism) are known to cause infertility. Adrenocortical tumors and hyperplasia may also cause infertility.

Approach to the Diagnosis

The workup of infertility first involves doing a sperm count on the male. If that is normal, then, provided the examination of the female discloses no gross abnormality, a temperature chart is kept by the patient or the Spim–Barkeit test is used to determine if the female

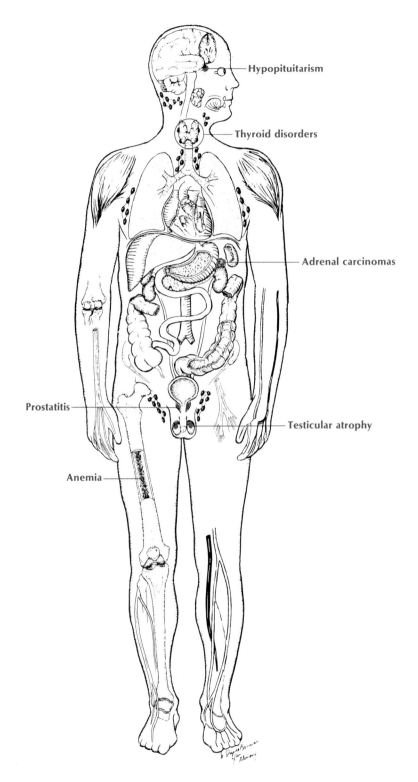

Hypopituitarism

Thyroid disorders

Adrenal carcinomas

Prostatitis

Testicular atrophy

Anemia

INFERTILITY

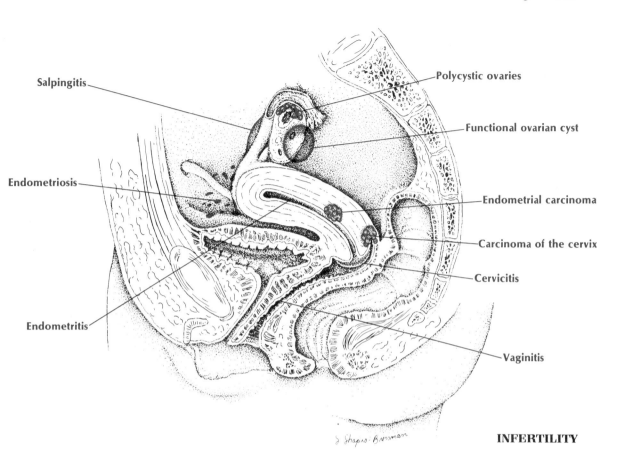

Salpingitis

Endometriosis

Endometritis

Polycystic ovaries

Functional ovarian cyst

Endometrial carcinoma

Carcinoma of the cervix

Cervicitis

Vaginitis

J Shapiro-Brennan

INFERTILITY

ovulates. Thyroid function studies, serum/prolactin, FSH and LH, and estradiol and progesterone levels may all be done if ovulation is proved not to take place. Other tests such as tubal insufflation, hysterosalpingogram, and a trial of clomiphene will be useful in selected cases. Often establishing the time of ovulation and assuring copulation at that time solves the problem. Cauterizing a chronic cervicitis may lead to fertility. Counselling about emotional problems may be necessary. These and other procedures are summarized in Appendix I.

INSOMNIA

It is customary to assume that the cause of the disorder is psychogenic and simply to prescribe a sleeping pill to anyone suffering from insomnia, hoping that it will go away by itself. Although this may be true in many cases, the conscientious clinician should rule out organic disease and investigate the hygiene and psyche of the patient before he prescribes a medication that may launch him on a lifelong habit.

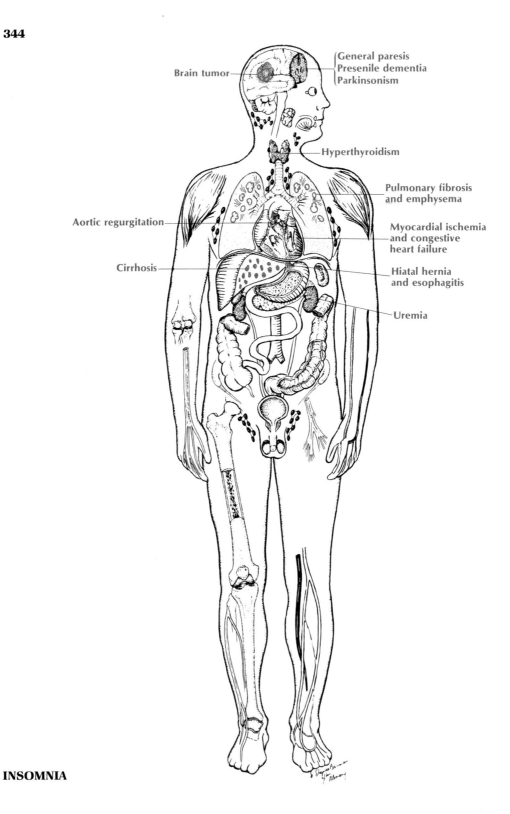

Brain tumor

General paresis
Presenile dementia
Parkinsonism

Hyperthyroidism

Pulmonary fibrosis
and emphysema

Aortic regurgitation

Myocardial ischemia
and congestive
heart failure

Cirrhosis

Hiatal hernia
and esophagitis

Uremia

INSOMNIA

Anatomy is the key to a differential of the many organic causes. Visualizing the many organs of the body, one can discover most of the significant causes. Beginning with the **stomach** and the **esophagus**, one should recall indigestion from alcoholic gastritis, overeating or reflux esophagitis, and hiatal hernia. Cirrhosis of the **liver** may cause insomnia because of nocturnal delirium. **Renal** diseases may cause insomnia because of nocturia or because of the toxic effects of uremia. **Heart** diseases, particularly those associated with pulmonary edema or arrhythmias, may awaken the patient with paroxysmal nocturnal dyspnea or palpitations. Aortic regurgitation in particular awakens the patient because of the noise of his own heart. **Lung** diseases such as emphysema interfere with breathing, and both the cerebral anoxia and the fear of not being able to breathe cause insomnia. Upper airway obstruction from rhinitis, snoring, and epiglottitis cause insomnia.

The **thyroid** may be the site of origin of insomnia, particularly in the thyroid storm of Graves' disease. Anemia of any kind will cause insomnia if it is severe enough to cause cerebral anoxia. Skeletal deformities such as rheumatoid spondylitis may cause insomnia by forcing the patient to sleep in a chair.

In the **nervous system** the many neurological disorders that can cause insomnia can be remembered by using **INSOMNIA** as a mnemonic.

I—Intoxication results from central nervous system (CNS) stimulants such as amphetamines and caffeine. Although drugs and alcohol initially sedate the drinker, they produce a subsequent period of excitation.

N—Neuropsychiatric disorders include neurosis, manic-depressive psychosis, and schizophrenia.

S—Syphilis, seizure disorders, and senile dementia are included.

O—Opiate addiction

M—Mental retardation and malformations such as hydrocephalus may be responsible for insomnia. The hyperactive child syndrome is just one example of a brain damaged child with potential insomnia.

N—Neoplasms of the brain may cause insomnia or somnolence. When the tumor leads to increased intracranial pressure there may eventually be coma.

I—Inflammatory diseases include viral encephalitis, tuberculosis, cryptococcosus, and various parasites.

A—Arteriosclerosis (cerebral and cerebral **arterial occlusions.**

Frequently the insomnia is related to some physiological or environmental problem. A sagging mattress, a room that is too hot or too cold, a poor pillow (or too many pillows), and excessive noise or light all are environmental factors that may cause insomnia. Lack of exercise, mental exhaustion, muscular aches and pain from hard work or exercise, hunger, and too much sleep in the afternoon are some of the physiological conditions that may cause insomnia.

Approach to the Diagnosis

In the approach to the diagnosis every physician should take the time to talk to the patient about possible reasons for fear or hostility. A nagging wife or mother-in-law, financial worries, a strict boss, or fear of losing his job are just a few examples of problems that can be handled with some sympathetic professional help. A good physical examination and neurological examination may reveal any organic cause. The laboratory evaluation will be based on suspicion of one or more of the diseases mentioned above and using Appendix I. A skull x-ray film, EEG, CT scan, and possibly a spinal tap are indicated if a neurological disorder is strongly suspected.

JAUNDICE

Jaundice is not to be confused with xantho-chromia, in which the skin turns orange from carotene deposits but the sclera remains normal in appearance. Carotenemia is often seen in hypothyroidism and diabetes mellitus, but jaundice is not usually a complication of these two conditions.

The causes of jaundice can best be estab-

lished by applying physiology (Table 5-13). Jaundice develops from hyperbilirubinemia and may not be noticed until the bilirubin exceeds 3 or 4 mg/dl. Hyperbilirubinemia is due to an increased production of bilirubin, impaired transport of bilirubin to the liver for excretion, and decreased excretion of bilirubin.

1. Increased production. Bilirubin is produced by the release of hemoglobin from

TABLE 5-13. JAUNDICE

	V Vascular	I Inflammatory	N Neoplasm	D Degenerative
Increased Production of Bilirubin	Pulmonary infarction	Septicemia Malaria Oroya fever Mycoplasma infection	Leukemia Myeloid Metaplasia	
Impaired Transport of Bilirubin	Congestive heart failure			
Decreased Excretion Due to Decreased Conjugation	Budd–Chiari syndrome Pyelophlebitis	Viral hepatitis Leptospirosis Amebic abscess Yellow fever Infectious mononucleosis	Metastatic carcinoma	Idiopathic cirrhosis
Decreased Excretion Due to Decreased Transfer of Conjugated Bilirubin		Syphilis	Metastatic carcinoma	
Decreased Excretion Due to Obstruction of the Bile Ducts		Cholecystitis and cholangitis Chronic pancreatitis	Carcinoma of pancreas Carcinoma of ampulla or ducts Hodgkin's disease	Biliary cirrhosis

the red cells and its subsequent break-down. Thus the hemolytic anemias are the principal cause of this category of jaundice. These include hereditary spherocytosis, Cooley's anemia, septicemia, autoimmune hemolytic anemia, and malaria.

2. **Impaired transport.** Congestive heart failure is the principal cause of this form of jaundice, but it must be advanced enough to cause cardiac cirrhosis.

3. **Decreased excretion.** This group of causes of jaundice is divided into conditions in which the liver is unable to transform unconjugated bilirubin to the conjugated form (Gilbert's disease, infectious hepatitis, and cirrhosis); conditions in which the liver cannot transfer the conjugated bilirubin into the bile ducts, such as the Dubin–Johnson syndrome; and conditions that obstruct the bile ducts, such as common duct stones, cholangitis, chloro-

I Intoxication	C Congenital	A Allergic and Autoimmune	T Trauma	E Endocrine

Alphamethyldopa,
  quinine
Primaquine
Other drugs
	Hereditary spherocytosis
	Cooley's anemia
		Lupus erythematosus
		Transfusion reaction
			Valve prosthesis
			Intra-abdominal
			  hemorrhage	

Toxic hepatitis Wilson's disease Alcoholic cirrhosis	Gilbert's disease	Periarteritis nodosa Sarcoid		Hyperthyroidism
	Dubin–Johnson syn- drome			
Toxic hepatitis Cholorpromazine	Biliary cirrhosis Congenital atresia of bile duct		Surgical ligation	

promazine toxicity, and carcinomas of the pancreas and ampulla of Vater.

Approach to the Diagnosis

The exact diagnosis of jaundice is established by the association of other symptoms and the performance of liver function and special diagnostic procedures (Appendix 1). For exam-ple, jaundice with fever, a prodromal phase of anorexia and malaise and a tender liver suggests hepatitis. Jaundice with itching suggests xanthomatous or primary biliary cirrhosis. Jaundice and anemia suggest hemolytic anemia. Jaundice, back pain, and an abdominal mass suggest a carcinoma of the pancreas.

When liver functions show only an elevated

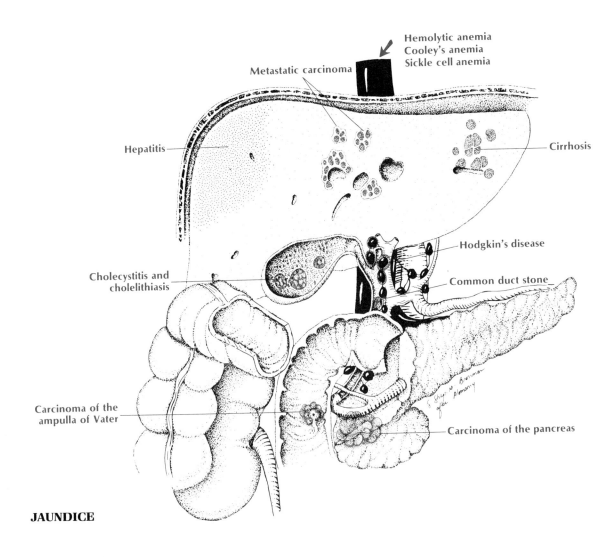

JAUNDICE

indirect bilirubin, Gilbert's disease or hemolytic anemia is suggested. A normal urine urobilinogen will make Gilbert's disease even more likely. Liver functions with only an elevated bilirubin and alkaline phosphatase suggest bile duct obstruction by a stone or tumor. Liver functions with an impressive elevation of the bilirubin, serum glutamic oxaloacetic transaminase (SGOT), and serum glutamic pyruvic transaminase (SGPT) suggest hepatitis.

In cases in which obstruction versus parenchymal disease remains a dilemma after routine tests, several newer procedures have been developed that may help avoid an exploratory laparotomy. Endoscopic retrograde cholangiography and pancreatography (ERCP), cutaneous transhepatic cholangiography, and peritoneoscopy are very useful in these cases. CT scans and ultrasonography are also valuable. The old steroid whitewash is still useful. This is done by administering 20 mg of prednisone daily for 5 days and watching the bilirubin. A positive test, indicating parenchymal diseases, is considered a drop of the bilirubin to one half its original value or more. Exploratory laparotomy may be necessary despite an extensive workup.

MEMORY LOSS AND DEMENTIA

Memory loss is a real symptom and sign, but organic brain syndrome should be dropped from usage because it is a waste-basket term. Unless the memory loss is functional ("supratentorial"), the cerebrum is the principal anatomical site of diseases that produce memory loss. Applying the mnemonic **VINDICATE** to this area provides a method for the prompt recall of causes.

V—Vascular disease includes cerebral arteriosclerosis, thrombi, emboli, and hemorrhages.

I—Inflammatory disorders include syphilis, chronic encephalitis (inclusion body encephalitis, and Jacob–Creutzfeldt disease), and cerebral abscess.

N—Neoplasms include primary and metastatic neoplasms of the brain and meninges.

D—Degenerative and deficiency diseases suggest senile and presenile dementia, Pick's disease, Wernicke's encephalopathy, and pellagra. Pernicious anemia may be associated with dementia.

I—Intoxication brings to mind alcoholism, bromism, lead poisoning, and a host of other toxic or drug-induced encephalopathies. "**I**" may stand for idiopathic and suggest normal pressure hydrocephalus.

C—Congenital disorders include the encephalopathies, Tay Sachs disease, cerebral palsy, mongolism, Wilson's disease, and Huntington's chorea. Congenital hydrocephalus and many other causes must be considered. Porphyria is often forgotten in the differential.

A—Autoimmune disease suggests lupus erythematosus and multiple sclerosis, although severe dementia is uncommon in the latter.

T—Trauma should prompt the recall of concussion and epidural, subdural, and intracerebral hematomas. Heat stroke may cause temporary memory loss. The dissociative reaction of psychoneurosis may be precipitated by trauma.

E—Endocrine disorders with memory loss are myxedema, insulinoma with chronic hypoglycemia, and hypoparathyroidism. If a pituitary tumor invades the hypothalamus there may be memory loss. Addison's disease and aldosteronism may affect memory by the associated disturbance in potassium balance.

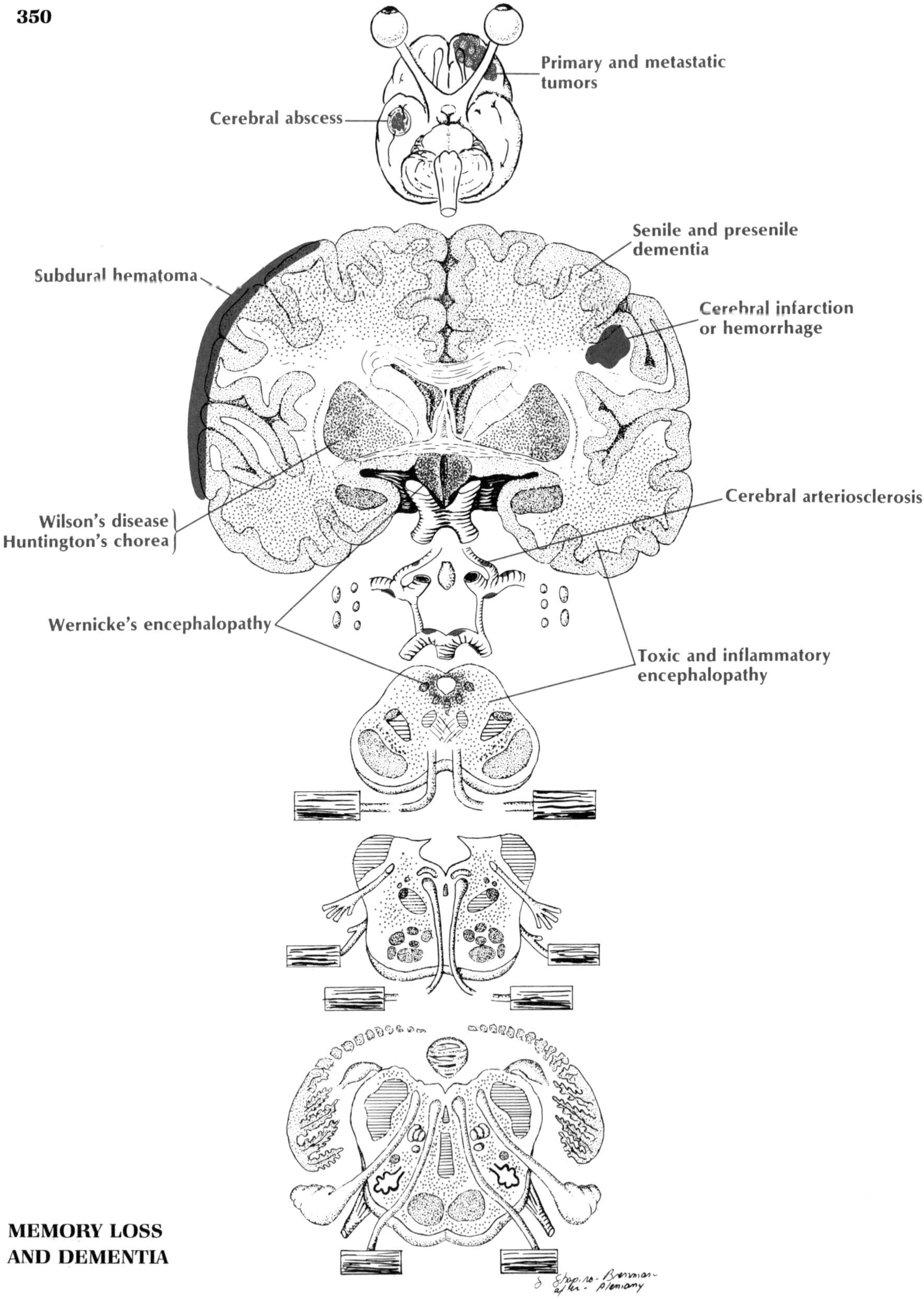

Primary and metastatic tumors

Cerebral abscess

Senile and presenile dementia

Subdural hematoma

Cerebral infarction or hemorrhage

Cerebral arteriosclerosis

Wilson's disease
Huntington's chorea

Wernicke's encephalopathy

Toxic and inflammatory encephalopathy

**MEMORY LOSS
AND DEMENTIA**

Approach to the Diagnosis

Once again the presence or absence of other neurological signs and symptoms is important. If one does not have the skills or the time for a complete neurological examination, immediate referral is indicated. Next, a careful drug history is done. Withdrawal of all drugs may clear the dementia. An EEG, skull x-ray film, CT scan, spinal tap (if there is no papilledema), and psychometric tests are basic to any workup. If the CT scan shows dilated ventricles, a spinal fluid nuclear flow study is indicated to exclude normal pressure hydrocephalus. In the absence of other neurological signs and a negative spinal fluid for syphilis and other chronic encephalopathies, one should do an endocrine workup and look for systemic diseases like porphyria. Drug screens for lead, intoxication, and bromism, for example, are wise. Other tests for memory loss are listed in Appendix I.

MURMURS ■

The first consideration on hearing a heart murmur is to determine whether the murmur is functional or organic. Certainly the low grade systolic murmurs tend to be functional; if the murmur changes or disappears on position, inspiration, or exercise it is likely to be functional. A diastolic murmur, however, is invariably organic. Perhaps the most significant question to ask is, "Are the heart sounds normal?" This is a decisive factor in many cases. If the heart sounds are normal, organic disease is unlikely. Once the murmur is determined to be organic, one needs to have a working differential diagnosis in mind to proceed efficiently. **VINDICATE** provides a mnemonic for this purpose.

V—Vascular suggests myocardia infarction, ball valve thrombi, mural thrombus, and congestive heart failure. Hypertensive cardiovascular disease may lead to cardiac dilatation and murmurs.

I—Inflammatory recalls acute and subacute bacterial endocarditis and viral myocarditis, as well as the myocarditis of trichinosis and Chagas' disease. Syphilis is also a prominent cause of aortic insufficiency.

N—Neoplasm includes atrial myxomas, the most significant disorder to remember here, but leukemic infiltration of the heart and all the neoplasms associated with anemia might be considered.

D—Degenerative disease recalls atherosclerotic heart disease, muscular dystrophy, and Friedreich's ataxia. Atherosclerotic heart disease should perhaps be emphasized as it frequently causes aortic murmurs. Medionecrosis may lead to murmurs when a dissecting aneurysm begins.

I—Intoxication reminds one that there may be no murmur in alcoholic myocardiopathy until failure develops, but it is a condition to consider nevertheless.

C—Congenital heart disease is a well-known cause of murmurs.

A—Autoimmune disease includes rheumatic fever, the best known of these disorders, although it is now a less frequent consideration in murmurs. Libman–Sacks mitral valvular disease occurs in lupus erythematosus.

T—Traumatic disorders recall a ventricular or aortic aneurysm and occasionally a coronary arteriovenous fistula or valvular insufficiency that may result from a stab wound.

E—Endocrinopathies indicate hyperthyroidism and hypothyroidism, particularly because the associated congestive heart failure may lead to cardiac dilatation and murmurs. Hyperthyroidism produces murmurs in some cases because of the rushing

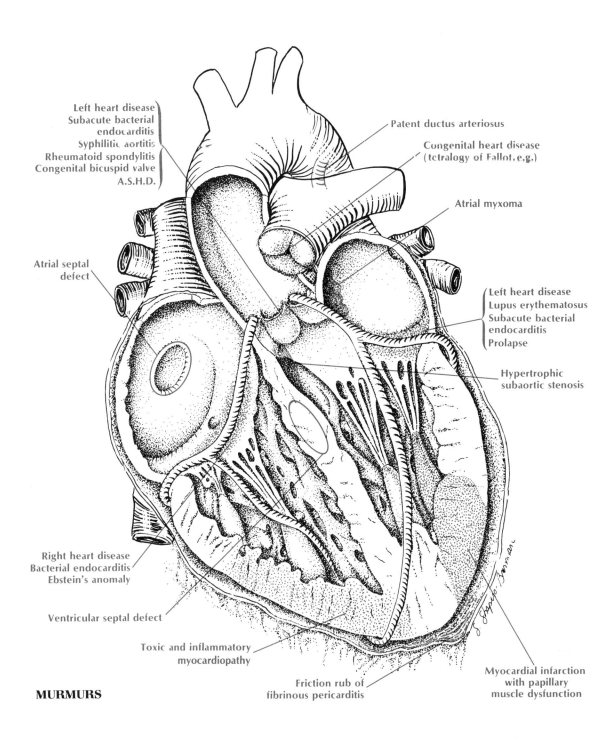

Left heart disease
Subacute bacterial
endocarditis
Syphilitic aortitis
Rheumatoid spondylitis
Congenital bicuspid valve
A.S.H.D.

Patent ductus arteriosus

Congenital heart disease
(tetralogy of Fallot, e.g.)

Atrial myxoma

Atrial septal
defect

Left heart disease
Lupus erythematosus
Subacute bacterial
endocarditis
Prolapse

Hypertrophic
subaortic stenosis

Right heart disease
Bacterial endocarditis
Ebstein's anomaly

Ventricular septal defect

Toxic and inflammatory
myocardiopathy

Friction rub of
fibrinous pericarditis

Myocardial infarction
with papillary
muscle dysfunction

MURMURS

blood and rapid rate, causing many eddy currents.

Approach to the Diagnosis

A chest x-ray film with anterior obliques during a barium swallow along with an ECG, sedimentation rate, a blood serology, and cbc are basic in the workup of a murmur. If there is a fever or if there is recent onset of the murmur, blood cultures, an antistreptolysin-O (ASO) titer and C-reactive protein (CRP) should be done. An ANA test, echocardiography, and phonocardiography are frequently done. Referral to a cardiologist is wise if the cause is obscure or if one is unable to spend the time for a careful workup. Angiocardiography and cardiac catheterization are the only sure ways to determine the location of the valvular disease, and, in many cases, the exact cause.

MYOCLONUS ■

The differential diagnosis of this sign is similar to the differential diagnosis of tremors (see p. 396), but a few additional possibilities should be kept in mind. Idiopathic myoclonus epilepsy, *petit mal* epilepsy (with the *petit mal* triad), *grand mal* epilepsy, and hysteria are the important ones to remember. Congenital hypsarrhythmia may present with saloam sali movements. Decerebrate states are associated with myoclonic jerks in which there is flexion of the arms and extension of the legs. Phenothiazine and some other tranquilizers may cause myoclonus. L-dopa will cause oculogyric crisis and smacking of lips. The workup of all of these conditions includes a skull x-ray film, EEG (preferably sleep), possibly a CT scan, and, if there is no evidence of increased intracranial pressure, a spinal tap. It is recommended that the patient be referred to a neurologist for this workup.

NAUSEA AND VOMITING ■

These two should be considered together, since nausea is just a *forme fruste* of vomiting. This symptom lends itself well to **anatomical** analysis, particularly by the target method illustrated on page 354. The main focus should be on the GI tract. Starting from the top and working to the bottom and at the same time cross-indexing this with etiologies (Table 5-14), one can review the most important causes of vomiting.

In the **nasopharynx** one encounters tonsillitis and foreign bodies. In the **esophagus,** achalasia, reflux esophagitis, and carcinoma are important, although they are more likely to produce dysphagia (see p. 277). In the **stomach,** gastritis, gastric ulcers, and gastric carcinoma are important causes of vomiting. A polyp, carcinoma, or ulcer at the pyloris is most likely to produce vomiting because of gastric outlet obstruction. In children one must not forget pyloric stenosis.

In the **duodenum,** one must consider not only ulcers and duodenitis but also the afferent loop obstructions that occur after Billroth II surgery and the "dumping syndrome" in Billroth I and II surgery. Bile gastritis is also a cause. Intestinal obstruction from a variety of causes (*e.g.,* volvulus, intussusception, malrotation, bezoar, carcinoma, and regional ileitis) must be considered in the jejunum and ileum. Parasites such as *Strongyloides, Ascaris,* and *Taenia solium* must also be considered in this part of the GI tract.

An obstructed Meckel's **diverticulum** or **appendix** may present with vomiting. In the large bowel, ulcerative colitis, amebiasis, and neoplasms should be considered. Mesenteric thrombosis can cause vomiting regardless of which portion of the intestine it involves. Acute viral or bacterial enteritis is associated with nausea and vomiting, but almost invariably there is diarrhea in botulism, salmonella, and shigellosis.

(*Text continues on p. 358*)

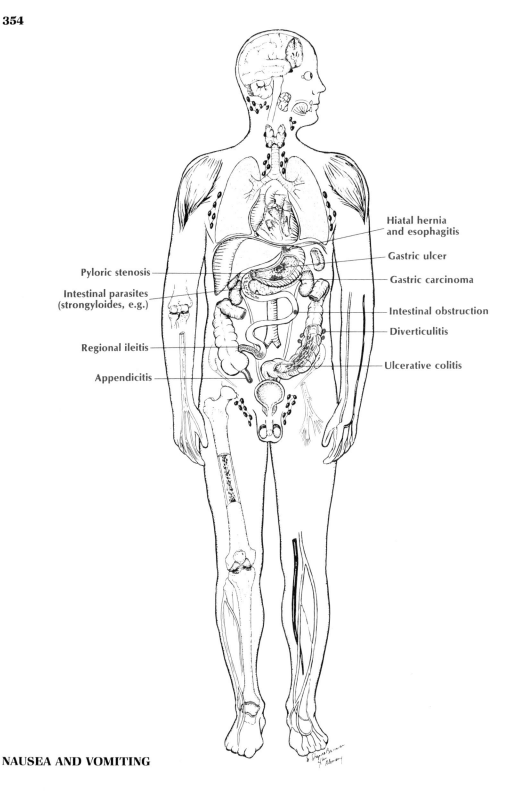

Hiatal hernia
and esophagitis

Gastric ulcer

Gastric carcinoma

Intestinal obstruction

Diverticulitis

Ulcerative colitis

Pyloric stenosis

Intestinal parasites
(strongyloides, e.g.)

Regional ileitis

Appendicitis

NAUSEA AND VOMITING

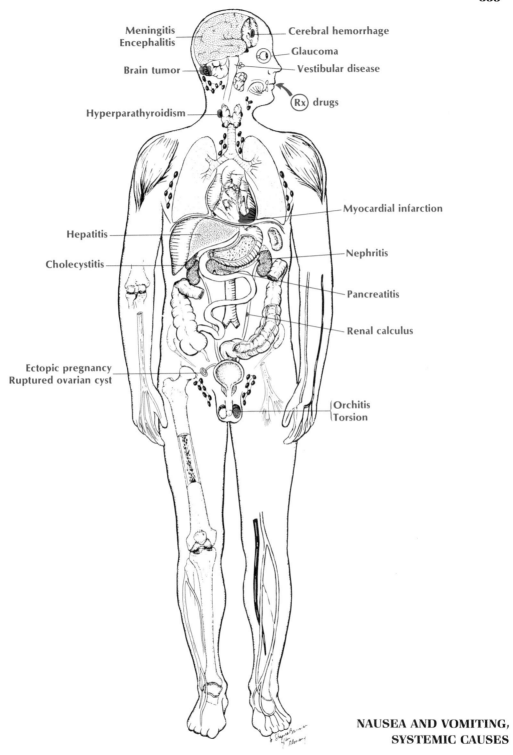

Meningitis
Encephalitis

Cerebral hemorrhage

Glaucoma

Brain tumor

Vestibular disease

(Rx) drugs

Hyperparathyroidism

Myocardial infarction

Hepatitis

Nephritis

Cholecystitis

Pancreatitis

Renal calculus

Ectopic pregnancy
Ruptured ovarian cyst

Orchitis
Torsion

**NAUSEA AND VOMITING,
SYSTEMIC CAUSES**

TABLE 5-14.   NAUSEA AND VOMITING

	V Vascular	I Inflammatory	N Neoplasm	D Degenerative and Deficiency
Pharynx		Tonsillitis Diptheria		Plummer–Vinson syndrome
Esophagus	Aortic aneurysm	Esophagitis Chagas' disease	Carcinoma	
Stomach		Gastritis Ulcers	Carcinoma	Pernicious anemia
Duodenum		Ulcers Duodenitis Strongyloides		
Jejunum and Ileum	Mesenteric thrombosis	Tinea solium and other parasites (*e.g.,* salmonella, shigella)	Carcinoid Sarcomas	Pellagra Malabsorption syndrome
Appendix		Appendicitis	Carcinoid	
Colon	Mesenteric thrombosis	Amebic colitis Staph colitis	Carcinoma	
Gallbladder		Cholecystitis	Cholangioma	
Pancreas		Pancreatitis	Pancreatic cysts and carcinomas	
Kidneys	Renal artery thrombosis	Pyelonephritis	Carcinomas with obstruction	
Pelvic Organs	Torsion of ovary or cyst	PID	Ectopic pregnancy	
Blood		Chronic anemia	Leukemia Multiple myeloma	Iron deficiency anemia

I Intoxication	C Congenital and Collagen	A Autoimmune Allergic	T Trauma	E Endocrine
		Vincent's angina	Foreign body	
Lye stricture	Achalasia sclerodema		Foreign body	
Aspirin, Reserpine	Pyloric stenosis Cascade stomach			Gastrinomas Hyperparathyroidism
				Gastrinomas
Botulism	Whipple's disease Meckel's diverticulum	Regional enteritis	Ruptured viscus	VIP syndrome
			Rupture Fecolith	
	Malrotation Diverticulum	Ulcerative colitis Granulomatous colitis	Ruptured viscus	
			Stones	
	Mucoviscoidosis			
Drug neuropathy	Polycystic kidneys	Glomerulonephritis	Ruptures Stones Obstruction	
			Induced abortion	
Uremia				

In the next circle in the target one encounters cholecystitis and cholelithiasis, pancreatitis, gastrinomas and pancreatic cysts, peritonitis, and myocardial infarction. In the next circle are the kidneys (*e.g.*, renal stones), the thyroid, the pelvic organs (*e.g.*, ectopic pregnancy), and the lungs (pneumonia with gastric dilation). The next circle contains the vestibular apparatus (Meniere's disease), the brain (*e.g.*, tumors) and the testicles (*e.g.*, torsion and orchitis).

The target method has served us well, but a biochemical evaluation of vomiting should also be done because many foreign substances or natural body substances occurring in high or low concentrations in the blood may affect the vomiting centers or cause a paralytic ileus. Thus uremia, increased ammonia and nitrogen breakdown products in hepatic disease, and hypokalemia and hyperkalemia may cause vomiting. Alterations in sodium, chloride, and CO_2 may also cause vomiting. More important is hypercalcemia due to hyperparathyroidism or other causes.

In summary, vomiting is best analyzed anatomically. Physiologically the symptoms of vomiting should suggest obstruction, either functional or mechanical. When all studies (see p. 507) are normal, consider a neuropsychiatric disorder.

Approach to the Diagnosis

The association of other symptoms and signs is essential in pinpointing the diagnosis of vomiting. For example, vomiting with tinnitis and vertigo suggests Meniere's disease, whereas vomiting with hematemesis suggests gastritis, esophageal varices, and gastric ulcers. The laboratory workup should include a flat plate of the abdomen, upper GI series and esophagram, cholecystogram, gastric analysis, serum electrolytes, and amylase and lipase. Stools for occult blood, ova, and parasites are usually indicated. Gastroscopy and esophagoscopy are often indicated in the acute case, but an exploratory laparotomy should not be delayed if the patient's condition is deteriorating and pancreatitis has been excluded. Other tests that may be useful in the workup are listed in Appendix I.

NOCTURIA ■

The differential diagnosis of nocturia is similar to that of polyuria. A pathophysiological analysis of the symptom would indicate that the patient is producing excessive urine at night, or that there is an obstruction to the output of urine so that the bladder cannot be emptied fully on one voiding, or that there is an irritative focus in the urinary tract stimulating the patient to urinate more frequently.

1. **Excessive urine production at night.** In this category are included all the causes of polyuria: diabetes insipidus, diabetes mellitus, hyperthyroidism, diuretic drugs, nephrogenic diabetes insipidus, and chronic nephritis. In addition, the one condition that produces excessive urine output almost exclusively at night—congestive heart failure—must be considered. In heart failure edema accumulates in the extremities during the day while the patient is in the upright position and is returned to the circulation and poured out through the kidney at night while the patient is in the recumbent position.

2. **Obstructive uropathy.** Bladder neck obstruction by a calculus, enlarged or inflamed prostate, median bar hypertrophy, or urethral stricture is a condition to consider here. Neurogenic bladder from poliomyelitis, multiple sclerosis, and other spinal cord diseases must also be considered here.

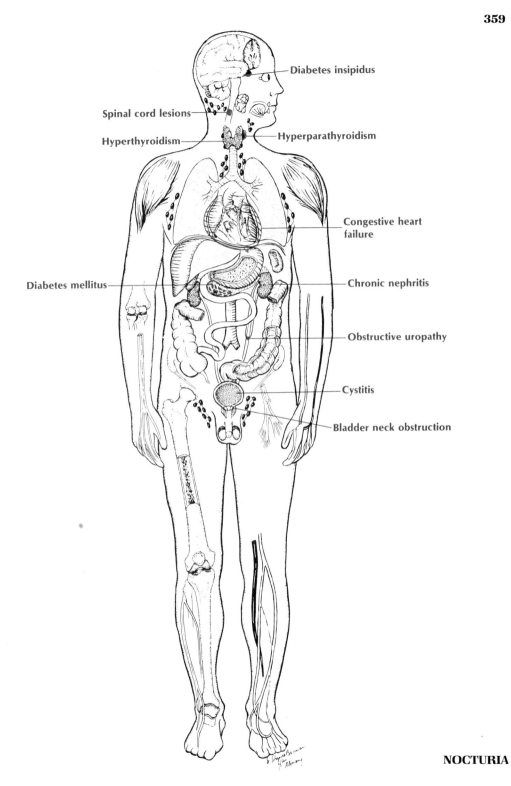

Diabetes insipidus

Spinal cord lesions

Hyperthyroidism

Hyperparathyroidism

Congestive heart failure

Diabetes mellitus

Chronic nephritis

Obstructive uropathy

Cystitis

Bladder neck obstruction

NOCTURIA

3. **Irritative focus in the urinary tract.** Nocturia may result from inflammation of the bladder, prostate, urethra, and kidney on this basis. Occasionally a bladder tumor or prostatic carcinoma may be the irritative focus. Inflammation of the vagina, fallopian tubes, and rectum are also occasionally responsible.

Approach to the Diagnosis

The workup of nocturia is essentially the same as the working of polyuria and urinary frequency (Appendix I). Obviously the search for obstruction and infection are most important. A venous pressure and circulation times and pulmonary function studies to rule out congestive heart failure ought to be done if the urinary tract is clean.

NYSTAGMUS

Why not consider the differential diagnosis of nystagmus under vertigo, because **anatomical pathophysiology** is the key to the differential in both? The reason is that there are two forms of nystagmus (ocular and cerebellar) which do not necessarily occur with vertigo. In addition to these two categories, nystagmus that usually occurs with vertigo is divided into nystagmus of middle ear diseases, nystagmus of inner ear diseases, nystagmus due to auditory nerve involvement, and nystagmus due to brain stem and cerebral diseases.

1. **Ocular nystagmus.** This is a pendular to-and-fro nystagmus with no fast component, which is usually due to congenital visual defects but which may be due to working in poor lighting (miner's nystagmus). It is really an effort of the eye to find a better visual image. Infants with *spasmus nutans* have this type of nystagmus.

2. **Middle ear disorders.** Nystagmus may result from otitis media, which causes associated inflammation of the labyrinth.

3. **Inner ear diseases.** Labyrinthitis may be viral, postinfectious, traumatic, or toxic (*e.g.,* from salicylates, quinine, streptomycin, or gentamycin). A cholesteatoma also causes nystagmus, as does Meniere's disease.

4. **Auditory nerve.** Acoustic neuromas, internal auditory artery occlusions, or aneurysms and basilar meningitis may be considered in this category. Diabetic neuritis is another cause.

5. **Brain stem.** Transient ischemic attacks (TIA) from basilar artery insufficiency, multiple sclerosis, gliomas, syphilis, and tuberculosis are the major conditions to consider here. Thrombi, emboli, and hemorrhages in the branches of the basilar artery are important too. With TIA the possibility of migraine and emboli from subacute bacterial endocarditis or atrial fibrillation should be investigated. Dissemination encephalomyelitis and other forms of encephalitis should not be overlooked. Degenerative disease such as syringobulbia and olivopontinocerebellar atrophy are real possibilities.

6. **Cerebellum.** In addition to the causes of nystagmus mentioned under brain stem, the physician should consider cerebellar tumors, abscesses, posterior fossa subdural hematomas, and diphenylhydantoin toxicity, as well as Friedreich's ataxia and other forms of hereditary cerebellar ataxia. Alcoholic cerebellar degeneration is a significant cause of nystagmus. Acute cerebellar ataxia of children cannot be forgotten. Platybasia may compress the cerebellum and cause nystagmus. Cerebellar

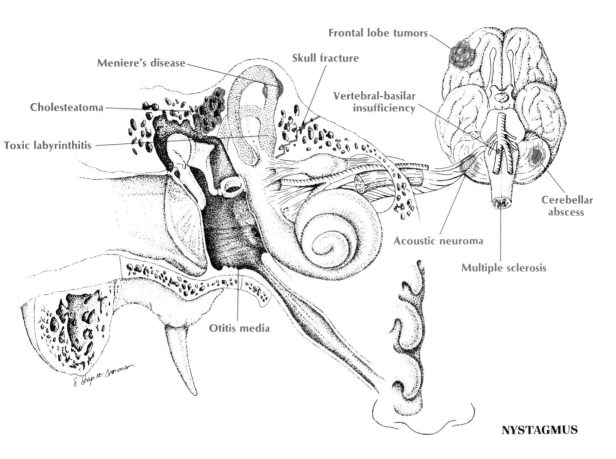

Frontal lobe tumors

Meniere's disease

Skull fracture

Cholesteatoma

Vertebral-basilar
insufficiency

Toxic labyrinthitis

Cerebellar
abscess

Acoustic neuroma

Multiple sclerosis

Otitis media

NYSTAGMUS

degeneration associated with carcinoma of the lung is often misdiagnosed.

7. **Cerebrum.** Curiously enough, frontal lobe tumors may cause nystagmus. Head injuries, encephalitis, chronic subdural hematomas, occipital meningiomas, and the aura of an epileptic seizure may also cause nystagmus.

Approach to the Diagnosis

The workup here is similar to the workup of vertigo. Nystagmus without other signs of central nervous system disease is usually ocular or peripheral in the middle or inner ear. Vertigo is almost invariably present in nystagmus of aural origin. Nystagmus with long tract signs such as hemiplegia or hemianesthesia is invariably brain stem in origin. Purely cerebellar nystagmus is not easily fatigued and is associated with dyskinesia and dyssynergia of the extremities as well as ataxia. There are no long tract or cranial nerve signs. Nystagmus with vertigo, nausea, vomiting, tinnitis, and deafness suggest Meniere's disease.

Confirmation of the diagnosis is made by audiograms, caloric tests, skull roentgenograms, with special views of the mastoids and petrous bones, angiography, CT scans, any myelography. MRI scans are useful, especially in diagnosing brain stem lesions and multiple sclerosis. A spinal tap will help in the diagnosis of multiple sclerosis and neurolues as well as acoustic neuromas.

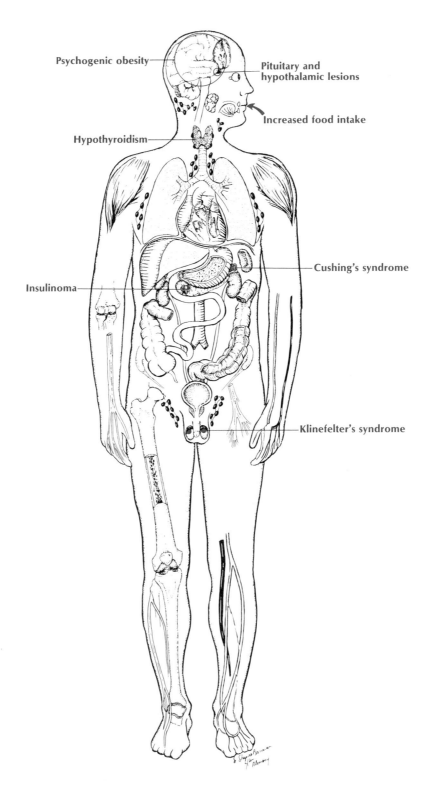

Psychogenic obesity

Pituitary and
hypothalamic lesions

Increased food intake

Hypothyroidism

Cushing's syndrome

Insulinoma

Klinefelter's syndrome

OBESITY

OBESITY

The differential diagnosis of obesity, like that of weight loss, is best developed using **physiology** because most cases of obesity are caused by an absolute increased intake of calories or a relative increased intake of calories over output of energy. Fluid retention may also be associated with weight gain.

1. **Increased intake of calories.** This type of obesity is due to an increased appetite. Under this heading are idiopathic obesity, psychogenic obesity, hypothalamic obesity (due to pituitary tumors and other lesions affecting the hypothalamus), islet cell adenomas and carcinomas (causing hypoglycemia and, consequently, a big appetite), early stages of diabetes mellitus when functional hypoglycemia is common, Cushing's syndrome and exogenous corticosteroids (which increase appetite), and alcoholism, which stimulates the appetite but which also adds calories in the alcohol (up to 250 calories per cocktail).
2. **Decreased output of energy.** Under this heading should be listed hypothyroidism and possibly hypogonadism (such as Klinefelter's syndrome), where the motivation to work or exercise may be impaired. Mild pituitary insufficiency (as in Sheehan's or Frölich's syndrome) may also cause obesity by this mechanism. This type of obesity may be occupational (*e.g.,* white collar workers) or environmental (*i.e.,* watching television all day).
3. **"Obesity" due to fluid retention.** This increase is in reality an increase in weight from fluid retention. Inappropriate ADH syndromes such as occur in carcinoma of the lung, hypothalamic lesions, and drugs are the most important obscure causes. Congestive heart failure, nephrosis, cirrhosis, beriberi, and myxedema rank as significant among more obvious causes.

4. **Miscellaneous causes.** Heredity is definitely a cause of obesity, but the physiological mechanism is uncertain.

Approach to the Diagnosis

It would be ridiculous to do a complete endocrine workup on every case of obesity, but thyroid function studies may be worthwhile. Patients who fail to lose weight on a strict diet may require hospitalization with observation. If they still fail to lose weight, a complete endocrine workup would seem to be indicated, (Appendix I).

PARESTHESIAS, DYSESTHESIAS, AND NUMBNESS

Anatomically, tingling and numbness or other abnormal sensations in the extremities result from involvement of either the peripheral nerve, the nerve plexus (brachial or sciatic), the nerve root, the spinal cord, or the brain. When each of these is cross-indexed with the etiologies suggested by the mnemonic **VINDICATE** most of the causes can be developed (Table 5-15). Only the most important conditions are mentioned in this discussion.

1. **Peripheral nerve.** Peripheral neuropathies from alcohol, diabetes, and other causes are important causes here, but one should not forget the vascular diseases such as peripheral arteriosclerosis, Raynaud's syndrome, and Buerger's disease that may cause paresthesias. In addition, the metabolic disorders such as tetany and uremia should be considered. Finally, the nerve entrapments like the carpal tunnel syndrome need to be checked.
2. **Nerve plexus.** The brachial plexus may be involved by the scalenus anticus syndrome

and a cervical rib or Pancoast's tumor. The sciatic plexus may be compressed by pelvic tumors.

3. **Nerve root.** Herniated discs, spondylosis, tabes dorsalis, and infiltration of the spine by tuberculosis, metastatic tumors, and multiple myeloma need to be remembered here.
4. **Spinal cord.** Spinal cord tumors, pernicious anemia, and tabes dorsalis are the most important conditions to recall here.
5. **Brain.** Transient ischemic attacks, emboli, and migraine are vascular diseases to re-

member in addition to the diseases that affect the spinal cord. The aura of epilepsy is also important. One would not want to miss brain tumors, abscesses, and toxic encephalopathy because these are potentially treatable.

Approach to the Diagnosis

This would be the same as the workup of weakness in one or more extremities. If the condition is in the hand one would check for Tinel's sign, Adson's signs, and roentgeno-

TABLE 5-15. PARESTHESIAS, DYSESTHESIAS, AND NUMBNESS

	V Vascular	I Inflammatory	N Neoplasm	D Degenerative
Peripheral Nerve	Causalgia Raynaud's disease Buerger's disease Arteriosclerosis Ischemic neuritis			Pellagra Beriberi Nutritional neuropathy
Nerve Plexus	Leriche's syndrome		Pancoast's tumor	
Nerve Root		Tabes dorsalis Turberculosis	Metastatic and primary tumors of the cord and spine (multiple myeloma)	Herniated disc Cervical and lumbar spondylosis
Spinal Cord	Anterior spinal artery occlusion Aortic aneurysm	Poliomyelitis Epidural abscess Tuberculosis Syphilis	Metastatic and primary tumors of the cord and spine	Spondylosis Disc disease Pernicious anemia
Brain	Cerebral emboli thrombi, hemor- rhage Carotid or basilar artery insufficiency Migraine	Neurosyphilis Encephalitis Brain abscess	Brain tumors	Senile dementia Presenile dementia

graph the cervical spine for a cervical rib or disc degeneration. The next step is nerve conduction studies and electromyography. Objective signs of radiculopathy are a clear indication for cervical myelography preferably combined with a CT scan. MRI may pick up tiny disc herniations. With associated pain in certain roots, diagnostic nerve blocks may be indicated. If there is coldness in the hand, a stellate ganglion block may be helpful.

If the condition is in the lower extremity a careful examination of the arterial pulses is made, particularly the femoral. If these are abnormal perhaps a flow study or femoral angiography would be indicated. X-ray films of the spine to rule out a herniated disc or tumor of the spine are done routinely. One must not forget a pelvic examination in a female. If other neurological signs are present, a myelogram or CT scan examination may be necessary. When a disc herniation is still likely, thermography should be ordered. EMG has the same usefulness here as in the upper extremity. When a cerebral lesion is suspected, a CT scan, EEG, and four-vessel angiography should be considered.

(Text continues on p. 369)

I Intoxication	C Congenital	A Autoimmune Allergic	T Trauma	E Endocrine

Alcoholic neuropathy
Isoniazid toxicity
Lead and arsenic
  neuropathy
	Porphyria	Infectious neuronitis
		Periarteritis nodosa
			Trauma
			Hematoma
			Laceration
			Neuromas
			Frostbite
				Tetany of hypopara-
				  thyroidism
				Aldosteronism

	Scalenus anticus Cervical rib	Infectious neuronitis	Contusion Laceration Fractures	Diabetic neuropathy
	Spondylolisthesis		Fracture Herniated disc	

Transverse myelitis
  from radiation
	Spina bifida
	Myelocele
	Syringomyelia
		Guillain–Barré
		  syndrome
		Multiple sclerosis
			Fracture
			Herniated disc
			Hematoma	

Alcoholism Bromism Encephalopathy Opiates, barbiturates, etc.	A-V anomalies Aneurysm Epilepsy Cerebral palsy	Lupus cerebritis Multiple sclerosis	Depressed fracture Subdural hematoma	Pituitary tumors Acromegaly

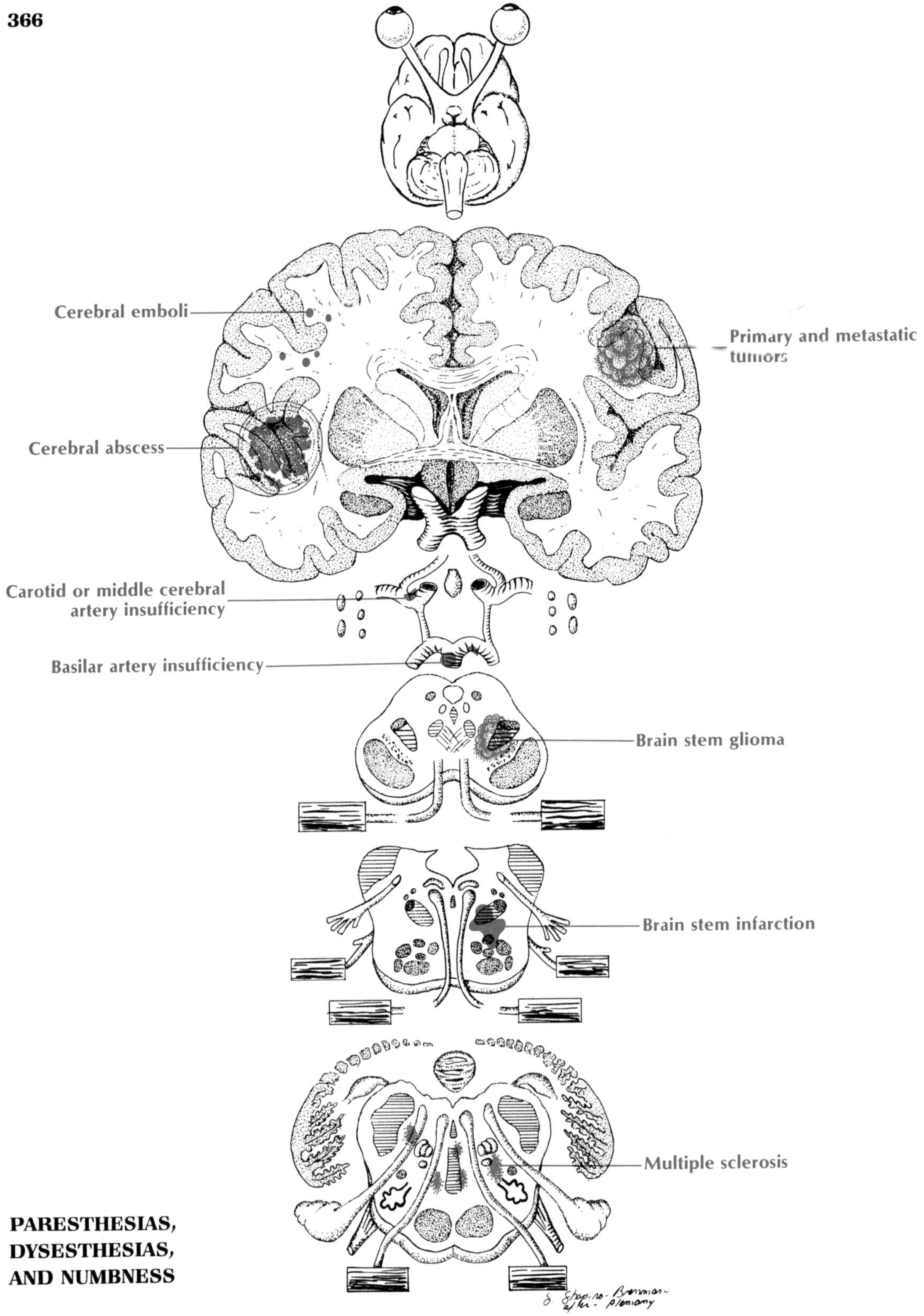

Cerebral emboli

Primary and metastatic tumors

Cerebral abscess

Carotid or middle cerebral artery insufficiency

Basilar artery insufficiency

Brain stem glioma

Brain stem infarction

Multiple sclerosis

PARESTHESIAS, DYSESTHESIAS, AND NUMBNESS

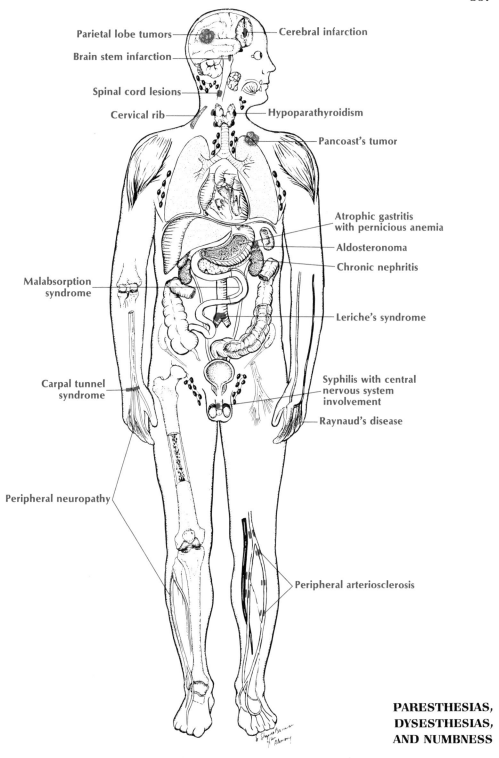

Parietal lobe tumors

Cerebral infarction

Brain stem infarction

Spinal cord lesions

Cervical rib

Hypoparathyroidism

Pancoast's tumor

Atrophic gastritis
with pernicious anemia

Aldosteronoma

Chronic nephritis

Malabsorption
syndrome

Leriche's syndrome

Carpal tunnel
syndrome

Syphilis with central
nervous system
involvement

Raynaud's disease

Peripheral neuropathy

Peripheral arteriosclerosis

**PARESTHESIAS,
DYSESTHESIAS,
AND NUMBNESS**

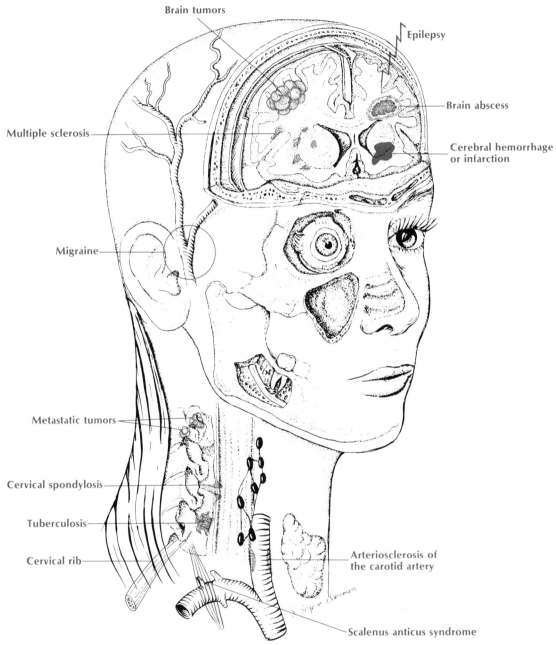

Brain tumors

Epilepsy

Brain abscess

Multiple sclerosis

Cerebral hemorrhage or infarction

Migraine

Metastatic tumors

Cervical spondylosis

Tuberculosis

Cervical rib

Arteriosclerosis of the carotid artery

Scalenus anticus syndrome

PARESTHESIAS, DYSESTHESIAS, AND NUMBNESS

PHOTOPHOBIA ■

Sensitivity to light may be due to local eye disease or systemic disease, but in both cases it is usually due to inflammation, with three exceptions: albinism because there is poor pigmentation of the iris and choroid, allowing more light to get in; migraine, where the explanation is still not available; and eye strain from astigmatism and especially from hyperopia.

1. **Local.** Following the path of light from the conjunctiva to the retina, one may easily recall the causes of photophobia. Conjunctivitis (chemical, allergic, and infectious), keratitis, and foreign bodies of the cornea, iritis, retinitis, chorioretinitis, and optic neuritis may all be associated with photophobia.
2. **Systemic.** All the febrile states, especially those associated with conjunctival infection, cause photophobia. Measles, meningitis, encephalitis, hay fever, influenza, the common cold, and trichinosis are just a few. Certain toxins can cause photophobia, notably iodism, bromism, and atropine derivatives. Simply staying in the dark will cause photophobia. Hysteria and simple fear or annoyance with crowds will also cause this condition.

Approach to the Diagnosis

The approach to the diagnosis of photophobia is the same as that for blurred vision (see p. 236).

POLYDIPSIA ■

Excessive thirst is best analyzed by the application of **physiology**. Increased desire for water may be due to a **decreased intake,** as in prolonged abstinence, vomiting of pyloric stenosis and intestinal obstruction, and diarrhea of any cause. **Poor transport** of fluid in hemorrhagic or vasomotor shock and congestive heart failure may be the cause. Anything that decreases the effective circulatory volume, such a hypoalbuminemia, may cause retention of salt and consequent thirst through the renin–angiotensin–aldosterone mechanism. **Increased output** of water may be responsible for polydipsia. The increased output may result from a solute diuresis in diabetes mellitus and hypercalcemic states (*e.g.*, hyperparathyroidism); an increased glomerular filtration rate in hyperthyroidism; inability of the kidney to respond to antidiuretic hormone in chronic glomerulonephritis, aldosteronism, and renal diabetes insipidus; or a lack of antidiuretic hormone in diabetes insipidus. **Increased output** of salt and water in excessive sweating of work or fever will lead to thirst. This mechanism is an additional factor in hyperthyroidism and diabetes mellitus where diaphoresis is common.

A neurosis may be responsible for polydipsia in neurogenic diabetes insipidus. Drugs such as lithium and demeclocycline (Delcomycin) can damage the distal tubule and cause a renal diabetes insipidus. Drugs such as belladonna alkaloids, amitriptyline, parasympatholytic drugs, and gallic acid may cause a dry mouth and an excessive thirst. Alcohol may cause excessive thirst by inhibiting the antidiuretic hormone.

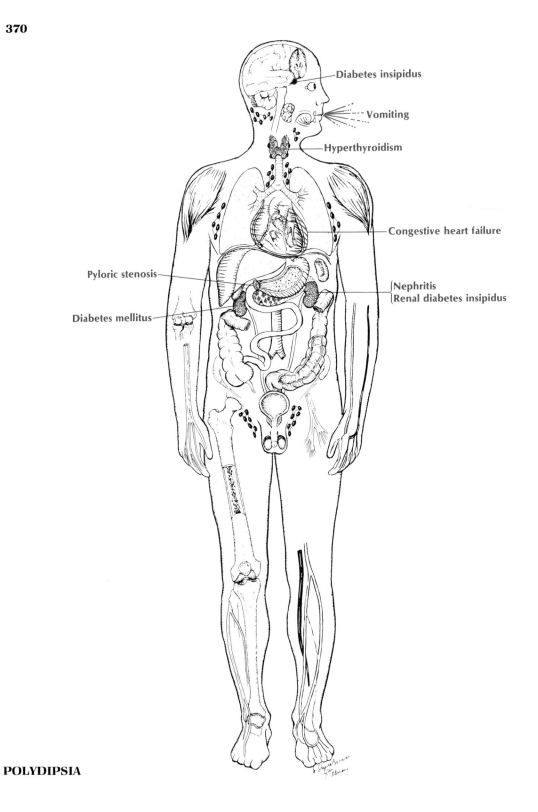

Diabetes insipidus

Vomiting

Hyperthyroidism

Congestive heart failure

Pyloric stenosis

Nephritis
Renal diabetes insipidus

Diabetes mellitus

POLYDIPSIA

Approach to the Diagnosis

The approach to the diagnosis of polydipsia involves establishing the presence or absence of other symptoms, such a polyuria, polyphagia, weakness, and weight loss. Polydipsia with polyuria and excessive appetite (polyphagia) should suggest diabetes mellitus or hyperthyroidism, whereas polydipsia with polyuria alone should suggest a form of diabetes insipidus (pituitary, renal, or psychogenic). The laboratory workup involves checking intake and output, blood sugars, electrolytes, and T_3, T_4, and T_7. Additional tests for this disorder are found in Appendix I.

POLYPHAGIA

The causes of increased appetite are similar to those of obesity and can be recalled with the help of **physiology.** The appetite may be based on a psychic desire for food, a lack of food or a particular vitamin, impaired intake of food, an increased metabolism of the body (and consequently an increased need for food), increased uptake of food by the cell, and inability of the cell to absorb food, causing "cell starvation."

1. **Psychic desire for food.** This occurs in many chronic anxiety and depressed states and is frequently associated with obesity.
2. **Lack of food or particular ingredient in food.** Starvation and avitaminosis can cause polyphagia.
3. **Impaired uptake of food.** Rapid mobility of food in gastric hypersection and intestinal bypass as well as preempting of food by intestinal worms may cause polyphagia on this basis.
4. **Increased body metabolism.** Hyperthyroidism, rapid growth of adolescence, and gigantism are included in this category.
5. **Increased uptake of food by the cell.** Any condition associated with hyperinsulinism (functional hypoglycemia and **insulinomas**) is recalled in this category.
6. **"Cell starvation."** Here diabetes mellitus and acromegaly are associated with diabetes where the cell cannot absorb glucose.

Approach to the Diagnosis

Association with other symptoms is the key to a definitive diagnosis of polyphagia. Thus polyphagia and obesity suggest an islet cell adenoma. Polyphagia with polyuria, polydipsia, weakness and weight loss suggest hyperthyroidism or diabetes mellitus.

The laboratory workup should include thyroid function studies, a skull x-ray film for pituitary size, glucose tolerance tests, and possibly a 48-hour fast with frequent blood sugar determinations.

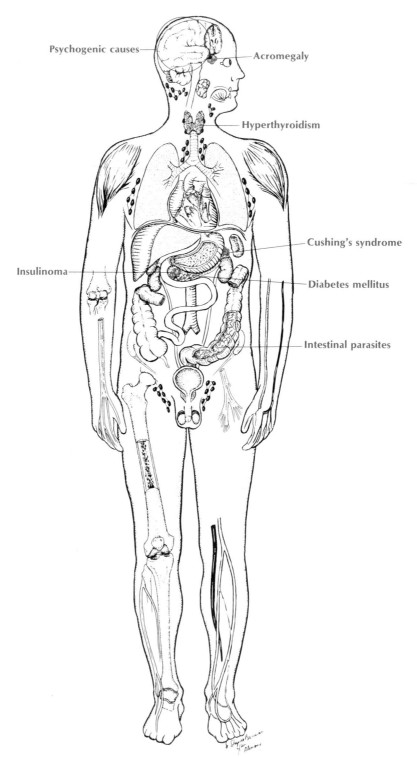

Psychogenic causes

Acromegaly

Hyperthyroidism

Cushing's syndrome

Insulinoma

Diabetes mellitus

Intestinal parasites

POLYPHAGIA

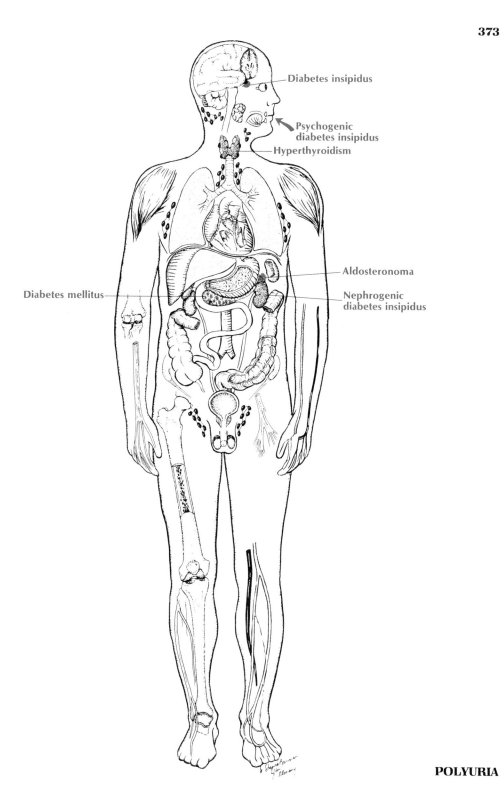

Diabetes insipidus

Psychogenic
diabetes insipidus

Hyperthyroidism

Aldosteronoma

Nephrogenic
diabetes insipidus

Diabetes mellitus

POLYURIA

POLYURIA

Polyuria is an absolute increase in the urine output in a 24-hour period. The average individual excretes 1500 ml of urine a day. Many physiological conditions increase the output of urine (stress, exercise, and warm weather associated with copious drinking). From a pathophysiological standpoint polyuria results from one of four mechanisms: (1) Increased intake of fluids; (2) Increased glomerular filtration rate; (3) Increased output of solutes such as sodium chloride and glucose; (4) Inability of the kidney to reabsorb water in the distal tubule.

1. **Increased intake of fluid.** As already mentioned this can occur under stress and nervous tension. It becomes pathological in psychogenic diabetes insipidus when 6 to 10 liters of fluid may be ingested each day.
2. **Increased glomerular filtration rate.** This is a factor in the polyuria of hyperthyroidism and fever of any cause.
3. **Increased output of solutes.** Uncontrolled diabetes mellitus (where the solute is glucose) and hyperthyroidism (where the solute may be glucose or urea) are examples of this type of polyuria. Hyperparathyroidism is another important cause (increased calcium output). Diuretics are a significant cause of this type of polyuria because they increase the amount of solute arriving at the distal tubule and hold onto the water that would otherwise be absorbed.
4. **Decreased reabsorption of water in the distal tubule.** This, the most common cause of polyuria, is divided into two groups: those conditions where there is inadequate or blocked output of ADH, and those conditions where the distal tubule and collecting ducts are unable to respond

to the ADH. Decreased output of antidiuretic hormone occurs in diabetes insipidus from pituitary tumors, infarcts, Hands–Schuller–Christian disease, and sarcoidosis, among other things. It also results from alcohol intoxication and hypothalamus lesions. The inability of the distal tubule to respond to ADH occurs in aldosteronism, chronic glomerulonephritis, polycystic kidneys and pyelonephritis, lithium and demeclocycine (Declomycin) therapy, and idiopathic nephrogenic diabetes insipidus. Diuretics operate somewhat in this manner.

Cases of myxedema are reported with polyuria, but the mechanism is unclear.

Approach to the Diagnosis

The diagnosis of polyuria depends largely on the association of other symptoms Polyuria, polyphagia, and polydypsia suggest diabetes mellitus and hyperthyroidism. Polyuria with only polydipsia suggests psychogenic or idiopathic diabetes insipidus; the Hickey–Hare test will differentiate these two. Polyuria with polydipsia and weakness but with no significant weight loss suggests hypercalcemia and possible hyperparathyroidism. Chronic nephritis will be diagnosed by examination of the urine sediment and a specific gravity that remains at 1.010. Nephrogenic diabetes insipidus can be differentiated from neurogenic diabetes insipidus by the inability of the kidney to respond to a pitressin injection. Other useful diagnostic tests are listed in Appendix I.

PRIAPISM

This unfortunate condition may be humorous to everyone but the one who is "blessed" with it The common causes are few and the mne-

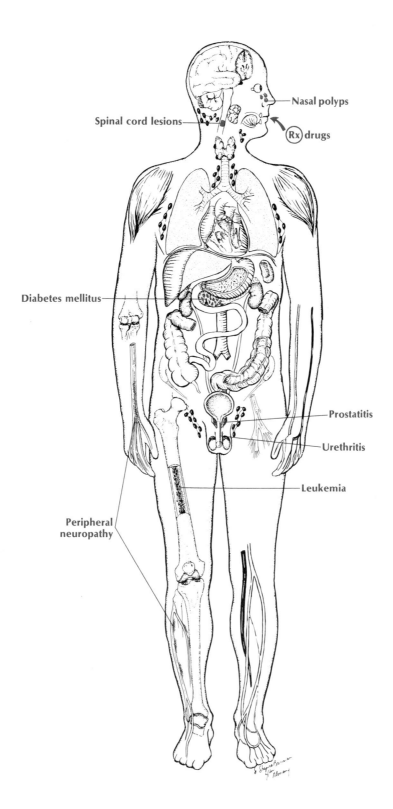

Nasal polyps

Spinal cord lesions

Rx drugs

Diabetes mellitus

Prostatitis

Urethritis

Leukemia

Peripheral neuropathy

PRIAPISM

monic MINT is an easy method for recall of these.

M—Malformation suggests phimosis and other deformities of the penis.

I—Inflammation and **intoxication** suggest posterior urethritis, prostatitis, and cystitis, as well as aphrodisiac drugs such as alcohol, cannabis, indica, camphor, and damiana.

N—Neoplasms suggest two common causes of priapism—chronic lymphatic or myeloid leukemia and nasal polyps. The **N** also suggests neurological disorders such as neurosyphilis, multiple sclerosis, and diabetic neuropathy.

T—Trauma recalls not only direct trauma to the penis producing a local hematoma but also trauma to the spinal cord with fractures or contusion.

Approach to the Diagnosis

The diagnosis of priapism usually depends on the association of other symptoms and signs (*e.g.,* boggy prostate), but a blood smear or bone marrow examination may be necessary to exclude leukemia. A careful history of the patient's sexual activities to rule out too frequent masturbation or sexual excesses may be indicated.

PRURITUS

The differential diagnosis of pruritus is best developed by **anatomy.** Local conditions such as bites and parasitic infestations (*e.g.,* scabies, hookworms, and schistosomiasis) usually reveal an obvious lesion. Generalized skin conditions such as dermatitis herpetiformis, atopic dermatitis, and exfoliative dermatitis are also more likely to show obvious skin manifestations and severe itching. These conditions are to be distinguished from cutaneous syphilis, where there is no itching at all, and psoriasis and pemphigus, where the itching is minimal. Numerous other skin conditions cause pruritus, but we are more concerned with the systemic causes because they are more difficult to diagnose.

Jaundice, particularly obstructive jaundice, is associated with marked pruritus. Primary biliary cirrhosis may begin with pruritus without jaundice because the liver must turn over 30 grams of bile salts (the cause of the itching) a day to only one gram of bilirubin. Thus, although there may be enough function left to turn over the bilirubin, there is not enough to turn over the bile salts.

Diabetes, mellitus may cause pruritus, particularly vulvar, where it predisposes to moniliasis. Renal disease may also cause pruritus, presumably because of the retention of toxic wast products. Finally, leukemia and Hodgkin's disease are systemic causes of pruritus. Of course, psychoneurosis and malingering must be considered.

In addition to systemic conditions mentioned above, one should search for local conditions in the anus and rectum (pruritus ani), especially hemorrhoids (internal ones may not be obvious), anal fissure, and anal abscess or fistulae. Condyloma acuminatum may contribute to pruritis; anal moniliasis or pinworms should be sought for.

Any vaginal discharge may cause pruritus vulvae. Thus, *Trichomonas* and moniliasis should be looked for. One should also consider lack of estrogen leading to atrophic vaginitis and dermatitis.

Approach to the Diagnosis

It should be obvious that the clinical approach to pruritus without an obvious dermatological manifestation should be to order appropriate tests (Appendix I) to rule out the above systemic disorders.

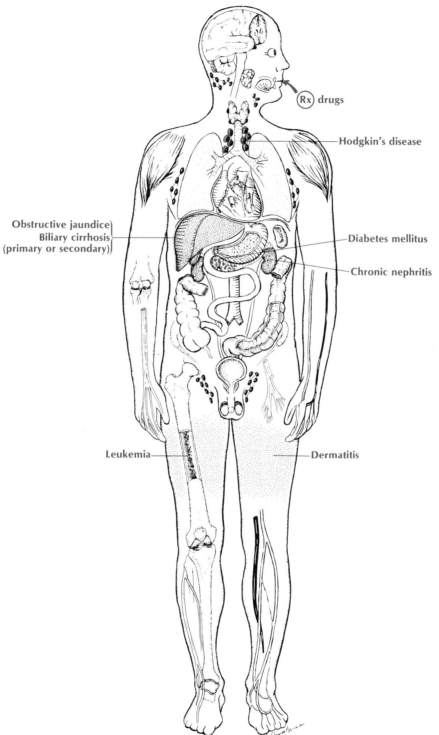

Rx drugs

Hodgkin's disease

Obstructive jaundice
Biliary cirrhosis
(primary or secondary)

Diabetes mellitus

Chronic nephritis

Leukemia

Dermatitis

PRURITUS

PTOSIS ◼

A drooping eyelid may result from direct involvement of the levator palpebrae superioris muscle (end organ) or from involvement of the sympathetic or oculomotor nerve pathways from the muscle to the central nervous system. Consequently, visualizing **neuroanatomy** is the key to a differential diagnosis.

1. **End organ** (levator palpebrae superioris muscle). The end organ can be involved in congenital ptosis (defective development of the muscle), injury to the tendon of the muscle, neoplasms of the eye or orbit, or dermatomyositis.
2. **Sympathetic pathway.** If the sympathetic pathways are involved there is almost invariably an associated miosis and enophthalmos (Horner's syndrome). The lesion may be along the intracranial pathways of the postganglionic fibers around the carotid artery in internal carotid aneurysms, thrombosis, and migraine. Orbital cellulitis or tumors may rarely affect the sympathetic nerve pathways here. The lesion may be in the stellate ganglion and its connections in cervical rib, scalenus anticus syndrome, Pancoast's tumors, cervical Hodgkin's disease, and brachial plexus injuries. The lesion may be in the spinal cord or nerve roots in spinal cord tumors, syringomyelia, syphilis, thoracic spondylosis, metastatic carcinoma, myeloma, or tuberculosis of the spinal column. Finally, the lesion may be in the brain stem in gliomas, posterior inferior cerebellar artery occlusions syringobulbia, and encephalitis.
3. **Oculomotor nerve pathways.** When the ptosis is due to involvement in this pathway there is usually other extraocular muscle palsies as well. The levator muscle may be affected by myotonic dystrophy. The myoneural junction may be affected by myasthenia gravis. The oculomotor nerve may be involved by orbital tumors or cellulitis by compression from herniation of the uncus in cerebral tumors or subdural hematomas, by cavernous sinus thrombosis or carotid aneurysms, and occasionally by syphilitic or tuberculous meningitis or pituitary and suprasellar tumors. Diabetic neuropathy may cause ptosis due to oculomotor nerve involvement. In the brain stem the nuclei or supranuclear connections of the oculomotor nerve may be involved by syphilis (*e.g.*, general paresis), gliomas, pinealomas, basilar artery occlusions, encephalitis, botulism, and progressive muscular atrophy.

Approach to the Diagnosis

As always the diagnosis is usually established by the presence or absence of other neurological signs and symptoms. Bilateral partial ptosis suggests myotonic dystrophy, a congenital origin, or progressive muscular dystrophy. Unilateral ptosis without miosis or extraocular muscle palsy suggests injury to the levator palpebrae superioris muscle or myasthenia gravis. A Tensilon test should always be considered. When all the components of a Horner's syndrome are present, x-ray films of the skull, cervical and thoracic spine, and chest should be done. A spinal tap and arteriography should be considered.

If oculomotor involvement is certain, a glucose tolerance test, skull roentgenograms, serological tests for syphilis, spinal tap (if no contraindications), CT scans, and possibly arteriography would be indicated. Other tests would depend on the presence of other neurological signs. An ophthalmologist and neurologist should probably be consulted in all cases of unilateral ptosis.

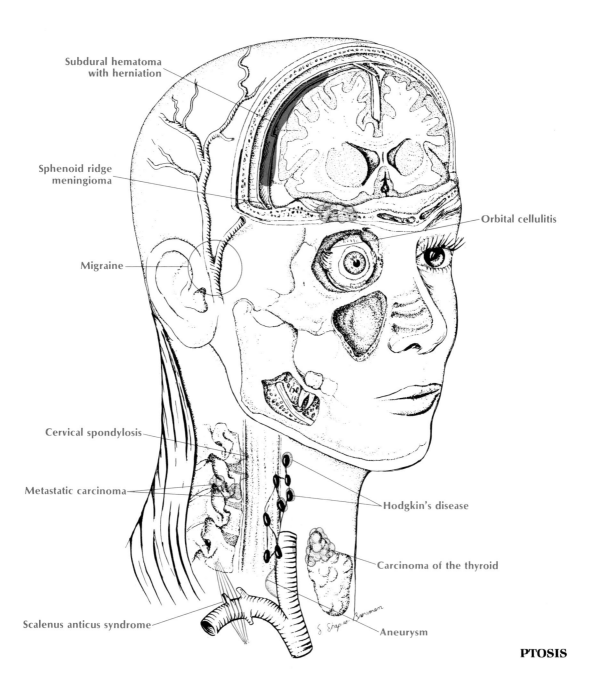

Subdural hematoma
with herniation

Sphenoid ridge
meningioma

Migraine

Cervical spondylosis

Metastatic carcinoma

Scalenus anticus syndrome

Orbital cellulitis

Hodgkin's disease

Carcinoma of the thyroid

Aneurysm

PTOSIS

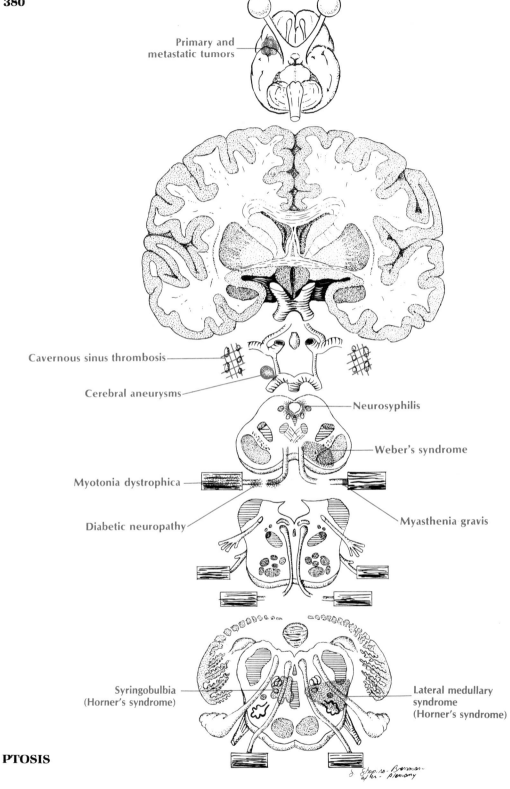

Primary and metastatic tumors

Cavernous sinus thrombosis

Cerebral aneurysms

Neurosyphilis

Weber's syndrome

Myotonia dystrophica

Myasthenia gravis

Diabetic neuropathy

Syringobulbia
(Horner's syndrome)

Lateral medullary syndrome
(Horner's syndrome)

PTOSIS

SNEEZING ▪

Allergic rhinitis (hay fever) is the most common cause of this condition and perhaps any patient with sneezing as his chief complaint needs to have this excluded first. Other conditions, however, may present with sneezing and the clinician needs to be able to recall these while examining the patient. The mnemonic **MINT** forms a good method for recalling these conditions.

M—Malformations include a deviated septum, a cleft palate that allows food to enter the nose, and large tonsils and adenoids.
I—Inflammation suggests pertussis, acute viral influenza, the common cold, chronic rhinitis, and measles, among other upper respiratory infections. The **I** also suggest **immunological** disorders; allergic rhinitis and bronchial asthma head the list.
N—Neoplasms suggest nasal polyps and carcinomas of the nasopharynx.
T—Toxic disorders include pepper, tear gas, phosphine, chlorine, and iodism.

Approach to the Diagnosis

The workup of sneezing involves a careful (ENT) examination to exclude foreign bodies, polyps, and malformations. The typical mucoid bluish mucosa of allergic rhinitis may be spotted. A nasal smear for eosinophils will clinch the diagnosis of allergic rhinitis, and skin testing or a radio-allergosorbent test (RAST) can be undertaken, although a good allergy history may be more important.

STRIDOR AND SNORING ▪

Both these symptoms are the result of the same pathophysiological mechanism: obstruction in the upper air passages. That obstruction may be due to any one of the etiologies recalled by the mnemonic **MINT.**

M—Malformations that may cause snoring or stridor include a large tongue, large tonsils and adenoids, a large soft palate, a cleft palate, congenital webs of the glottis, and malformation of the epiglottis (causing the well-known congenital laryngeal stridor). Foreign bodies must be considered here, as well as laryngeal stenosis.
I—Inflammatory conditions obstructing the upper airway include purulent sputum, acute laryngitis of diphtheria, acute tonsillitis, epiglottitis as in *H. influenza*, rhinitis, hay fever, acute laryngotracheitis (usually of viral origin), Ludwig's angina, and angioneurotic edema. Whooping cough should also be remembered here.
N—Neoplasms and neurological disorders causing stridor or snoring include laryngeal polyps and carcinomas and bulbar or pseudobulbar palsy from basilar artery occlusions or hemorrhage, poliomyelitis or encephalitis, myasthenia gravis, and tabes dorsalis.
T—Traumatic disorders include the passage of an endotracheal tube, tracheotomies, and karate chops to the larynx.

Approach to the Diagnosis

The approach to the diagnosis involves a careful examination of the air passage with the laryngoscope and bronchoscope (if necessary under anesthesia). If these are negative a thorough neurological examination should be performed and a Tensilon test may be indicated. Laryngismus stridulus in children may be terminated by putting the child in a steambath; this helps establish that diagnosis. Skin testing for allergies may be necessary. A sleep study is often necessary to rule out neurogenic or obstructive sleep apnea.

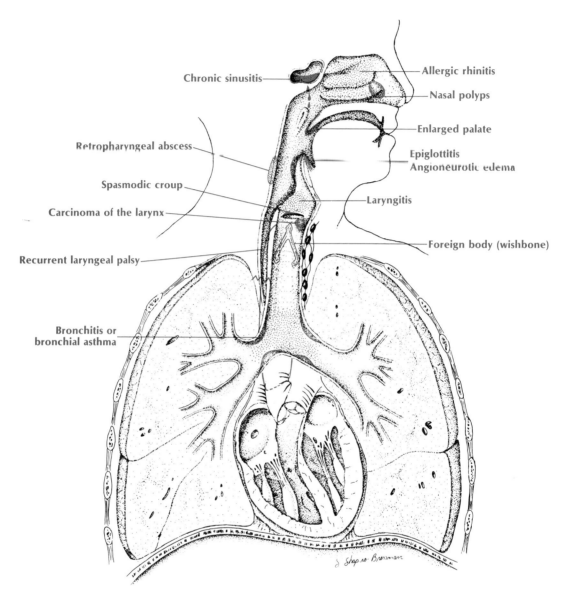

Chronic sinusitis

Allergic rhinitis

Nasal polyps

Enlarged palate

Retropharyngeal abscess

Epiglottitis
Angioneurotic edema

Spasmodic croup

Laryngitis

Carcinoma of the larynx

Foreign body (wishbone)

Recurrent laryngeal palsy

Bronchitis or
bronchial asthma

STRIDOR AND SNORING

SYNCOPE

The differential of syncope or a brief loss of consciousness is best developed with the use of **physiology** and, to a lesser extent, anat-

omy. Like convulsions (see p. 258), syncope is due to a diminished supply of oxygen and glucose in the brain cell. Anything that produces hypoglycemia (see p. 384) may lead to episodes of syncope, but the most common

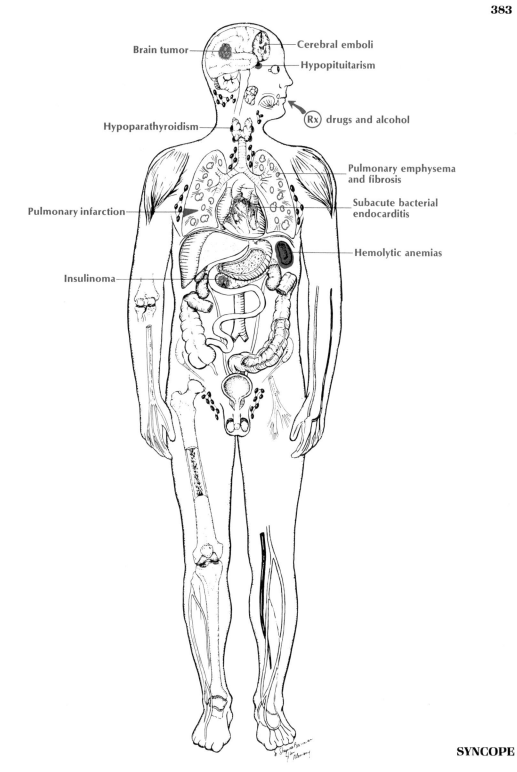

Brain tumor

Cerebral emboli

Hypopituitarism

(Rx) drugs and alcohol

Hypoparathyroidism

Pulmonary emphysema and fibrosis

Pulmonary infarction

Subacute bacterial endocarditis

Hemolytic anemias

Insulinoma

SYNCOPE

cause is overdose of insulin. It is also important to include insulinomas and overdose of the oral hypoglycemic agents (Table 5-16).

Actually, a reduced delivery of oxygen to the brain cell accounts for most cases of syncope. Oxygen must get into the body through the lungs with adequate ventilation. It must then be absorbed through the alveolar-capillary membrane and picked up by an adequate number of red cells. It must then be delivered to the brain by a good functioning heart and unobstructed carotid and vertebral-basilar system. Retracting the above physiology and anatomy will develop the disease entities that

must be considered in the differential diagnosis of syncope.

Thus, mechanical obstructions of the larnyx (foreign body), the bronchi, or bronchioles (asthma and emphysema), or the alveolar capillary membrane (pulmonary fibrosis, sarcoidosis, or pulmonary embolism) may cause anoxia and syncope. Severe anemia prevents the adequate transport of oxygen. Oxygen transport from the heart to the brain may be obstructed mechanically or functionally. It is functionally obstructed by congestive heart failure of Stoke's–Adams syndrome (heart block) and other arrhythmias, particularly

---

TABLE 5-16.   SYNCOPE

	V Vascular	I Inflammatory	N Neoplasm	D Deficiencies or Degenerative
Hypoglycemia			Insulinoma Oat-cell carcinoma	Cirrhosis of liver
Lungs	Pulmonary embolism	Pneumonia Chronic bronchitis		Pulmonary fibrosis Emphysema
Blood		Chronic anemia Septemic shock	Leukemia	Aplastic anemia
Heart	Myocardial infarction Ball valve thrombi	Syphilitic aortitis	Atrial myxoma	Myocardopathies
Carotid Arteries	Thrombosis Embolism			Atherosclerosis
Arteriole	Thrombosis	Subacute bacterial endocarditis		

ventricular tachycardia and sick sinus syndrome. Functional obstruction may result from a drop in blood pressure from carotid sinus syncope (see p. 330), postural hypotension (see p. 332), and vasovagal syncope. True vertigo (see p. 282) may lead to syncope by way of the latter mechanism.

Mechanical obstruction may occur at the aortic valve (aortic stenosis or insufficiency), at the carotid arteries (thrombi or plaques), or focally in the smaller arteries from ischemia due to arterial thrombi or emboli. Rarer mechanical obstruction may occur from ball valve thrombi in the mitral or tricuspid valve,

large pulmonary emboli, or cough syncope in which poor venous return to the heart is the cause.

Approach to the Diagnosis

Clinical differentiation of the various forms of syncope is made by combinations of symptoms. Thus syncope with marked sweating and tachycardia is more likely due to hypoglycemia. Syncope with sweating and bradycardia is more likely due to vasovagal syncope. Focal neurological signs during the attack suggest transient cerebral ischemia (TIA) and

I Intoxication	C Congenital	A Autoimmune Allergic	T Trauma	E Endocrine
Tolbutamide Hypoglycemic drugs and insulin				Insulinomas Addison's Hypopituitarism
Pneumoconiosis	Cystic fibrosis	Sarcoidosis Anemia	Pneumothorax	
Drug-induced anemia	Sickle cell anemia	Hemolytic anemia ITP	Blood loss	
Cardiac arrhythmias from drugs and alcohol		Rheumatic valvular disease		
Drug-induced postural hypotension	Anomalous circle of Willis			
	Migraine	Vasculitis Purpura		

prompts a search for sources of emboli or thrombosis (sickle cell disease, polycythemia, or macroglobulinemia). A family history of syncope suggests migraine, epilepsy, or vaso-vagal attacks. Epilepsy is a strong possibility in the young, whereas heart block is more likely in the aged. Consequently an EEG and Holter monitoring are useful in the workup. The laboratory workup of syncope is discussed on page 502.

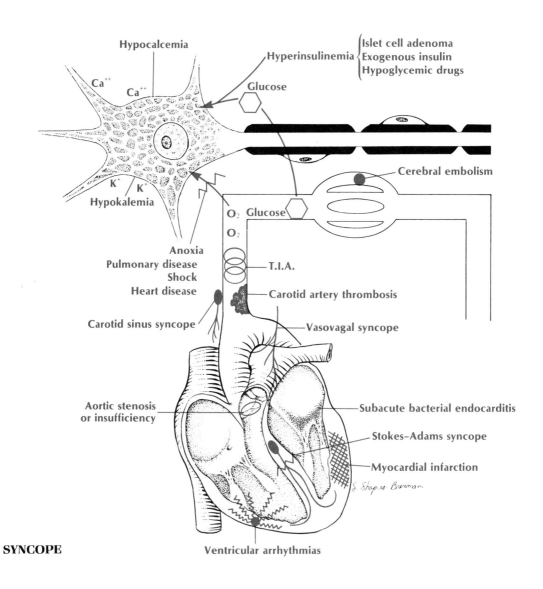

Hypocalcemia

Hyperinsulinemia { Islet cell adenoma / Exogenous insulin / Hypoglycemic drugs

Ca^{++} Ca^{++} Glucose

K^+ / K^+
Hypokalemia

Cerebral embolism

O_2 Glucose
O_2

Anoxia
Pulmonary disease
Shock
Heart disease

T.I.A.

Carotid artery thrombosis

Carotid sinus syncope

Vasovagal syncope

Aortic stenosis
or insufficiency

Subacute bacterial endocarditis

Stokes–Adams syncope

Myocardial infarction

S. Shapiro-Brennan

SYNCOPE

Ventricular arrhythmias

TACHYCARDIA ◼

Tachycardia, like dyspnea, is usually a sign that the tissues are not getting enough oxygen to meet their demands. To recall a list of causes **pathophysiology** is applied. If tachycardia results from anoxia then the causes can be developed on the basis of the causes for anoxia, which may result from a decreased intake of oxygen, a decreased absorption of oxygen, and inadequate transport of oxygen to the tissues. Tachycardia also results when the tissues' demand for oxygen increases. Another cause is peripheral arteriovenous shunts. In addition, anything that stimulates the heart directly, such as drugs or electrolyte imbalances or disturbances in the cardiac conduction system, will cause tachycardia. Let us review the conditions that may fall into each of these categories.

1. **Decreased intake of oxygen.** Anything that obstructs the airway and prevents oxygen from getting to the alveoli should be recalled in this category. Bronchial asthma, laryngotracheitis, chronic bronchitis, and emphysema are most important to recall. In addition, if the "respiratory" pump (thoracic cage, intercostal and diaphragmatic muscles, and respiratory centers in the brain stem) is affected by disease, especially acutely, there will be tachycardia. Poliomyelitis, myasthenia gravis, barbiturate intoxication and intoxication by other central nervous system depressants are examples of disorders in this category. Finally, the intake of oxygen may decrease if there is a low atmospheric oxygen tension. High altitude is an obvious cause but hazardous working conditions must also be considered.

2. **Decreased oxygen absorption.** This may result from three mechanisms.

    A. **Alveolar-capillary block** in sarcoidosis, pneumoconiosis, pulmonary fibrosis, congestive heart failure, alveolar proteinosis, and shock lung.

    B. **Diminished perfusion of the pulmonary capillaries** in pulmonary emboli and pulmonary and cardiovascular arteriovenous shunts.

    C. **Disturbed ventilation–perfusion ratio** in which alveoli are perfused but not well ventilated, in alveoli that are not well ventilated, or in alveoli that are ventilated but not well perfused. This is typical of pulmonary emphysema, atelectasis, and many chronic pulmonary diseases.

3. **Inadequate oxygen transport.** Severe anemia, shock, and congestive heart failure (regardless of the cause) fall into this category, as do methemoglobinemia and sulfhemoglobinemia.

4. **Increased tissue oxygen demands.** Fever, hyperthyroidism, leukemia, metastatic malignancies, polycythemia, and certain physical or emotional demands.

5. **Peripheral arteriovenous shunts.** These shunts may occur in the popliteal fossa following a gunshot wound, in the sellar area following the rupture of a carotid aneurysm into the cavernous sinus, and in Paget's disease.

6. **Disorders that directly affect the heart.** Stimulants of the heart like caffeine, adrenalin (pheochromocytomas), thyroid hormone (hyperthyroidism), amphetamines, theophylline, and other drugs fall into this category. Nervous tension and neurocirculatory asthenia may be the cause. Electrolyte disturbances such as hypocalcemia and hypokalemia may precipitate ventricular tachycardia. Excessive amounts of digitalis may also provoke atrial or ventricular tachycardia.

Tachycardia of various types may occur from disturbances in the conducting system of the heart. Digitalis has already been mentioned, but the Wolff–Parkinson–White syndrome, focal myocardial anoxia from emboli or infarction, and distention of various chambers of the heart (atria in mitral stenosis, ventricles in essential hypertension and cor pulmonale) are also etiologies of this mechanism. Anticholinergic drugs such as atropine block the ability of the vagus to slow the heart and may cause or contribute to tachycardia.

All of the above categories are outlined in Table 5-17 where a few more specific diseases are mentioned.

Approach to the Diagnosis

The association of other clinical signs and symptoms will often help pinpoint the diagnosis. Tachycardia with tremor and an en-

TABLE 5-17. TACHYCARDIA

	V Vascular	I Inflammatory	N Neoplasm	D Degenerative
Decreased Intake of Oxygen	Aortic aneurysm with compression of bronchi	Laryngitis Bronchitis	Carcinoma of the lung	Pulmonary emphysema
Increased Oxygen Absorption	Pulmonary embolism	Pneumonia	Hemangioma Carcinoma of the lung	Pulmonary emphysema Fibrosis
Inadequate Oxygen Transport	Shock from myocardial infarcts Congestive heart failure	Septicemic shock		Aplastic anemia
Peripheral Arteriovenous Shunts				Paget's disease
Increased Tissue Demands for Oxygen		Septicemia Fever of any infection	Leukemia Hodgkin's disease Polycythemia vera	
Disorders Affecting the Heart Directly	Myocardial infarction Essential hypertension	Myocarditis Tuberculosis Pericarditis	Rhabdomyosarcoma	Muscular dystrophy

larged thyroid suggests hyperthyroidism. Tachycardia with respiratory wheezes suggests bronchial asthma. Tachycardia with a black stool suggests a bleeding peptic ulcer. If the blood pressure is low the workup will proceed as that of shock (Appendix I). On the other hand, tachycardia with a normal blood pressure should prompt thyroid function studies, pulmonary function studies, arterial blood gases, and a venous pressure and circulation time. Electrolyte determinations, a drug screen, and 24-hour urine for catecholamine determinations may be indicated if there is hypertension as well. Other tests for the workup of tachycardia are listed in Appendix I.

I Intoxication	C Congenital	A Allergic and Autoimmune	T Trauma	E Endocrine
Pneumoconiosis	Alpha-I trypsin deficiency Cystic fibrosis	Bronchial asthma	Pneumothorax	
Nitrofurantoin Pneumoconiosis Shock lung Lipoid pneumonia	Congenital cysts	Scleroderma Wegener's granulomatosis	Shock lung	Fat emboli
Drug-induced shock Methemoglobinemia	Sickle cell anemia Cooley's anemia	Hemolytic anemia (autoimmune)	Hemorrhagic shock	
	Carotidcavernous shunt		Popliteal aneurysm	
				Hyperthyroidism
Caffeine Amphetamines Alcohol Hyperkalemia Digitalis	Wolff–Parkinson– White syndrome Glycogen storage disease	Lupus erythematosus	Traumatic aneurysm	Hyperthyroidism Pheochromocytomas

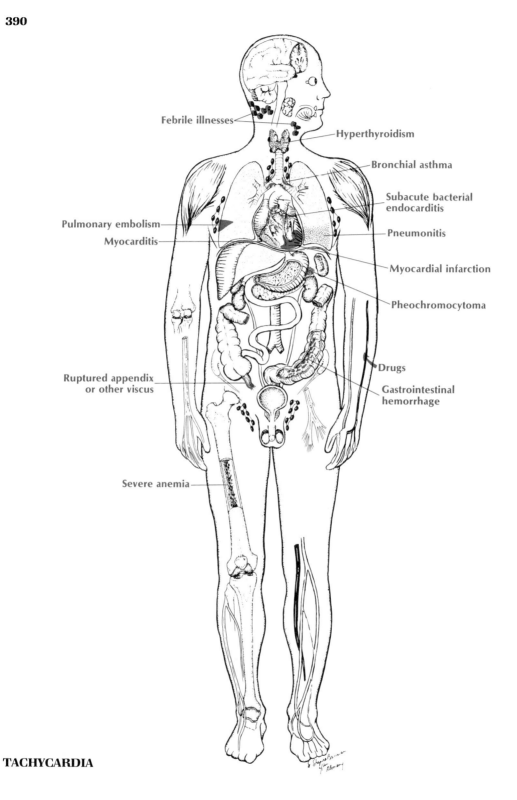

Febrile illnesses

Hyperthyroidism

Bronchial asthma

Subacute bacterial
endocarditis

Pulmonary embolism

Pneumonitis

Myocarditis

Myocardial infarction

Pheochromocytoma

Drugs

Ruptured appendix
or other viscus

Gastrointestinal
hemorrhage

Severe anemia

TACHYCARDIA

TINNITUS AND DEAFNESS ■

If one dissects the **anatomy** of the external, middle, and internal ear one can obtain an excellent list of conditions to be considered in the differential diagnosis of tinnitus and deafness (Table 5-18).

Beginning in the **external canal,** impacted cerumen and foreign bodies are occasionally the cause. Next, visualizing the **drum,** one is reminded of otitis media, herpes zoster oticus, myringitis bullosa, and traumatic rupture of the drum. Behind the drum are the **audi-**

tory ossicles; these little bones should prompt the recall of otosclerosis. The **chordae tympani nerve** passes behind the drum on its way to the jaw and tongue. This structure should suggest the tinnitus of Costen's temporomandibular joint syndrome. The **eustachian tube** should remind one of the aerotitis connected with flying and the serous otitis connected with blockage of the tube from upper respiratory infections and allergies. Behind the middle ear the connecting passages of the **mastoid bones** suggest mastoiditis.

Moving deeper to the **inner ear,** one is re-

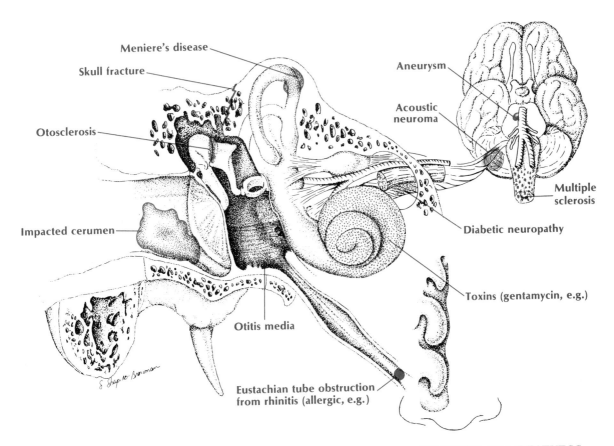

TINNITUS AND DEAFNESS

minded of toxic labyrinthitis from salicylates, quinine, streptomycin, gentamycin, and a host of other drugs. Classified here is also the "toxic" labyrinthitis of uremia, anemia, and leukemia. Syphilis, typhoid, and other bacteria may occasionally invade the inner ear but most infections here are viral. The chronic granulomatous cholesteatoma should be recalled. In visualizing the **labyrinth,** one cannot help but recall Meniere's disease, a prominent cause of tinnitus and deafness. Severe head injuries may cause tinnitus and traumatic labyrinthitis.

Connecting the auditory apparatus to the brain is the **auditory nerve** and acoustic neuromas are quickly brought to mind in the differential diagnosis. The **nerve, brain stem,** and **brain,** however, are affected by numerous conditions and it would be well to recall them with the mnemonic **VINDICATE.**

V—Vascular lesions include aneurysms and occlusions of the vertebral–basilar or internal auditory arteries. Hypertension and migraine may cause intermittent spasms of these arteries with tinnitus and occasional deafness.

I—Inflammatory lesions include syphilis, tuberculous and bacterial meningitis of other organisms, and many febrile illnesses that may lead to transient tinnitus and deafness. Viral encephalitis, rubella *in utero*, and mumps may cause tinnitus and deafness.

N—Neoplasms include acoustic neuroms, meningiomas, and occasional gliomas or metastatic carcinomas and sarcomas.

D—Degenerative disorders remind one of the idiopathic symmetrical tinnitus and deafness in the aged (presbycusis) and the dominant progressive nerve deafness dis-

TABLE 5-18. TINNITUS AND DEAFNESS

	V Vascular	I Inflammatory	N Neoplasm	D Degenerative
External Canal		Otitis externa	Papillomas	
Middle Ear		Otitis media		Otosclerosis
Inner Ear	Spasm of internal auditory artery (migraine)	Petrositis Labyrinthitis or cochleitis	Cholesteatoma	Senile deafness Meniere's disease
Acoustic Nerve	Aneurysms		Acoustic neuromas	
Brain Stem	Basilar artery insufficiency and occlusion	Syphilis Viral encephalitis	Gliomas Meningiomas	Syringomyelia

eases considered under the congenital category. Paget's disease might also be considered here.

I—Intoxication. It is uncertain whether drugs and certain poisons such as lead, phosphorus, mercury, and aniline dyes affect the nerve or cochlea more, but it is well to remember them here also.

C—Congenital disorders that may cause tinnitus and deafness include maternal rubella and all the hereditary causes of sensorineural deafness. Hallgren's disease, Alstrom's disease, Refsum's disease, and Treacher–Collins disease are only a few of these. Some of these are associated with lesions in other organs. For example, Alport's syndrome is the combination of hereditary deafness and nephritis. The aura of tinnitus in epilepsy should be recalled here.

A—Autoimmune diseases that cause involve-

ment of the acoustic nerve and its tributaries include multiple sclerosis and postinfectious encephalomyelitis.

T—Traumatic conditions include skull fractures and the postconcussion syndrome. The occupational tinnitus and deafness of continuous noise must also be considered here.

E—Endocrine diseases include hypothyroidism, acromegaly, and diabetic neuritis.

Approach to the Diagnosis

When a patient complains of tinnitus and deafness, a good occupational history is essential. Gradual onset of unilateral deafness should be considered an acoustic neuroma until proven otherwise. The combination of other symptoms and signs is the key to a clinical diagnosis. Thus tinnitus, deafness, and

I Intoxication	C Congenital	A Autoimmune Allergic	T Trauma	E Endocrine
	Congenital obstruction or absence of canal		Impacted cerumen Foreign body	
		Serous otitis media	Rupture of drum	
Streptomycin Gentamycin INH Other toxins		Meniere's disease	Skull fracture Contusion	Myxedema
			Skull fracture	Diabetic neuropathy
		Mutiple sclerosis	Hemorrhage	

vertigo suggest Meniere's disease. Almost total unilateral deafness (sudden in onset in a diabetic) suggests diabetic neuritis. A similar episode can occur in syphilis but vertigo is also often present. Tinnitus and vertigo following a head injury suggest either traumatic myringitis, labyrinthitis, or a postconcussion syndrome. If there is total deafness with the above, a basilar skull fracture should be considered. Tinnitus and headache suggest migraine.

Diagnostic studies that should be done in all cases are audiograms, caloric tests, and roentgenograms of the skull, petrous bones, and mastoids. If an acoustic neuroma is suspected, tomography of the petrous bones, a CT scan and basilar myelography may be indicated. Syphilis and multiple sclerosis require a spinal tap to assist in diagnosis. Angiography and EEGs may be required in selected cases.

TORTICOLLIS

Torticollis is relatively infrequent; when seen in the adult it is thought to be "supratentorial." There are, however, organic diseases that actually may be responsible. The best approach to recalling these instantly is **anatomical,** beginning with the muscle and proceeding along the nerve pathways to the brain and "supratentorium."

1. **Muscle.** These may be divided into intrinsic and extrinsic lesions.
   A. Intrinsic. Hematomas of the sternocleidomastoid muscle follow trauma, but congenital torticollis is thought to be due to injury or hematoma of the muscle at birth. Another intrinsic lesion is cervical fibromyositis. In this condition the head is usually held in one position.
   B. Extrinsic. Cervical ribs, scars of the neck, tonsillitis, dental abscess, or cervical adenitis may cause torticollis.
2. **Nerve and nerve root.** Conditions of the spinal column such as cervical spondylosis, tuberculosis of the cervical vertebrae, dislocation or fracture of the cervical spine, and cord tumors can cause this disorder.
3. **Central nervous system.** Tumors of the brain stem and cerebellum can cause torticollis. Some cases are due to postinfectious encephalitis and cerebral palsy. Drugs such as phenothiazines and L-dopa may be the culprits.
4. **Supratentorium.** Spasmotic torticollis would seem to fall into this category. I have seen cases begin while a patient is under the pressure of litigation for an occupational injury, especially if he is wearing a cervical collar. Hysteria may also cause torticollis.

Approach to the Diagnosis

An x-ray film of the cervical spine and a thorough neurological examination are axiomatic before one considers the problem psychogenic. A Minnesota Multiphasic Personality Inventory (MMPI) will help support the diagnosis of psychoneurosis, depression, and even malingering. Referral to a psychiatrist may be best if the patient is willing.

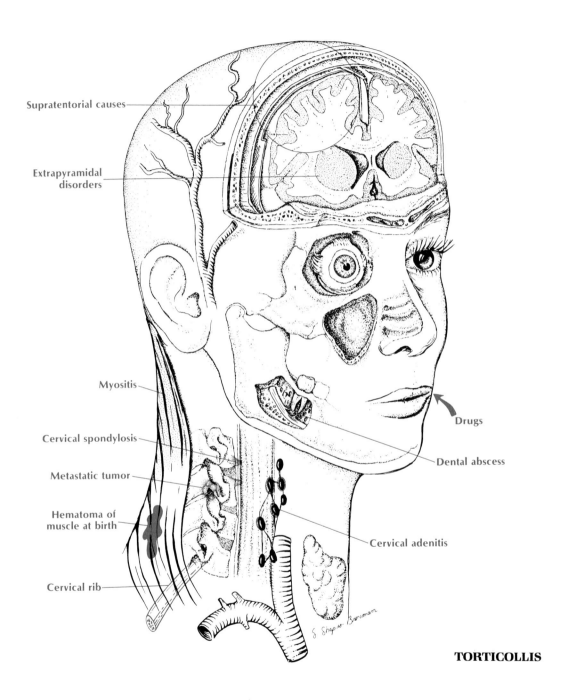

Supratentorial causes

Extrapyramidal disorders

Myositis

Cervical spondylosis

Metastatic tumor

Hematoma of muscle at birth

Cervical rib

Drugs

Dental abscess

Cervical adenitis

TORTICOLLIS

TREMOR AND OTHER INVOLUNTARY MOVEMENTS ■

Anatomy can assist one greatly in formulating a differential diagnosis of tremor of hepatic coma, Wilson's disease, and alcoholism. The **thyroid** brings to mind the tremor of Graves' disease. The **kidneys** signify the tremor of uremia and electrolyte disturbances. The **heart** suggests the choreiform movements of rheumatic fever (Sydenham's chorea). Finally, the **nervous system** indicates a host of other causes that can be further differentiated by considering the tracts and nuclei of the brain. The substantia nigra and globus pallidus are the sites of Parkinson's disease and other related diseases, especially chlorpromazine toxicity. The putamen is the site of gross cavitation and atrophy in Wilson's disease. The red nucleus may be involved in the syndrome of Benedikt, a vascular occlusion of a branch of the basilar artery. The thalamic syndrome produces a unilateral tremor in the extremities and is caused by an occlusion of the thalamogeniculate artery. Manganese, carbon monoxide poisoning, cerebral palsy, and general paresis all affect the brain and basal ganglia leading not only to a tremor but also to an organic brain syndrome in many cases. Huntington's chorea produces bizarre choreiform movements; it can be recalled by its association primarily with atrophy of the caudate nucleus.

Intention tremor is associated primarily with cerebellar disease. The tremor of cerebellar ataxia, olivopontocerebellar atrophy, multiple sclerosis, Dilantin toxicity, and cerebellar neoplasms can be recalled in this fashion.

Considering the entire **brain** and **brain stem** will bring to mind viral encephalitis and postinfectious encephalitis. If one includes the spinal cord and peripheral nerves, Jakob–Creutzfeldt disease will be recalled. Other rare causes of tremor can be recalled by visualizing the tracts or nuclei of the brain that are most significantly involved.

A second method to recall quickly the causes of tremor is to apply the mnemonic **VINDICATE.**

V—Vascular suggests thalamic syndrome and arteriosclerosis.

I—Inflammatory signifies encephalidites.

N—Neoplasms signify neoplasms of the cerebellum and brain stem.

D—Degenerative brings to mind Parkinson's disease, Wilson's disease, Friedreich's ataxia, and a host of other central nervous system disorders.

I—Intoxication recalls alcoholism, manganese toxicity, Dilantin, carbon monoxide, and lead toxicity, as well as hepatic and renal coma with tremors.

C—Congenital suggests dystonia muscularum deformans and cerebral palsy.

A—Autoimmune suggests Sydenham's chorea.

T—Trauma suggests the tremor in post-traumatic and postconcussion syndrome and in post-traumatic necrosis.

E—Endocrine brings to mind hyperthyroidism.

Approach to the Diagnosis

The workup of tremor and other involuntary movements involves most of all a good history. The neurological exam is important as it will determine the type of tremor. Rapid fine tremors (8 to 20 per second) are suggestive of hyperthyroidism and emotional disorders. Coarser tremors at rest suggest Parkinsonism, whereas a flapping tremor of 4 to 8 per second suggests Wilson's disease. The association of other neurological signs helps pin down the diagnosis. Spasms of pain suggest a thalamic syndrome, whereas ataxia suggests Friedreich's ataxia and loss of memory suggests manganese toxicity. Laboratory tests will be

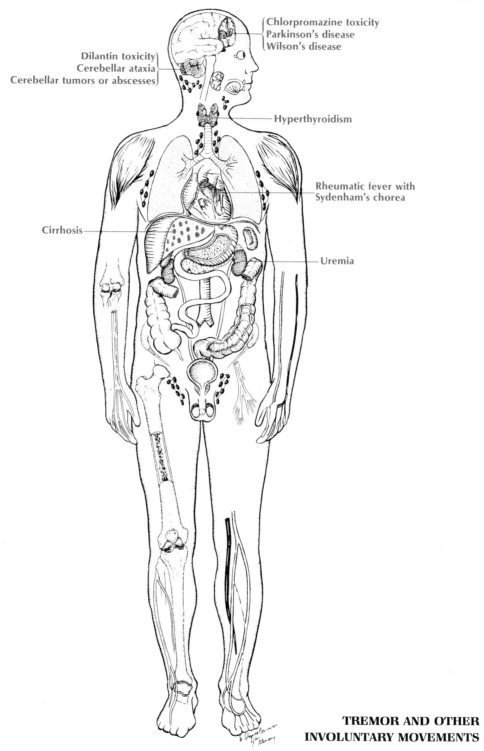

Chlorpromazine toxicity
Parkinson's disease
Wilson's disease

Dilantin toxicity
Cerebellar ataxia
Cerebellar tumors or abscesses

Hyperthyroidism

Rheumatic fever with
Sydenham's chorea

Cirrhosis

Uremia

**TREMOR AND OTHER
INVOLUNTARY MOVEMENTS**

useful in selected cases. Blood lead levels, manganese levels, copper and ceruloplasmin levels may be necessary. A T_3, T_4 and free thyroxine index will confirm the diagnosis of Grave's disease. Other tests that may be helpful may be found in Appendix I and Appendix II.

WALKING DIFFICULTIES

When a patient complains of difficulty walking, visualize the **anatomical** components of the leg: skin, muscle, arteries, veins, bones, joints, and peripheral nerves. Going one step further, follow the peripheral artery to its origin (femoral artery, aorta, and so forth) and the peripheral nerve to its origin in the spinal cord, and then follow its secondary connections to the cerebellum and cerebrum. Now it is possible to recall the causes of difficulty walking as the patient is being examined.

1. **Skin.** Look for calluses, infectious ulcers, and deformities of the feet.
2. **Muscle.** Check for possible myositis, contusions, and muscular atrophy or dystrophy. The gait of muscular dystrophy is slapping and waddling and there is a pelvic tilt forward.
3. **Arteries.** Peripheral arteriosclerosis and Buerger's disease will often be detected by palpation of the dorsalis pedis and tibialis pulses. However, do not forget to feel the femorals (to rule out Leriche's syndrome) and popliteals. Listening to the heart may determine a cause for a peripheral embolism.
4. **Veins.** Dilated varicose veins will be obvious but checking for a positive Homan's sign will be necessary to rule out deep vein phlebitis.
5. **Bones.** Osteomyelitis and sarcomas or metastatic disease of the bone will usually present with the worst pain and make the patient extremely reluctant to walk. A mass or deformity in the bone is usually palpable.
6. **Joints.** Osteoarthritis, gout, and rheumatoid arthritis of the knee are not hard to detect. The gait in diseases in any joint in the leg is a limp. The cause of pain in the other joints may be more difficult to appraise even with an x-ray film. Nevertheless these and a full joint disease workup will help (see p. 486). An osteoarthritic spur of the heel may be found. Bursitis in numerous areas should be looked for. Congenital lesions such as slipped epiphysis, dislocation of the hip, and aseptic necrosis should be considered in children.
7. **Peripheral nerves.** A peripheral neuropathy from alcohol or diabetes will cause a steppage gait (due to moderate or severe foot drop) and traumatic or lead neuropathy may cause an overt foot drop. The atrophy of the muscles without fasciculations will help in the diagnosis of these as well as in Dejerine–Sottas hereditary neuropathy and Charcot–Marie–Tooth disease. Sensory changes (glove and stocking anesthesia and analgesia) are also useful.
8. **Spinal cord.** These diseases present with different types of gaits. There may be a wide-based ataxic gait with a positive Romberg's sign in dorsal column and dorsal root involvement, suggesting tabes dorsalis and pernicious anemia. There may be a wide-based reeling ataxia with a negative Romberg's sign, suggesting cerebellar disease like Friedreich's ataxia. A spastic gait suggests amyotrophic lateral sclerosis, multiple sclerosis, and diseases with diffuse spinal cord involvement such as anterior spinal artery occlusion. A spastic ataxic gait is typical of multiple sclerosis. Other causes of a spastic gait are compression by tumors, cervical spondylosis, or

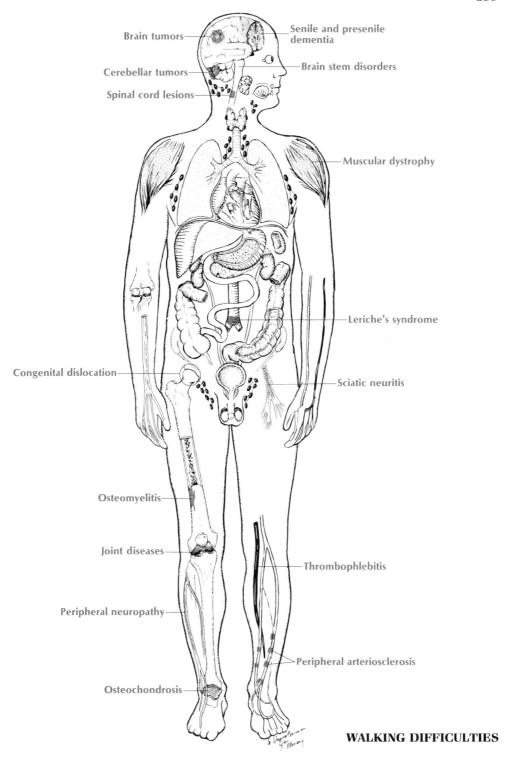

Brain tumors

Senile and presenile dementia

Cerebellar tumors

Brain stem disorders

Spinal cord lesions

Muscular dystrophy

Leriche's syndrome

Congenital dislocation

Sciatic neuritis

Osteomyelitis

Joint diseases

Thrombophlebitis

Peripheral neuropathy

Peripheral arteriosclerosis

Osteochondrosis

WALKING DIFFICULTIES

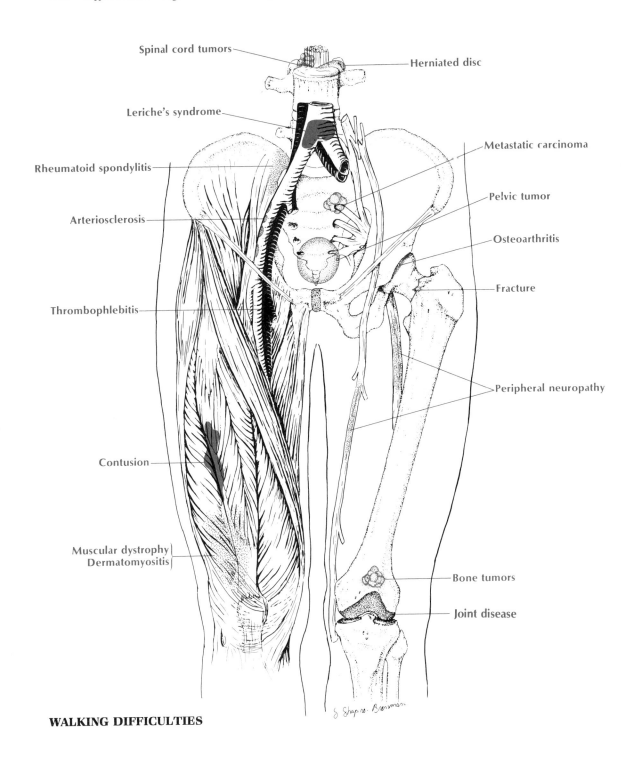

Spinal cord tumors

Herniated disc

Leriche's syndrome

Metastatic carcinoma

Rheumatoid spondylitis

Pelvic tumor

Arteriosclerosis

Osteoarthritis

Fracture

Thrombophlebitis

Peripheral neuropathy

Contusion

Muscular dystrophy
Dermatomyositis

Bone tumors

Joint disease

S. Shapiro-Brenman

WALKING DIFFICULTIES

discs and transverse myelitis, traumatic conditions like fractures, and hematomas and epidural abscesses. The gait of herniated discs of the lumbosacral spine is usually a list to the left or right or a limp. Loss of the ankle or knee jerk, dermatomal sensory loss, and erector spinae muscle spasm will help in this diagnosis. If there is a cauda equina tumor or poliomyelitis, bladder symptoms are usually present as well. Other conditions of the lumbosacral spine disturb the gait (limp) and include osteoarthritis, rheumatoid spondylitis, spondylolisthesis, metastatic tumors, tuberculosis, and multiple myeloma.

9. **Secondary connections to the brain.** Involvement of the pyramidal tracts in the brain often produce a hemiplegic gait where the weak or spastic leg is dragged along the floor. The gait of vestibular disease is ataxic and reeling during an attack. Cerebellar disease has already been discussed. Tumors or abscesses here and alcoholic and phenylhydantoin toxicity may cause a cerebellar ataxia. Multiple sclerosis is another condition that may result in this type of a gait. Bilateral cerebral involvement in cerebral arteriosclerosis or presenile and senile dementia produces the short-stepped gait of *marche à petits pas.* Cerebral palsy may cause a scissor gait. The spastic, shuffling gait of Parkinsonism with propulsion and retropulsion is not easily missed.

Approach to the Diagnosis

The clinical diagnosis depends on the presence or absence of other symptoms and signs. If the extremities check out normally on appearance, a thorough neurological examination should be done. Roentgenograms of the spine and skull, CT scans, a spinal tap, and myelography all have their place. Appendix I presents a more complete list of tests that should be considered in the workup.

WEAKNESS AND FATIGUE, GENERALIZED

The analysis of the causes of weakness depends on a knowledge of both **anatomy** and **biochemistry.** Strength depends on an intact healthy muscle, a functioning myoneural junction, an intact peripheral nerve, lower and upper motor neuron pathways. Thus general weakness may develop in **muscle disease** (analyzed according to etiologic categories in Table 5–19), **myoneural junction disease** (myasthenia gravis), **peripheral neuropathies** (Table 5–19), **anterior horn disease** (poliomyelitis, lead poisoning, and spinal muscular atrophy), and **diffuse disease of the pyramidal tracts,** such as multiple sclerosis. Parkinson's disease fatigues the muscles by the tremor and spasticity it induces.

But this is only half the story. A muscle cannot be strong unless there is adequate intake and absorption of glucose or proper tissue use of glucose (insulin action). Malnutrition and malabsorption syndrome are excellent examples of the former, whereas diabetes mellitus, acromegaly, Cushing's disease, and insulinomas are good examples of the latter. The muscle must also have an adequate supply of oxygen. Thus chronic lung disease (see p. 266) of any cause, congestive heart failure of any cause, and chronic anemias may all produce weakness because of decreased supply of oxygen to the muscles. It is also vital to have the proper minerals surrounding the muscle fiber. Most important are proper sodium, potassium, and calcium balance. Thus any condition causing a low sodium syndrome (congestive heart failure or diuretics) a high or low potassium syndrome (Addison's disease, diuretics, aldosterone tumors), or a high or low calcium balance (hyperparathyroidism, metastatic carcinoma of the bone, and hypoparathyroidism) may produce weakness.

(Text continues on p. 404)

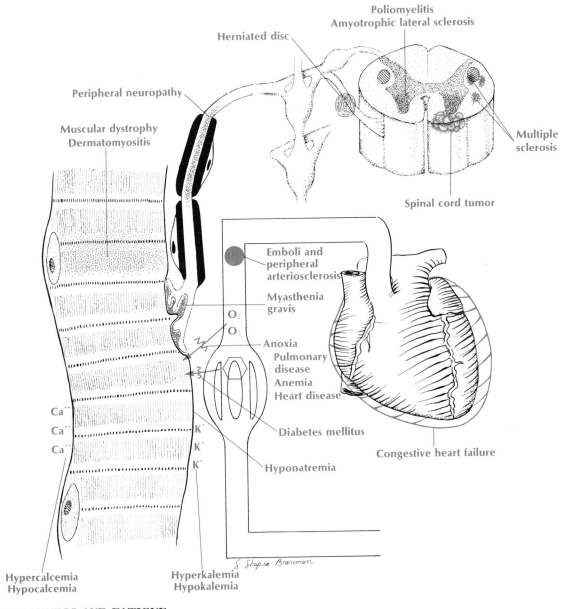

Poliomyelitis
Amyotrophic lateral sclerosis

Herniated disc

Peripheral neuropathy

Multiple sclerosis

Muscular dystrophy
Dermatomyositis

Spinal cord tumor

Emboli and peripheral arteriosclerosis

Myasthenia gravis

O_2

O_2

Anoxia
Pulmonary disease
Anemia
Heart disease

Ca^{++}
Ca^{++}
Ca^{++}

K^+
K^+
K^+

Diabetes mellitus

Hyponatremia

Congestive heart failure

Hypercalcemia
Hypocalcemia

Hyperkalemia
Hypokalemia

S. Shapiro-Brenman

WEAKNESS AND FATIGUE

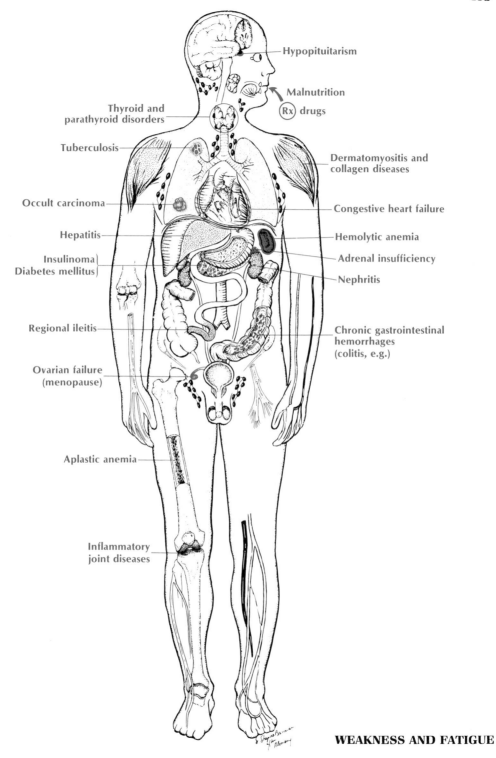

Hypopituitarism

Malnutrition
(Rx) drugs

Thyroid and
parathyroid disorders

Tuberculosis

Dermatomyositis and
collagen diseases

Occult carcinoma

Congestive heart failure

Hepatitis

Hemolytic anemia

Insulinoma
Diabetes mellitus

Adrenal insufficiency

Nephritis

Regional ileitis

Chronic gastrointestinal
hemorrhages
(colitis, e.g.)

Ovarian failure
(menopause)

Aplastic anemia

Inflammatory
joint diseases

WEAKNESS AND FATIGUE

TABLE 5-19.   WEAKNESS AND FATIGUE—GENERALIZED

	V Vascular	I Inflammatory	N Neoplasm	D Degenerative
Muscle	Congestive heart fail- ure	Epidemic myalgia		Malnutrition
Myoneural Junction				
Peripheral Nerve			Metastatic carci- noma	Pellagra Beriberi
Spinal Cord	Anterior spinal artery occlusion	Poliomyelitis Epidural abscess	Spinal cord tu- mors	Progressive muscular atrophy
Brain	Carotid or basilar in- sufficiency or occlusion	Encephalitis Meningitis	Brain tumors (pri- mary and meta- static)	Parkinson's disease Amyotrophic lateral sclerosis Senile dementia

Weakness develops in liver disease because of intermittent hypoglycemia or inability to dispose of toxins. In uremia the problem is not only poor ability to get rid of toxins, but the altered electrolyte media of sodium, potassium, calcium, and magnesium. In hypermetabolic states there may be breakdown of muscle to release protein for nutrition when intake is not adequate to meet demands of vital organs. Thus, in hyperthyroidism, chronic inflammatory and febrile disease, and diffuse neoplastic disease, weakness is a common manifestation.

No discussion of weakness would be complete without mentioning the psychogenic causes of weakness such as depression and chronic anxiety states. Finally, smoking and chronic ingestion of coffee, toxins, and various proprietary drugs (*e.g.,* aspirin) are, of course, related to psychogenic disturbances and should always be considered in the differential diagnosis.

Approach to the Diagnosis

The presence of other symptoms and signs will obviously help pin down the organ-system involved and the diagnosis. However, one is often faced with a negative history and physical examination, and extensive laboratory workup is the only avenue of escape. Or is it? Perhaps the busy diagnostician accepts

I Intoxication	C Congenital	A Allergic and Autoimmune	T Trauma	E Endocrine
Diuretics	McArdle's syndrome	Dermatomyositis	Multiple contusion	Diabetes mellitus Acromegaly Cushing's disease Insulinomas Addison's disease Hyperthyroidism
Cholinergic drugs	Familial periodic paralysis	Myasthenia gravis		
Lead arsenic Alcohol Porphyria	Hypertrophic poly- neuritis Charcot–Marie– Tooth disease	Periarteritis nodosa		Diabetic neuro- pathy Hypothyroidism
		Multiple sclerosis		
Manganese intoxica- tion Tranquilizers	Wilson's disease	Lupus erythematosus Multiple sclerosis	Concussion Postconcussion syndrome	Hypopituitarism

this option too soon when a heart-to-heart talk with the patient or referral to a psychiatrist may be less expensive and more productive. Appendix I lists the necessary tests to work up weakness and fatigue.

WEAKNESS OR PARALYSIS OF ONE OR MORE EXTREMITIES ■

This symptom, as opposed to generalized weakness and fatigue (see p. 401), is almost invariably due to a neurological disorder.

Consequently, a comprehensive list of causes is developed using *neuroanatomy.* Muscle weakness or paralysis may be due to disease of the muscle, myoneural junction, peripheral nerve, nerve roots and anterior horn cells, and pyramidal tract involvement in the spinal cord, brain stem, or cerebrum. Table 5-20 has been constructed with these anatomical components cross-indexed with the various etiologies suggested by the word **VINDICATE.** The most important of these will be covered in the following discussion.

1. **Muscle.** This should suggest muscular dystrophy and dermatomyositis.
2. **Myoneural junction.** Primary and symp-

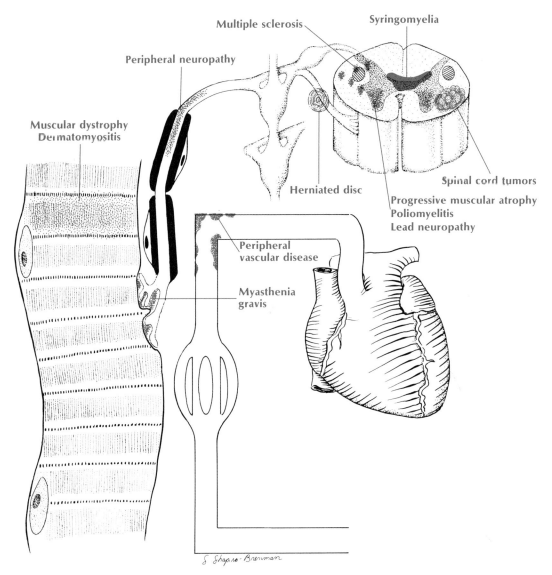

**WEAKNESS OR PARALYSIS
OF ONE OR MORE EXTREMITIES**

tomatic myasthenia gravis are promptly brought to mind here. The toxic effects of succinylcholine chloride (Anectine), cholinergic drugs, and antispasmodics should also be mentioned.

3. Nerve. The many causes of peripheral neuropathy should be recalled here. The most important are diabetic neuropathy, alcoholic and nutritional neuropathy, Buerger's disease, periarteritis nodosa,

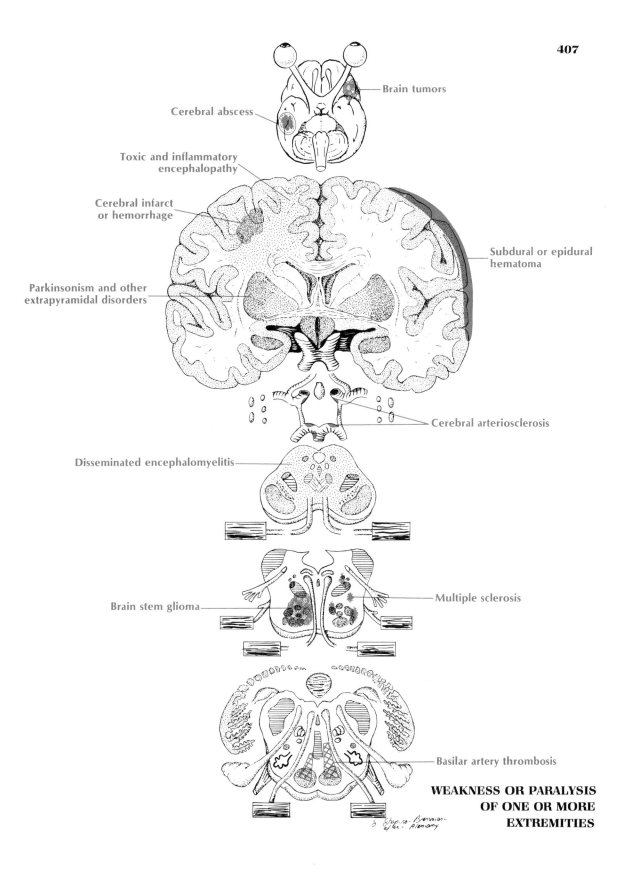

Brain tumors

Cerebral abscess

Toxic and inflammatory
encephalopathy

Cerebral infarct
or hemorrhage

Subdural or epidural
hematoma

Parkinsonism and other
extrapyramidal disorders

Cerebral arteriosclerosis

Disseminated encephalomyelitis

Multiple sclerosis

Brain stem glioma

Basilar artery thrombosis

**WEAKNESS OR PARALYSIS
OF ONE OR MORE
EXTREMITIES**

porphyria, peroneal muscular atrophy, and lacerations or contusions from blunt trauma or surgery.

4. **Nerve root or anterior horn.** Poliomyelitis, lead neuropathy, and progressive muscular atrophy are a few diseases that specifically attack the anterior horn and roots; the roots may also be compressed by her-

niated discs, fractures, tuberculosis, or metastatic carcinomas of the spine. The spinal cord is often involved in the compression too. Cervical spondylosis and spondylolisthesis may also compress the nerve root.

5. **Spinal cord.** The pyramidal tracts are involved in **malformations** such as syrin-

TABLE 5-20. WEAKNESS OR PARALYSIS OF ONE OR MORE EXTREMITIES

	V Vascular	I Inflammatory	N Neoplasm	D Degenerative
Muscle	Peripheral vascular disease	Trichinosis	Rhabdomyosarcoma Wasting of carcinoma	Muscular dystrophy
Myoneural Junction			Myasthenia of Eaton–Lambert syndrome Thymomas	
Nerve	Buerger's disease Ischemic neuropathy Leriche's syndrome	Diphtheria Infectious mononucleosis Leprosy Leptospirosis	Neuromas Neurofibromas Metastasis	
Spinal Cord	Anterior spinal artery occlusion Aortic aneurysms	Epidural abscess Transverse myelitis Syphilis	Primary and metastatic tumors Myeloma	Syringomyelia Amyotrophic lateral sclerosis
Brain Stem	Basilar artery occlusions and aneurysms	Syphilis TB Viral encephalitis Arachnoiditis	Primary and metastatic tumors	Syringobulbia Amyotrophic lateral sclerosis
Cerebrum	Emboli Thrombi Hemorrhage Aneurysms A-V anomaly	Syphilis Encephalitis Cerebral abscess Venous sinus thrombosis Tuberculosis	Primary and metastatic tumors	Senile and presenile dementia

gomyelia, arteriovenous anomalies, and Friedreich's ataxia; in **inflammatory** diseases like syphilis, tuberculosis of the spine, and transverse myelitis; in **neoplasms** (both primary and metastatic); and in **traumatic** lesions such as fractures, herniated discs, and hematomas. Thus the mnemonic **MINT** is helpful in recalling

these lesions. Cervical spondylosis, amyotrophic lateral sclerosis, syringomyelia, pernicious anemia, and multiple sclerosis may be forgotten, however, if only this mnemonic is used.

6. **Brain stem.** Brain stem gliomas and multiple sclerosis are important causes of pyramidal tract disease, but vascular occlu-

I Intoxication	C Congenital	A Allergic and Autoimmune	T Trauma	E Endocrine
	Muscular dystrophy Familial periodic paralysis	Dermatomyositis	Contusions	Hypothyroid myopathy
Cholinergic antispasmodic drugs		Myasthenia gravis		
Lead and alcoholic neuropathy Furadantin and other drugs	Peroneal muscular atrophy Hypertrophic neuritis Porphyria	Periarteritis nodosa Thrombotic thrombocytopenia purpura	Contusion Laceration surgery Carpal tunnel syndrome	Diabetic neuropathy
Spinal anesthesia Radiation	Friedreich's ataxia	Multiple sclerosis	Epidural hematomas Fractures Ruptured discs Decompression sickness	
	Platybasia	Multiple sclerosis Lupus erythematosus		
Bromism Lead intoxication Alcoholism	Schilder's disease Cerebral palsy Lipoidosis	Multiple sclerosis Lupus erythematosus	Concussion Epidural and subdural hematomas Cerebral hemorrhage	

sions of the basilar artery and its branches far exceed these in number.

7. **Cerebrum.** Any space-occupying lesion such as neoplasms, cerebral abscess, subdural hematomas, and large aneurysms may cause focal monoplegia, hemiplegia, or paraplegia (parasaggital meningioma). Occlusions and hemorrhages of the cerebral arteries, however, are much more common causes of focal paralysis. Diffuse paralysis may result from the toxic and inflammatory encephalidites, presenile dementia, lipoidosis, and diffuse sclerosis. Multiple sclerosis and lupus erythematosus may also attack the cerebral peduncles.

Approach to the Diagnosis

The site of weakness is determined by associated symptoms and signs. Fasciculations suggest nerve root or anterior horn cell involvement, whereas sensory changes suggest peripheral nerve or spinal cord involvement. A combination of spasticity in the lower extremities and flaccid and atrophic weakness in the upper extremities suggests cervical cord involvement. Cranial nerve lesions in association with paraplegia or quadriplegia usually indicate a brain stem lesion.

The workup will depend on the site in which the pathology is suspected to be located. If muscle is the site, then an EMG or biopsy is indicated. If the myoneural junction is involved a Tensilon test is done. Peripheral nerve lesions require a more extensive workup, including a glucose tolerance test, blood lead level, urine for porphobilinogens, EMG, NCV, and possibly a muscle biopsy. Spinal cord lesions require x-ray films of the spine, CT scan, myelography, discography, and spinal fluid analysis. Brain stem and cerebral lesions are best screened with a skull roentgenogram, EEG, and CT scan before a spinal tap or arteriography is considered. These and other tests are listed in Appendix I.

WEIGHT LOSS

As noted in Table 5-21, the diagnostic analysis of weight loss is best accomplished by applying **physiology.** Food and oxygen must be properly and regularly brought into the body (intake), properly absorbed and circulated to the cells, and properly used; the waste products must then be excreted in order for weight to be maintained. The storage of food is essential to maintain weight when food is not being regularly ingested. Finally, there must be minimal excretion of sugar, protein, electrolytes, and water to maintain weight. Let us explore each of these physiological functions for possible alterations.

Decreased intake of food results from any disease associated with vomiting, upper intestinal obstruction (e.g., carcinoma of the pyloris), and esophageal obstruction (cardiospasm and carcinoma of the esophagus). Starvation is not uncommon even today, particularly in the elderly trying to stretch their social security checks. Depression, anorexia nervosa, and other psychiatric disturbances may cause weight loss by decreased intake. Central nervous system diseases such as cerebral arteriosclerosis may cause disinterest in food and poor chewing and swallowing. Chronic alcoholics do not eat. The absence of one vitamin as in scurvy or pellagra may cause weight loss. **Decreased intake of oxygen** occurs in asthma, emphysema, and other respiratory disorders as well as in central nervous system diseases that may cause hypoventilation (poliomyelitis). **Decreased absorptions of food and electrolytes** are common in malabsorption syndrome, pancreatitis, intestinal parasites, and blind loop syndrome. Regional ileitis and tapeworms will reduce the absorption of vitamins. The **decreased circulation of oxygen** is probably the main cause of wasting in congestive heart failure, but certainly congestion of the liver and decreased excretion of

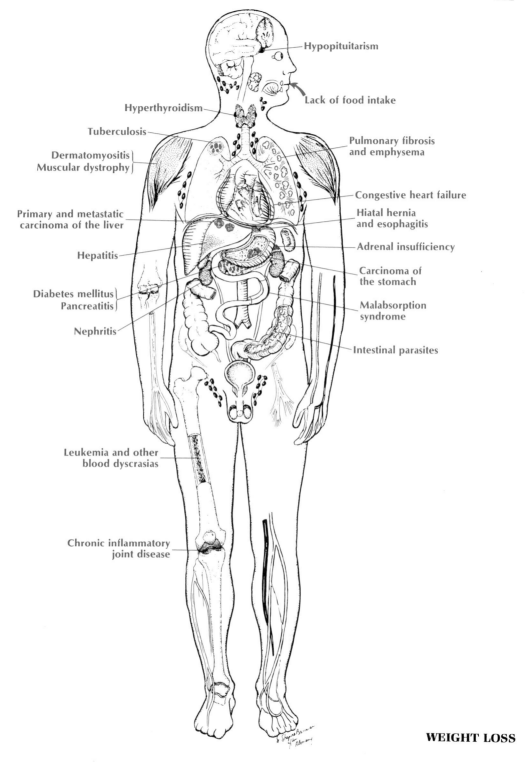

Hypopituitarism

Lack of food intake

Hyperthyroidism

Tuberculosis

Dermatomyositis
Muscular dystrophy

Pulmonary fibrosis
and emphysema

Congestive heart failure

Hiatal hernia
and esophagitis

Primary and metastatic
carcinoma of the liver

Adrenal insufficiency

Carcinoma of
the stomach

Hepatitis

Malabsorption
syndrome

Diabetes mellitus
Pancreatitis

Nephritis

Intestinal parasites

Leukemia and other
blood dyscrasias

Chronic inflammatory
joint disease

WEIGHT LOSS

TABLE 5-21. WEIGHT LOSS

		Physiological Analysis	
Decreased Intake	*Decreased Absorption*	*Decreased Circulation*	*Impaired Storage*
		Oxygen	
Asthma	Sarcoidosis	Anemia of various causes	
Emphysema	Pulmonary fibrosis of	Congestive heart failure	
Central nervous system hypoventilation	other causes		
		Food and Drink	
Vomiting of various causes	Sprue		Cirrhosis
Kwashiorkor	Nontropical sprue		Glycogen storage disease
Obstruction by carcinomas of esophagus or stomach cardiospasm	Intestinal parasites		Hypopituitarism
	Scleroderma		
	Blind loop syndrome		
Anorexia nervosa	Pancreatitis		
Cerebral arteriosclerosis or degenerations			
Chronic alcoholism			
		Vitamins	
Scurvy	*D. latum*		
Pellagra	Regional ileitis		
Alcoholism	Gastric atrophy		
	Pernicious anemia		
	Sprue		

waste products may play a role. Severe anemia of various causes will inevitably decompensate the delivery of oxygen to the tissues.

The weight loss of cirrhosis (numerous etiologies) is probably due to **impaired storage of fat and sugar** for use when it is most needed, but the ability to convert protein to sugar and vice versa is also impaired. In glycogen storage and lipid storage diseases, a one-way trip of sugar or fat into the liver is a prominent factor contributing to weight loss. Probably the most common causes of weight loss today are due to the **increased use of food** in hyperthyroidism and malignancies, but the hypermetabolism of fever and any inflammatory condition (rheumatoid arthritis) is also common.

Neurological and muscular diseases cause wasting and thus **decrease the use of sugar. Impaired use of sugar** in diabetes mellitus and other endocrinopathies is a significant cause of weight loss. Various toxins and electrolyte disorders may block the tissue uptake of oxygen (cyanide poisoning, and so forth)

Physiological Analysis

Increased Utilization	Impaired Utilization	Decreased Excretion	Increased Excretion
	Oxygen		
	Cyanide poisoning and other exogenous toxins Electrolyte disorders	Pulmonary disease, chronic obstructive	
	Food and Drink		
Hyperthyroidism Fever due to infection or neoplasm Hypermetabolism in malignancy, chronic infections (e.g., tuberculosis) Chronic inflammation of rheumatoid arthritis	*Decreased utilization* Various muscle and central nervous system diseases	Jaundice	Aminoacidurias/renal glycosuria Hypocalcemia of various causes Hypokalemia Diabetes insipidus Albuminuria

and cause weight loss. **Disorders of excretion,** also commonly play a role, thus one should always look for uremia, pulmonary emphysema, and jaundice.

Finally, there are many disorders already mentioned associated with albuminuria and glycosuria that may be classified under increased excretion of metabolic substances; these, of course contribute to weight loss. The numerous aminoacidurias and diabetes insipidus should be remembered in this regard.

Approach to the Diagnosis

The clinical approach to weight loss involves a careful search for associated symptoms and signs. It is combinations of these that shed light on the diagnosis. For example, weight loss, weakness, polyuria, polydypsia, and polyphagia suggest diabetes mellitus and hyperthyroidism. Weight loss, polydypsia, and weakness suggest diabetes insipidus. The laboratory workup is essential in most cases (Appendix I).

MISCELLANEOUS SYMPTOMS AND SIGNS

Chapter 6

GENERAL DISCUSSION

This group of symptoms and signs includes changes in the color of the skin, urine, stools and eyes; deformities of the trunk and extremities; and various lesions of the skin, nails, and mucous membranes that cannot be classified elsewhere.

In general no single basic science can be used to recall the many causes of these symptoms. Instead various mnemonics (*e.g.,* **VINDICATE** and **MINT**) are applied to bring to mind the many etiologies involved. Physiology is useful in analyzing the causes of changes in color, whereas anatomy is useful in analyzing such things as skin ulcers. There is no stereotyped pattern for the laboratory workup. The diagnosis is usually based on the presence or absence of other symptoms and signs and the workup of these when present.

CYANOSIS

The causes of cyanosis may be quickly recalled by applying the basic science of **physiology.** Cyanosis is due to **decreased oxygenation of the blood.** The decrease, however, cannot be mild; there must be at least 5 g of reduced hemoglobin per 100 ml of blood if cyanosis is to appear. It should be understood from the above that cyanosis will appear with less severe anoxia in polycythemia than it will in anemia. For example, a patient with 20 g of hemoglobin needs only one fourth of his blood unsaturated to show cyanosis, whereas a patient with 10 g of hemoglobin needs one half of his blood unsaturated to do the same.

Decreased oxygenation of the blood may result from **obstruction to the intake of oxygen** (*e.g.,* acute laryngotracheitis, chronic bronchial asthma, chronic bronchitis, and emphysema or foreign body); from the **decreased absorption of oxygen,** as in conditions with alveolar-capillary block (sarcoidosis, pulmonary fibrosis, pneumonia, pulmonary edema, and alveolar proteinosis); or from a ventilation–perfusion defect (*e.g.,* emphysema, pneumoconiosis, or sarcoidosis). Decreased oxygenation of the blood may also result from **decreased perfusion of the lung** with blood in shock, pulmonary embolism,

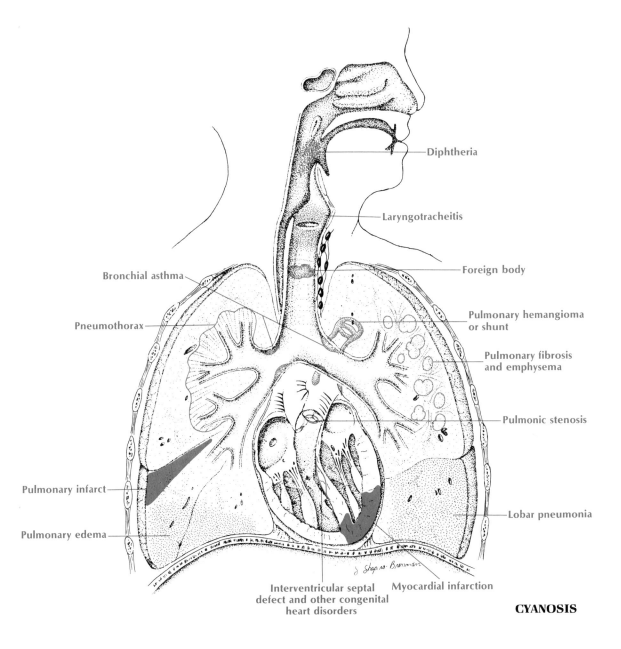

CYANOSIS

pulmonary vascular shunts or bypasses such as occur in pulmonary hemangiomas and congenital heart disease. Another cause of reduced intake of oxygen is an atmosphere with reduced concentration of oxygen. The hemoglobin may be unable to latch onto the oxygen in carbon monoxide poisoning and methemoglobinemia, but the cyanosis is associated with a cherry-red color to the lips and tongue in the former and a brownish hue in the latter; polycythemia vera may be associated with cyanotic hue to the face in cold weather, but the arterial oxygen saturation is not necessarily decreased (Table 6-1).

Another approach to developing a differential diagnosis of cyanosis is to apply the mnemonic **VINDICATE** to the heart and lungs. This is suggested as an exercise for the reader.

Approach to the Diagnosis

The workup of cyanosis includes pulmonary function studies before and after bronchodilators, arterial blood gases, routine and before-and-after breathing 100% oxygen; venous pressure and circulation times, chest roentgenogram, ECGs, and ventilation–perfusion scans. It is unusual not to be able to pinpoint the cause.

TABLE 6-1. CYANOSIS

	M Malformations	I Inflammatory Idiopathic	N Neoplasms	T Traumatic Toxication
Decreased Intake of Oxygen	Foreign body	Acute laryngotracheitis Chronic bronchitis and emphysema Asthma Whooping cough Emphysema		Pneumoconosis Lipoid pneumonia Drowning Pneumothorax Suffication
Decreased Absorption of Oxygen		Sarcoidosis Pulmonary fibrosis Alveolar proteinosis Emphysema	Oat cell carcinoma Metastatic carcinoma	
Decreased Perfusion of the Lungs	Congenital heart disease (Tetralogy of Fallot)		Hemangioma	
Decreased Oxygen Combining Power of Blood				Carbon monoxide Sulfhemoglobinemia Methemoglobinemia

DANDRUFF

The causes of dandruff are similar to the causes of baldness (see Chap. 5), but a brief review will be made here because certain skin conditions should be added. Pityriasis simplex capitis is probably the most common cause, although no definite etiology has been established. Autoimmune disorders such as lupus erythematosus should be considered. Inflammatory disorders include ringworm (tinea capitis), impetigo, and seborrheic dermatitis. Idiopathic skin disorders such as psoriasis and lichen planus cause dandruff. These disorders can all be recalled by the same mnemonic that was applied in baldness, that is, **HAIR.**

H—Heriditary lesions include eczema and psoriasis.

A—Autoimmune includes lupus.

I—Inflammatory diseases include ringworm, impetigo, and seborrheic dermatitis. **I** also stands for idiopathic and thus includes pityriasis simplex capitis.

R—Radiation dermatitis

The workup of dandruff is similar to that of baldness (see p. 235).

EXTREMITY, HAND, AND FOOT DEFORMITIES

Most deformities of the extremities are due to neurological or joint diseases, but because there are some exceptions to this rule the clinician needs a method for easy recall of all the causes when faced with the complaint. The mnemonic **VINDICATE** provides the key.

V—Vascular disease includes arteriosclerosis, Buerger's disease, and Raynaud's syndrome, which may lead to gangrene or loss of a foot or digit.

I—Inflammatory diseases that deserve special mention include the deformities of poliomyelitis, osteomyelitis, and septic arthritis. Syphilis of the bone causes the saber shin, rarely seen today.

N—Neurological disorders cover the largest group of deformities. The beefy red hand of syringomyelia, the wrist and foot drop of peripheral neuropathy (especially lead poisoning), the claw hand and foot of amyotrophic lateral sclerosis or progressive muscular atrophy, the preacher's hand of myotonic dystrophy, and the tight-fisted, flexed, and pronated hand of hemiplegia are the most important ones. Friedreich's ataxia causes a hammer toe and Charcot–Marie–Tooth disease causes a stork leg.

D—Degenerative diseases include the degenerative neurological diseases mentioned above and degenerative osteoarthritis. Deficiency diseases include the bow legs of rickets. Paget's disease causes bowing and hypertrophy of the tibia.

I—Intoxication should remind one of the toxic neuropathies such as lead and arsenic, but it also brings to mind the Dupuytren's contractures of alcoholic cirrhosis.

C—Congenital disorders are another large group, many of which have been mentioned under neurological disorders. However, congenital dislocation of the hip, talipes, equinovarus or valgus, and calcaneovarus or valgus should be remembered. These are often a sign that a congenital lesion exists elsewhere. Hallux valgus is a frequent deformity of the toes. Pes planus and pes cavus belong in this category, although they are not nearly as significant. The deformities of Marfan's syndrome (long fingers with syndactyly), monogolism (*e.g.,*

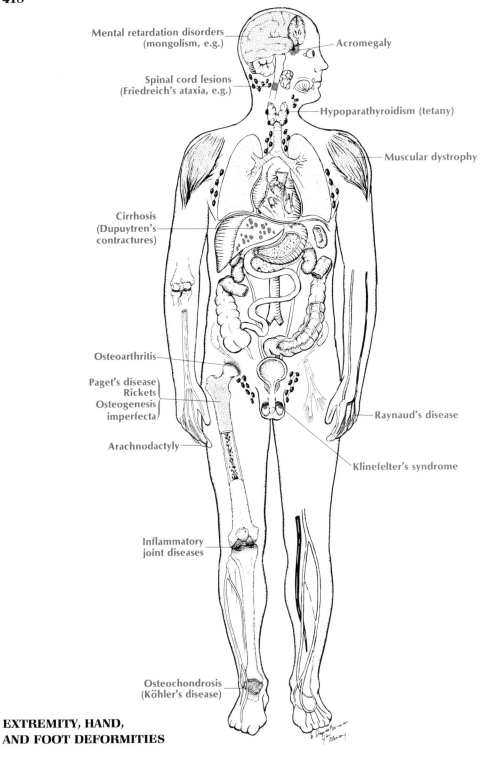

Mental retardation disorders (mongolism, e.g.)

Acromegaly

Spinal cord lesions (Friedreich's ataxia, e.g.)

Hypoparathyroidism (tetany)

Muscular dystrophy

Cirrhosis (Dupuytren's contractures)

Osteoarthritis

Paget's disease
Rickets
Osteogenesis imperfecta

Raynaud's disease

Arachnodactyly

Klinefelter's syndrome

Inflammatory joint diseases

Osteochondrosis (Köhler's disease)

EXTREMITY, HAND, AND FOOT DEFORMITIES

short fingers and simian crease), Laurence–Moon–Biedl syndrome, and achondroplasia are mentioned here.

A—Autoimmune diseases include the spindle deformities of lupus erythematosus and rheumatoid arthritis; the gangrene, autoamputation, and smooth-swollen hands of scleroderma; and the gangrene of periarteritis nodosa.

T—Traumatic lesions need little prompting to recall, but Pott's fracture with eversion of the foot and fracture of the neck of the femur that causes eversion of the entire leg are noteworthy. Dislocations of various joints should be easy to spot, but the mallet or baseball finger of ruptured tendons is tricky.

E—Endocrine disorders include the large hands of acromegaly, the short fingers of cretinism and pseudohypoparathyroidism, and the swollen hands of myxedema. The *accoucheur* hand ("pelvic exam hand") of tetany is appropriate to mention here.

Approach to the Diagnosis

It is usually a simple matter to decide whether the deformity is due to neurological disease or to joint or bone disease. An x-ray film of the hands or feet may be useful in acromegaly and many congenital disorders. Referral to the orthopedic or neurological specialist is usually indicated if bone or neurological involvement is probable. An arthritis workup can be done (see p. 486, Appendix I) if joint disease is the cause of the deformity.

FLUSHED FACE (PLETHORA) ■

Everyone with a red face should not be classified as an alcoholic. The causes of this symptom can best be established with the help of **physiology.** A flushed face may result from an increased amount of circulating blood (polycythemia) or from any factor that may dilate the blood vessels in the face.

Polycythemia may be primary, as in polycythemia vera, or secondary, as in Cushing's syndrome, unilateral renal disease, hypernephromas, and pulmonary or cardiovascular disease associated with chronic anoxia. Capillary dilatation may result from serotonin output in carcinoid syndrome, from vasomotor instability of menopause, from chronic alcoholism (which causes direct capillary dilatation), from sunburn or any burn that damages the capillaries and precapillary arterioles so that they cannot contract, and from mitral stenosis, where the back pressure from the heart causes congestion of the capillaries. It is less commonly found in the use of belladonna, alkaloids, histamine headaches (usually unilateral), and cirrhosis of the liver, but it is common in chronic skin diseases of the face like acne rosacea.

Approach to the Diagnosis

The approach to the diagnosis depends on associated symptoms and signs and the workup of diseases suggested in the differential diagnosis by using Appendix II.

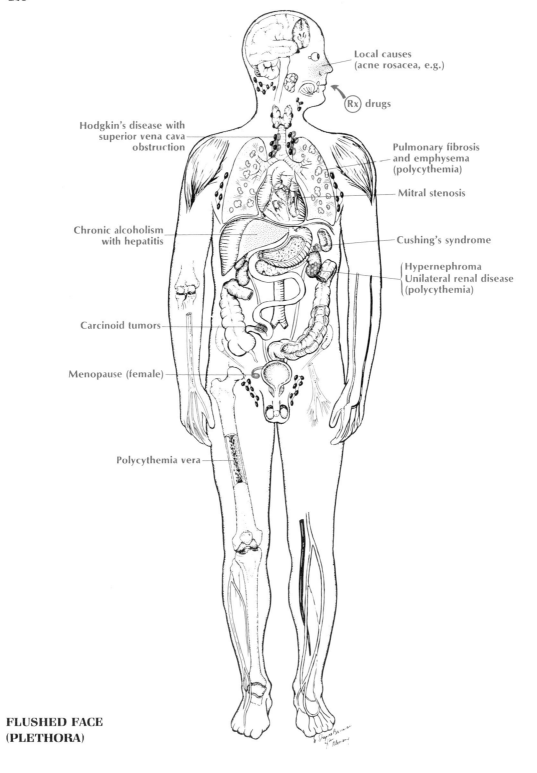

Local causes
(acne rosacea, e.g.)

Rx drugs

Hodgkin's disease with
superior vena cava
obstruction

Pulmonary fibrosis
and emphysema
(polycythemia)

Mitral stenosis

Chronic alcoholism
with hepatitis

Cushing's syndrome

Hypernephroma
Unilateral renal disease
(polycythemia)

Carcinoid tumors

Menopause (female)

Polycythemia vera

**FLUSHED FACE
(PLETHORA)**

HALITOSIS AND OTHER BREATH ODORS

What are the various causes of bad breath and how can they be recalled with ease? The best method is to visualize the respiratory and upper GI tree, because this is where the substances (mucus or sputum and vomitus or regurgitant material) that produce these odors may be found.

In the **mouth**, pyorrhea due to poor dental care and infection may cause halitosis. A stomatitis (*e.g.*, aphthous) may also be a cause. Sinusitis and atrophic rhinitis are causes in the **nasal passages.** Anyone who has a friend with large tonsils knows this is a frequent cause, especially when the tonsils become infected. Any form of pharyngitis may also cause halitosis. Carcinoma and tuberculosis of the larynx and lower respiratory tract may cause halitosis. More likely causes are bronchietasis and lung abscesses.

Proceeding down the **esophagus** to the **stomach**, one should recall the accumulation of food in diverticuli and cardiospasm of the esophagus and the frequent foul odor of chronic membranous or granulomatous esophagitis associated with a hiatal hernia. Carcinoma of the esophagus may also cause obstruction and allow putrifaction of food that accumulates there. A chronic gastritis or gastric carcinoma may also cause halitosis.

A sweet odor to the breath may be found in diabetes mellitus and alcoholism. Uremia will often present with an ammoniacal and urinous odor to the breath, while the breath of hepatic coma may be fishy (fector hepatus). The feculent odor of a gastrocolic fistula and late states of intestinal obstructions should also be recalled.

Approach to the Diagnosis

The workup of bad breath involves a careful examination of the mouth and nasal passages. If this is negative, chest and sinus roentgenograms and upper GI series with a barium swallow should be done. If the studies are still unrewarding, then endoscopy of the respiratory and upper GI tract would be indicated. Appropriate liver and renal function tests will be ordered when uremia or hepatic coma are suspected. If pyorrhea is suspected refer the patient to a dentist.

(Text continues on p. 424)

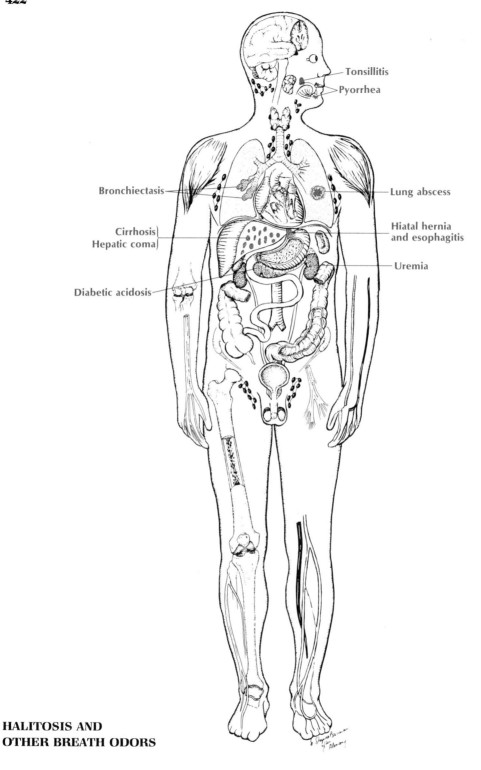

Tonsillitis

Pyorrhea

Bronchiectasis

Lung abscess

Cirrhosis
Hepatic coma

Hiatal hernia
and esophagitis

Uremia

Diabetic acidosis

**HALITOSIS AND
OTHER BREATH ODORS**

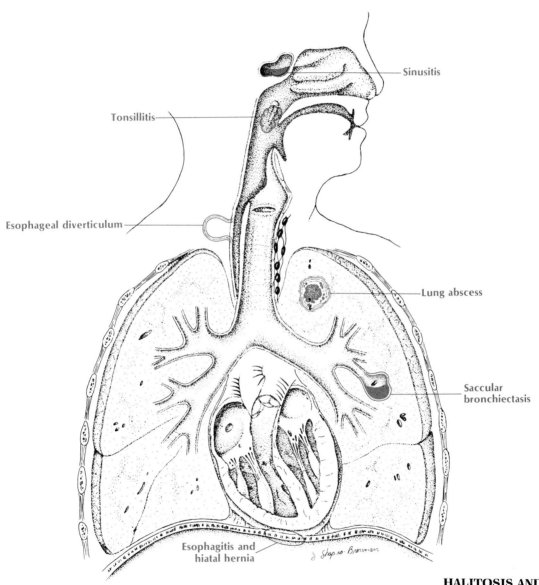

**HALITOSIS AND
OTHER BREATH ODORS**

HEAD DEFORMITIES   ■

The best method to recall the causes of head deformities is to think of the mnemonic **VIN-DICATE.**

V—Vascular suggests Cooley's anemia and the enlargement of head and cheek bones with a small bridge of the nose.

I—Infection recalls syphilis in which the head assumes the shape of a hot cross bun.

N—Neurological disease includes microcephaly (small underdeveloped brain) and hydrocephaly due to several causes); the most important from a treatable standpoint are subdural hematomas, brain abscesses, and neoplasms. Cerebral palsy should be included here too.

D—Deficiency disease suggests rickets, in which the head is elongated, square, and flattened at the vertex.

I—Idiopathic disease recalls Paget's disease. There is symmetrical enlargement (occasionally a triangular shape) because the bones of the face do not enlarge. In facial hemiatrophy one side of the head is smaller than the other half.

C—Congenital disorders include scaphocephaly (elongated from front to back), oxycephaly or tower skull, hypertelorism (increased breadth of the skull and eyes far apart), mongolism, and bradycephaly.

A—Achondrodysplasia suggests a large head with a broad nose and prognathism.

T—Trauma recalls injury to the skull, causing edema (caput succedaneum), hematomas, and fractures.

E—Endocrine disorders such as acromegaly, myxedema, and cretinism cause a large head. Acromegaly is usually easily distinguishable by the protruding jaw.

Approach to the Diagnosis

Obviously the most important thing in the workup of this symptom is a good neurological exam and a skull x-ray film. Other studies will be dictated by the findings of the above. A blood count and morphology study will be worthwhile if Cooley's anemia is suspected and a Wassermann or fluorescent treponemal antibody-absorption (FTA–ABS) test if congenital syphilis is suspected.

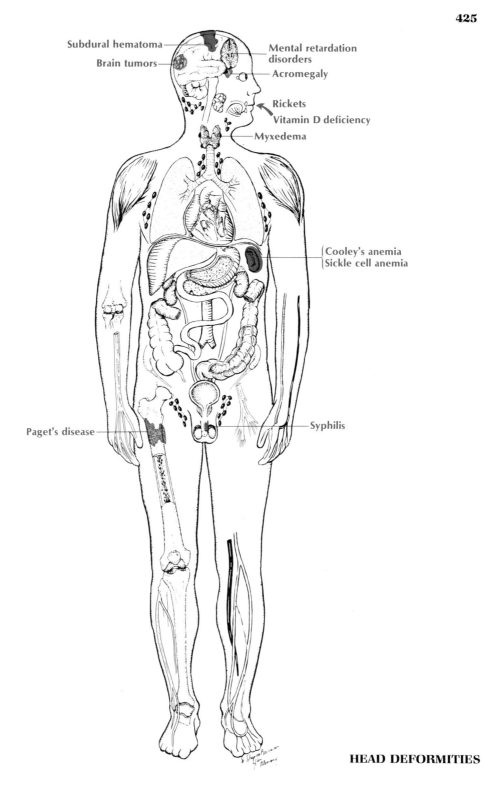

Subdural hematoma

Brain tumors

Mental retardation disorders

Acromegaly

Rickets

Vitamin D deficiency

Myxedema

Cooley's anemia

Sickle cell anemia

Paget's disease

Syphilis

HEAD DEFORMITIES

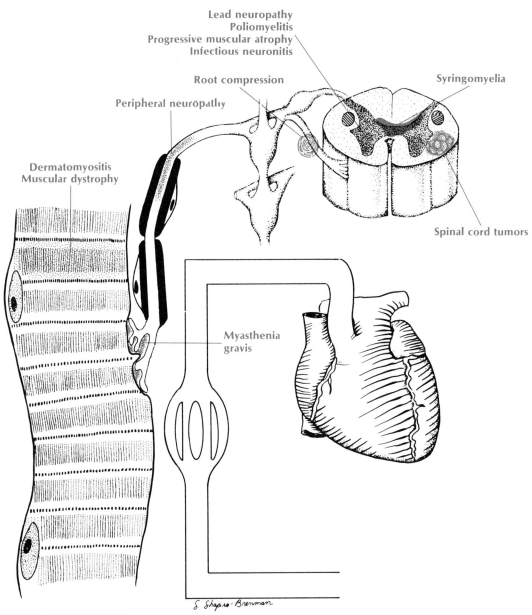

MUSCULAR ATROPHY

MUSCULAR ATROPHY ■

This symptom is developed using both **anatomy** and **physiology.** Atrophy of any muscle may develop in seven ways:

1. Lack of use of the muscle
2. Malnutrition or increased body metabolism
3. Primary muscle disease
4. Myoneural junction disease
5. Peripheral nerve disease
6. Nerve root disease
7. Spinal cord disease

When recalling the differential diagnosis of muscular atrophy, think of these seven factors and the causes will unfold.

1. **Lack of use of the muscle.** In focal or generalized bone or joint disease there is diminished use of the extremity or part involved, so the muscles atrophy. "Disuse" atrophy may also occur in compensation neurosis, hysteria, depression, and in many central nervous system diseases in which motivation is gone.
2. **Malnutrition or body hypermetabolism.** Starvation causes diffuse muscular wasting. Diffuse muscular wasting also occurs in anything that speeds up body metabolism, including hyperthyroidism, metastatic carcinoma and other diffuse neoplasms, chronic inflammatory conditions such as rheumatoid arthritis and collagen diseases, and chronic fever of any cause.
3. **Primary muscle disease.** Muscular dystrophy, dermatomyositis, trichinosis, and McArdle's syndrome should be considered here.
4. **Myoneural junction.** This category makes one think of *myasthenia gravis.*
5. **Peripheral nerve disease.** Diabetic neuropathy and the neuropathy from lead, arsenic, and other toxins should be considered here. Periarteritis nodosa and trauma to the nerve may give an asymmetrical neuritis. Hereditary neuropathies such as Charcot–Marie–Tooth disease and Dejerine–Sottas hereditary hypertrophic neuritis are also considered here. Porphyria is another cause to recall in this category.
6. **Nerve root disease.** Spinal column disorders that compress the root include fractures, herniated discs, spondylolisthesis, tuberculosis, metastatic tumors, and multiple myelomas.
7. **Spinal cord disease.** The degenerative diseases such as amyotrophic lateral sclerosis, progressive muscular atrophy, and syringomyelia must be considered here. In addition poliomyelitis, transverse myelitis of various areas, anterior spinal artery occlusion, infectious polyneuritis, and spinal cord tumors must be recalled.

Approach to the Diagnosis

Focal atrophy of a muscle often means a damaged peripheral nerve or root. If there are visible fasciculations, then a lesion of the spinal cord or root is most likely. Electromyography will determine which portion of the nerve is affected. It will also be helpful in diagnosing muscle disease. Muscle biopsy is valuable to rule out trichinosis, dermatomyositis, or muscular dystrophy. If there are fasciculations an x-ray film of the spine, spinal tap, and myelography may be necessary to establish the diagnosis. A sedimentation rate, CRP, R-A titer, ANA, and tuberculin test may be necessary.

NAIL CHANGES ■

There are various types of nail changes, such as thickening (onychogryposis), thinning, deformity, and separation from the nail bed

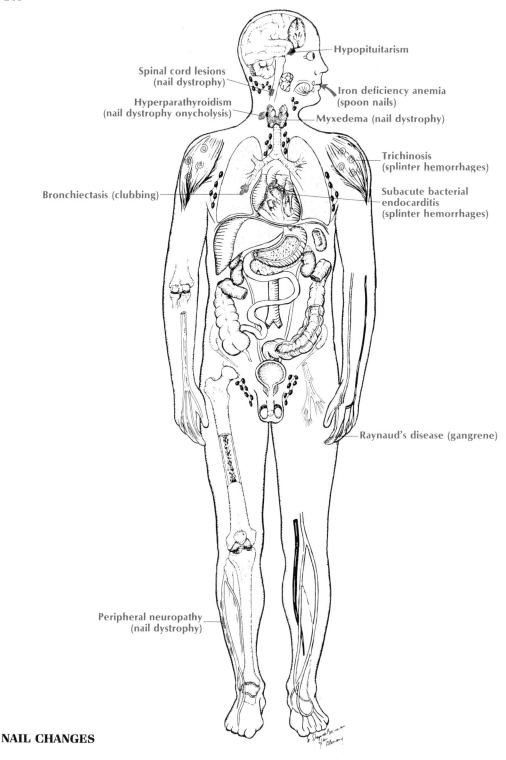

Hypopituitarism

Spinal cord lesions
(nail dystrophy)

Iron deficiency anemia
(spoon nails)

Hyperparathyroidism
(nail dystrophy onycholysis)

Myxedema (nail dystrophy)

Trichinosis
(splinter hemorrhages)

Bronchiectasis (clubbing)

Subacute bacterial
endocarditis
(splinter hemorrhages)

Raynaud's disease (gangrene)

Peripheral neuropathy
(nail dystrophy)

NAIL CHANGES

(onycholysis). Whenever a peculiarity of the nail exists, the mnemonic **VINDICATE** will help recall all the causes.

V—Vascular disease includes the anoxic disorders that cause clubbing (see p. 415), the iron deficiency anemia that causes spoon nails or koilonychia, Raynaud's disease, vasculitis (periarteritis nodosa), and peripheral arteriosclerosis, which causes dystrophy or onychogryposis of the nails.

I—Inflammatory diseases that involve the nail bring to mind fungus infections causing onychia (nail bed inflammation), paronychia, syphilis (which can cause almost any nail change), and subacute bacterial endocarditis or trichinosis, which causes splinter hemorrhages of the nail.

N—Neoplasms do not usually cause nail changes, with the exception of clubbing and pallor from secondary anemia. Chondromas, melanomas, and angiomas are a few neoplasms that do. Intestinal polyposis may cause nail atrophy. The **N,** however, can be used to recall **neurological** disorders such as peripheral neuropathy (dystrophy or onychogryposis), syringomyelia, and multiple sclerosis. The "**D**" suggests **deficiency** disease such as avitaminosis (B$_2$ and D).

I—Intoxication includes arsenic (white lines and transverse ridges across the nails) and radiodermatitis.

C—Congenital disorders include psoriasis, congenital ectodermal defects, absence of nails (ononychia), micronychia, and macronychia.

A—Autoimmune disorders suggest scleroderma, periarteritis nodosa, eczema, and lupus.

T—Trauma causes the familiar sublingual hematoma that causes the nail to turn dark red or black.

E—Endocrine disorders are probably some of the most important causes of nail changes. Hypothyroidism produces nail dystrophy, brittleness, and onycholysis; similar changes, plus spooning of the nails, occur in hyperthyroidism. In hypopituitarism these may be dystrophy, loss of the subcuticular moons, and spooning. Thickening and transverse grooving of the nails may be seen in hypoparathyroidism.

Approach to the Diagnosis

The diagnosis of nail abnormalities begins by correlating the nail changes with other findings (*e.g.,* neurological and endocrinological). Laboratory workup depends on the particular disease or diseases suggested by the nail changes (see Appendix II).

NUCHAL RIGIDITY

Finding nuchal rigidity on examination has almost invariably prompted the diagnosis of meningitis and lumbar puncture, but the astute clinician will want to consider other possibilities in order to avoid a potentially hazardous procedure. **Anatomy** is the key. Visualize the structures of the neck and the many causes come quickly to mind.

Cellulitis of the back of the neck or carbuncle may be the cause in the **skin.** The **muscles** of the neck may be rigid from Parkinsonism or pyramidal tract disease. Diseases of the **spine** such as cervical spondylosis, rheumatoid spondylitis, and tuberculosis may cause nuchal rigidity. An acute fracture of the cervical spine should be considered if no history can be obtained. The respiratory tree recalls retropharyngeal abscess, mediastinal emphysema, and endotrachial entubation. Finally, the spinal cord and meninges may be involved by meningitis, epidural abscess, subarachnoid hemorrhage, and primary and metastatic tumors resulting in nuchal rigidity.

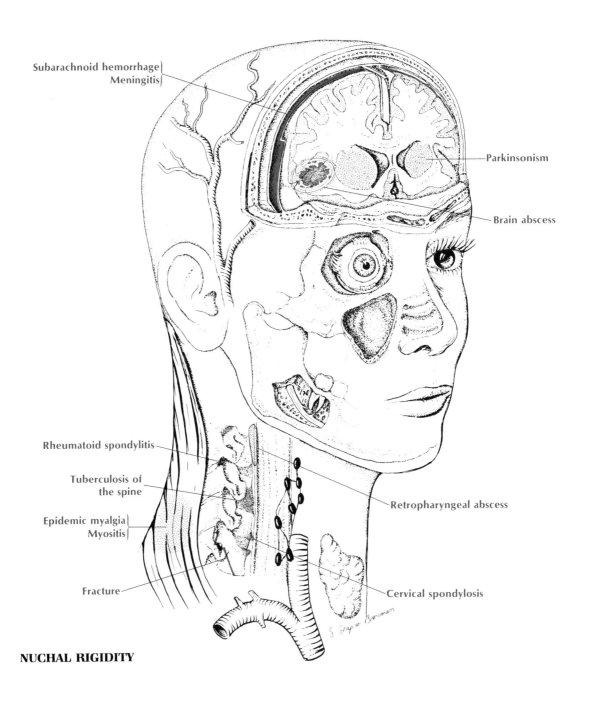

Subarachnoid hemorrhage
Meningitis

Parkinsonism

Brain abscess

Rheumatoid spondylitis

Tuberculosis of
the spine

Epidemic myalgia
Myositis

Retropharyngeal abscess

Fracture

Cervical spondylosis

NUCHAL RIGIDITY

Approach to the Diagnosis

The workup of nuchal rigidity requires a good history, but if one is unobtainable, no spinal tap should be performed until the cervical spine is roentgenographed and the eyegrounds are examined. Even with a good history, a spinal tap ought to be withheld if there is papilledema. A neurosurgeon should be consulted immediately under these circumstances. In a patient with fever, nuchal rigidity, no papilledema, and no focal neurological signs (particularly a dilated pupil), a spinal tap can be performed for diagnosis and immediate therapy. It is preferable, however, to have CT scan results in hand first. Meningitis or a subarachnoid hemorrhage is frequently found in these circumstances. Skull films, CT scans and x-ray films of the cervical spine will still be indicated in cases where the diagnosis remains obscure. (See Appendix I).

PALLOR OF THE FACE, NAILS, OR CONJUNCTIVA ■

Pallor is almost invariably caused by anemia and is best analyzed with the application of **pathophysiology.** Anemia may be caused by decreased production of blood, increased destruction of blood, or loss of blood. **Decreased production** results from poor nutrition particularly, poor absorption or intake of B_{12} (pernicious anemia), iron (iron deficiency anemia), and folic acid (malabsorption syndrome). It may also result from suppressed bone marrow (aplastic anemia) or infiltrated bone marrow (leukemia or metastatic carcinoma). **Increased destruction** is caused by hemolysis from intrinsic defects in the red cells (*e.g.*, sickle cell anemia and thalassemia) or extrinsic defects in the circulation (autoimmune hemolytic anemia of many disorders). **Blood loss** may result from peptic ulcers and carcinomas of the GI tract, excessive menstruation or metorrhagia from tumors of the uterus, or dysfunctional uterine bleeding. These are the principal causes of anemia, but the reader will be able to think of several more. What is important here is to have a systematic method to recall them.

If anemia is ruled out, the less frequent causes of pallor should be considered. Shock, congestive heart failure, and arteriosclerosis cause pallor by poor circulation of blood to the skin. Patients who have hypertension may be pale from reflex vasomotor spasms of the arterioles supplying the skin. Aortic regurgitation and stenosis, as well as mitral stenosis, cause pallor for the same reasons but the malar flush of mitral stenosis may negate this.

The reason that tuberculosis, rheumatoid arthritis, carcinomatosis, and glomerulonephritis cause pallor even when their victims are not anemic or hypertensive is not known.

Approach to the Diagnosis

The approach to the diagnosis of pallor is obviously to check for anemia first; then examination for the other chronic disorders may be carried out. Chest x-ray film, ECG, sedimentation rate and a check for rheumatoid factor are all appropriate in specific cases. Additional tests for the workup are provided in Appendix I.

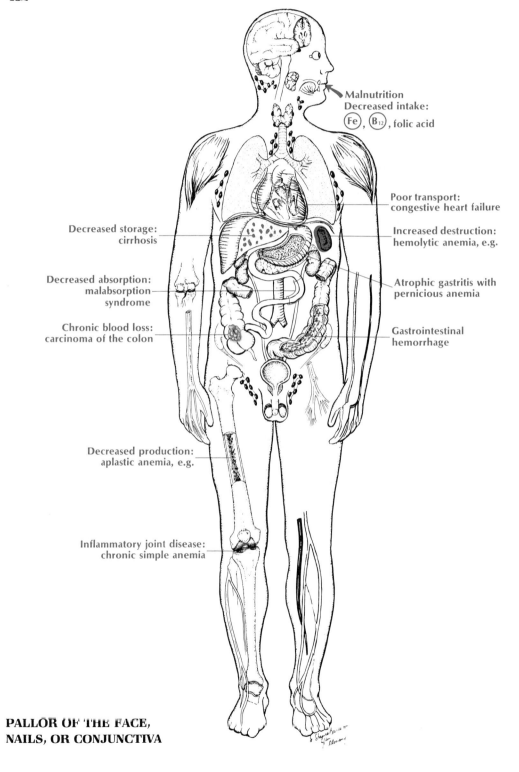

Malnutrition
Decreased intake:
Fe, B_{12}, folic acid

Poor transport:
congestive heart failure

Decreased storage:
cirrhosis

Increased destruction:
hemolytic anemia, e.g.

Decreased absorption:
malabsorption
syndrome

Atrophic gastritis with
pernicious anemia

Chronic blood loss:
carcinoma of the colon

Gastrointestinal
hemorrhage

Decreased production:
aplastic anemia, e.g.

Inflammatory joint disease:
chronic simple anemia

**PALLOR OF THE FACE,
NAILS, OR CONJUNCTIVA**

RASH, GENERAL ■

The best way to recall the causes of a general rash while still examining the patient is to think of the mnemonic **DERMATITIS.*** (See figures on pages 434, 435, 436, and 437.)

D—Deficiency diseases include pellagra, scurvy, and vitamin A deficiency.

E—Endocrine diseases recall the acne and plethora of Cushing's disease, the pretibial myxedema of hyperthyroidism, and the necrobiosis lipoidica diabeticorum of diabetes mellitus. Xanthoma diabeticorum should also be mentioned. Carcinoid tumors may cause a general erythema and cyanosis.

R—Reticuloendotheliosis suggests Niemann–Pick disease, Hand–Schüller–Christian disease, and Gaucher's disease, as well as Letterer–Siwe disease.

M—Malignancies suggest the rash of leukemia, Hodgkin's disease, and metastatic carcinoma. In addition, certain malignancies induce skin conditions like herpes zoster (lymphomas), dermatitis herpetiformis and dermatomyositis (GI malignancy), or acanthosis nigricans (abdominal malignancy). Multiple small metastasis to the skin may suggest a "rash." Neurofibromatosis is a cause of multiple skin fibromas.

A—Allergic and **autoimmune** disease includes angioneurotic edema, urticaria, allergic dermatitis, erythema nodosum and multiforme, and other skin lesions of rheumatic fever, dermatomyositis, scleroderma, lupus erythematosus, periarteritis nodosa, and pemphigus. Allergies to many foods and inhalants may cause a skin reaction. Thrombocytopenia purpura and allergic purpura belong in this category.

* Figures on pages 434, 435, 436, and 437 from Sauer GC: Manual of Skin Diseases, 4th ed. Philadelphia, JB Lippincott, 1980.

T—Toxic disorders include drug eruptions from sulfa, penicillin, and a host of other drugs. Serum sickness should be recalled here. Iodides, boric acid, and many toxins in the environment may be responsible.

I—Infectious diseases are perhaps the largest category to consider. They are best classified by the size of the organism working from the smallest on up.

1. **Viruses** include the exanthema of measles, infectious mononucleosis, rubella, smallpox, chickenpox, herpes zoster, viral hepatitis, and various Coxsackie and echo viruses.
2. **Rickettsiae** include Rocky Mountain spotted fever and typhus.
3. **Bacteria** include typhoid, meningococcemia, miliary tuberculosis (usually a focal lesion), Haverhill fever, brucellosis, leprosy, and subacute bacterial endocarditis.
4. **Spirochetes** include syphilis, which may present any form of a rash, but the lesions are usually small, indurated macules on the trunk, palm, and, to a lesser degree, the extremities. Rat-bite fever and Borrelia recurrentis may also cause a rash.
5. **Parasites** suggest *leishmaniasis americana*, hookworm, toxoplasmosis, and trichinosis.
6. **Fungi** suggest histoplasmosis, which is more likely to produce a general rash than coccidiomycosis, blastomycosis, and spirotrichosis, although all are associated on occasion with rash. Tinea versicolor is also responsible for a diffuse rash, but most of the other fungi cause a local rash.

T—Trauma suggests sunburn and other types of burns, such as radiation.

I—Idiopathic disorders account for a number of diseases. In this category one should remember psoriasis, lichen planus, epidermolysis bullosum, ichthyosis, porphyria,

(Text continues on p. 438)

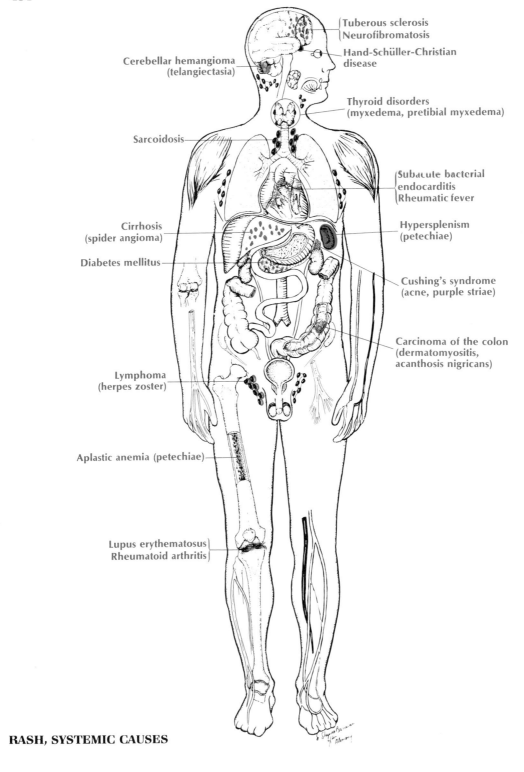

Tuberous sclerosis
Neurofibromatosis

Hand-Schüller-Christian disease

Cerebellar hemangioma (telangiectasia)

Thyroid disorders (myxedema, pretibial myxedema)

Sarcoidosis

Subacute bacterial endocarditis
Rheumatic fever

Cirrhosis (spider angioma)

Hypersplenism (petechiae)

Diabetes mellitus

Cushing's syndrome (acne, purple striae)

Carcinoma of the colon (dermatomyositis, acanthosis nigricans)

Lymphoma (herpes zoster)

Aplastic anemia (petechiae)

Lupus erythematosus
Rheumatoid arthritis

RASH, SYSTEMIC CAUSES

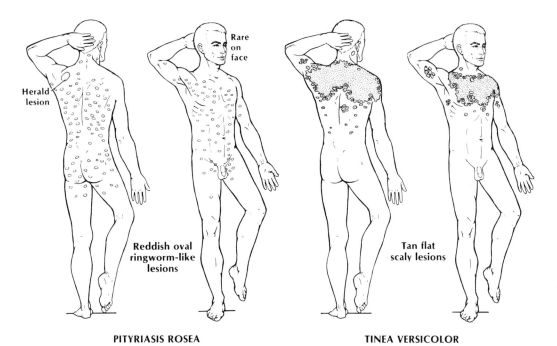

PITYRIASIS ROSEA

Herald lesion

Rare on face

Reddish oval ringworm-like lesions

TINEA VERSICOLOR

Tan flat scaly lesions

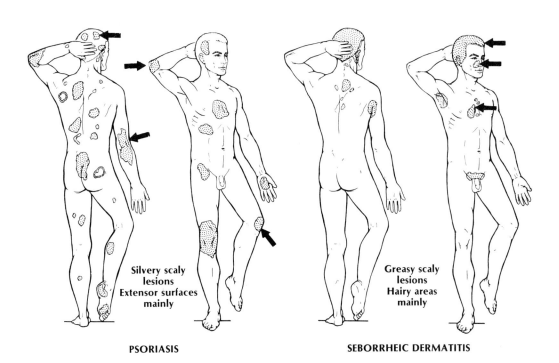

PSORIASIS

Silvery scaly lesions Extensor surfaces mainly

SEBORRHEIC DERMATITIS

Greasy scaly lesions Hairy areas mainly

RASH, GENERAL

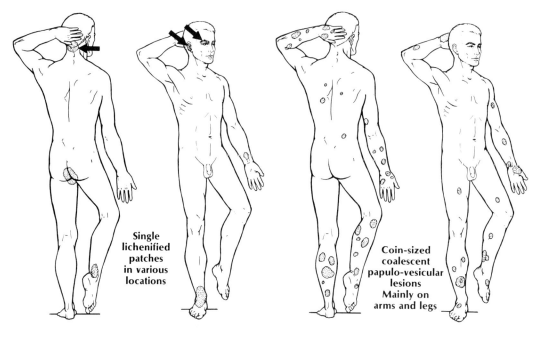

Single lichenified patches in various locations

NEURODERMATITIS

Coin-sized coalescent papulo-vesicular lesions Mainly on arms and legs

NUMMULAR ECZEMA

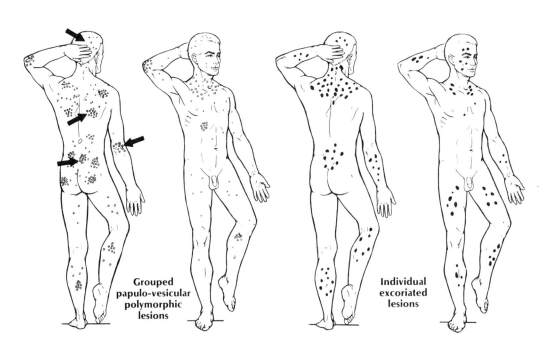

Grouped papulo-vesicular polymorphic lesions

DERMATITIS HERPETIFORMIS

Individual excoriated lesions

NEUROTIC EXCORIATIONS

RASH, GENERAL

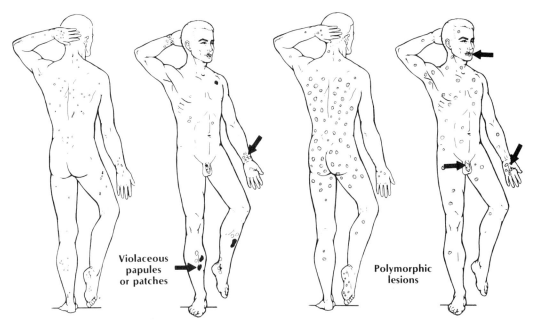

Violaceous papules or patches

LICHEN PLANUS

Polymorphic lesions

SECONDARY SYPHILIS

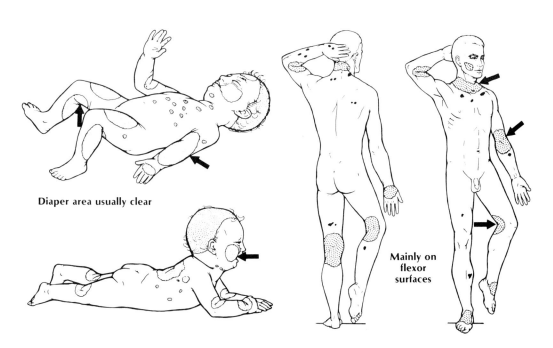

Diaper area usually clear

INFANTILE FORM OF ATOPIC ECZEMA

Mainly on flexor surfaces

ADULT FORM OF ATOPIC ECZEMA

RASH, GENERAL

neurodermatitis or eczema, the adenoma sebaceum of tuberous sclerosis, and keratosis pilaris. Pityriasis rosea may be due to a virus but this is not established yet.

S—Sweat gland and **sebaceous** gland disorders include miliaria (prickly heat) of the sweat glands and milia, folliculitis, and carbuncles and furuncles involving the base of the hair follicle and sebaceous glands. Acne rosacea and acne vulgaris can also be recalled here.

The diagnosis of a rash depends on a good history and a description of the type of rash and its distribution.

Description (only the most typical are listed):

1. **Macular rash.** Typhoid, syphilis, pityriasis rosea, variola (in early stages), rubella (first stages), and tinea versicolor fall in this group.
2. **Papular rash.** Measles, German measles, miliaria, scabies, drug eruptions, lichen planus, urticaria papulosa, warts, lupus erythematosus, erythema multiforme, rat-bite fever, and infectious mononucleosis generally present this way. Rocky Mountain spotted fever may have a maculopapular rash prior to the purpuric rash. Reticuloendotheliosis may also present this way.
3. **Purpural rash.** Meningococcemia, thrombocytopenic purpura from any cause, Henoch–Schonlein purpura, Letterer–Siwe disease, trichinosis, leukemia, subacute bacterial endocarditis, and Rocky Mountain spotted fever and other rickettsiae are in this category.
4. **Vesicles.** Contact or allergic dermatitis, miliaria, eczema, variola and varicella, dermatophytosis, tinea circinata, herpes zoster, poison ivy, scabies (one stage), and some drug allergies present this way. Impetigo may start as a vesicle but usually quickly becomes bullous.
5. **Bullae.** Pemphigus, impetigo contagiosa, hereditary syphilis, herpes zoster, dermatitis herpetiformis, and epidermyolysis bullosa are considered here.
6. **Scales.** Psoriasis, parapsoriasis, and lichen planus are the most typical causes of this lesion, but most dermatoses may get to this stage after chronic itching. Scarlet fever has a definite desquamative phase and pityriasis rosea will demonstrate scaling on scratching. Tinea versicolor, the dermatophytoses, and exfoliative dermatitis must be considered here.
7. **Pustules.** Furunculosis and impetigo are the most typical types of this lesion but they are usually focal rashes. Smallpox (variola) will demonstrate pustules in the late stages and chickenpox may do the same. It is unusual for pustular lesions to be generalized.
8. **Nodules.** Erythema nodosum, erythema induratum, and Weber–Christian disease fall into this category.

Distribution

1. **Trunk.** Pityriasis rosea, drug eruptions, herpes zoster, dermatitis herpetiformis, chicken pox, seborrheic dermatitis, and tinea versicolor occur typically on the trunk.
2. **Extremities.** Smallpox and Rocky Mountain spotted fever often begin on the extremities and work centripetally.
3. **Palms of the hands.** Four conditions typically occur here: Rocky Mountain spotted fever, penicillin allergy, syphilis, and erythema multiforme. Contact dermatitis, keratoderma, climacterium, warts, keratoderma palmaris, dyshidrosis, and psoriasis may also occur here.
4. **Feet.** Tinea pedis, warts, purpuras, psori-

asis, keratoderma plantaris, syphilis, penicillin allergy, Rocky Mountain spotted fever, acrodynia, varicose ulcers, diabetic ulcers, and ischemic ulcers may occur here more often than elsewhere. Contact dermatitis from leather is important to consider here.

5. **Face.** Acne vulgaris and rosacea, impetigo, seborrheic dermatitis, milia, lupus erythematosus, lupus vulgaris, basal cell and squamous cell carcinoma, eczema, contact dermatitis, and erythema multiforme have a predilection for the face.

6. **Groins and thighs.** Scabies, pediculosis, intertrigo, tinea cruris, moniliasis, and Weber–Christian disease occur here.

7. **Antecubital and popliteal spaces.** Eczema occurs here.

8. **Extensor surfaces of elbow and knees.** Psoriasis and epidermolysis bullosa should be considered.

9. **Shins.** Erythema nodosum occurs here.

The description and distribution of all the dermatological conditions would take volumes. Only the most common or important ones have been considered here.

Approach to the Diagnosis

The laboratory workup of a rash is considered in Appendix I. Any condition with pus should be cultured. If a fungus is suspected, a Wood's lamp examination and a fresh potassium hydroxide (KOH) preparation should be done. Skin biopsy is useful and is necessary in some cases. A dermatologist should be consulted if there is any question about a malignancy, if the condition persists, or if it causes systemic symptoms. It is foolish to persist in treatment without a definitive diagnosis for more than 2 or 3 weeks when one may be dealing with something serious.

RASH, LOCAL ■

The differential diagnosis of a local rash is best approached with the mnemonic **VINDICATE.**

V—Vascular suggests livedo reticularis, acrocyanosis, gangrene of Raynaud's syndrome, necrotic areas of periarteritis nodosa, and petechiae from emboli. Varicose and ischemic ulcers may also be considered here.

I—Inflammatory lesions include boils, caruncle, folliculitis, hydradenitis suppurativa, abscess, and erysipelas. Dermatophytosis, chancre, chanchroid, and yaws, pinta, and tularemia are important. Scabies, insect bites, anthrax, tuberculosis, or actinomycotic sinus fall in this category. The fistulous tracts of regional ileitis may belong here. Warts and moluscum contagiosa also need mentioning here.

N—Neoplasms of the skin include fibromas, melanomas, lipomas, basal cell and squamous cell carcinomas, and metastatic carcinoma. Kaposi's sarcoma and mycosis fungoides must also be considered.

D—Degenerative lesions like senile keratosis are considered here. Kraurosis vulvae may be recalled here.

I—Intoxication includes acid or alkaline burns of the skin. Fixed-drug eruptions should not be forgotten.

C—Congenital lesions include epidermolysis bullosa, eczema, neurofibromatosis, and lipomas.

A—Allergic and **autoimmune** diseases suggest pyoderma gangrenosum (ulcerative colitis), necrotic lesions of periarteritis nodosa, and subcutaneous fat necrosis of Weber–Christian disease.

T—Trauma suggests burns, contusions, lacerations, and hemorrhages.

E—Endocrine diseases immediately recall

(Text continues on p. 442)

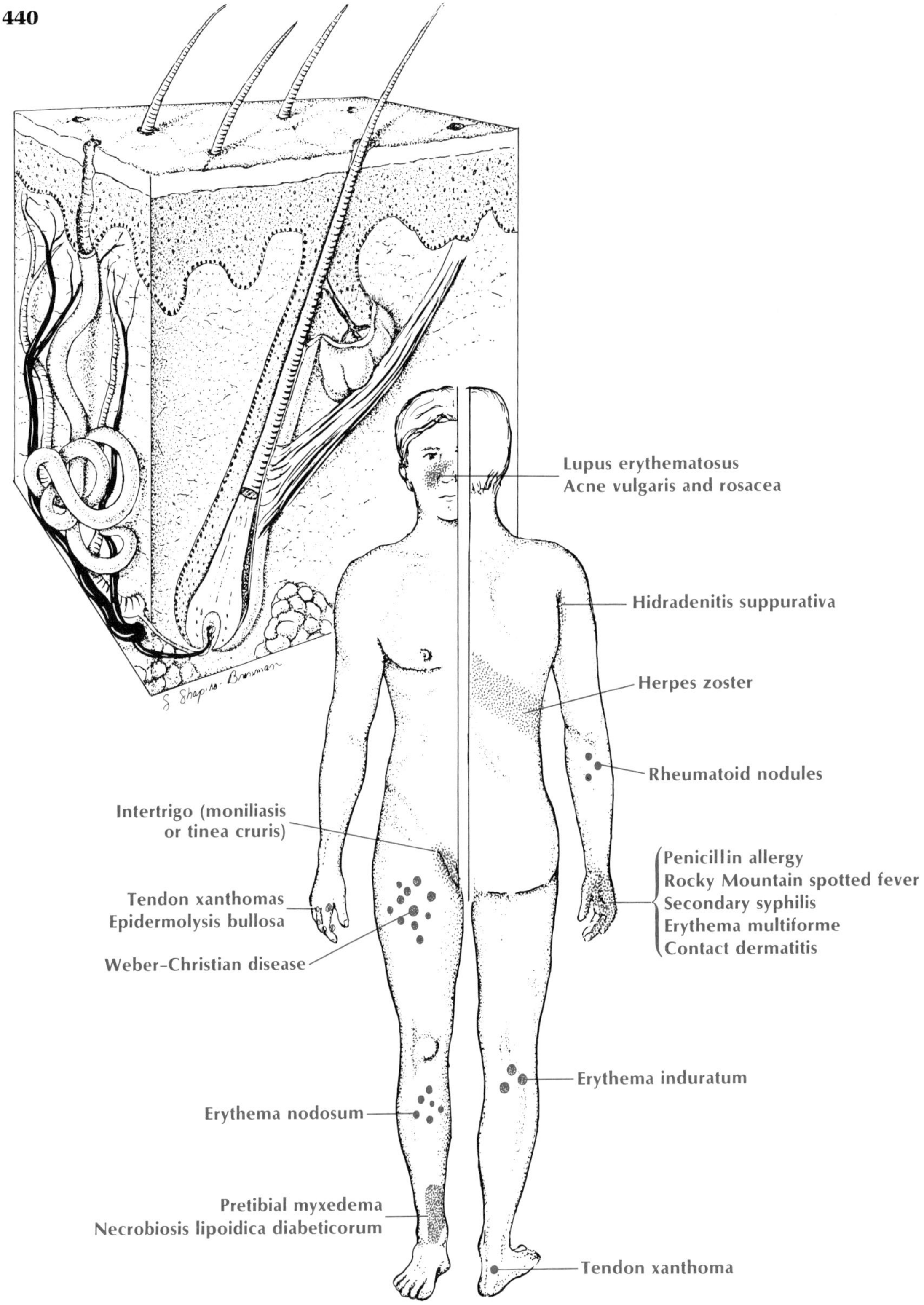

Lupus erythematosus
Acne vulgaris and rosacea

Hidradenitis suppurativa

Herpes zoster

Rheumatoid nodules

Penicillin allergy
Rocky Mountain spotted fever
Secondary syphilis
Erythema multiforme
Contact dermatitis

Intertrigo (moniliasis or tinea cruris)

Tendon xanthomas
Epidermolysis bullosa

Weber-Christian disease

Erythema induratum

Erythema nodosum

Pretibial myxedema
Necrobiosis lipoidica diabeticorum

Tendon xanthoma

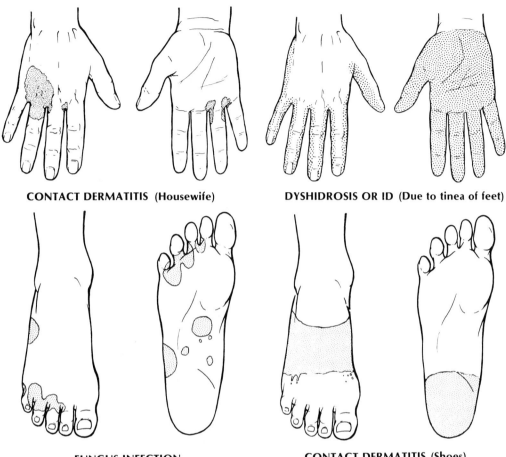

CONTACT DERMATITIS (Housewife)

DYSHIDROSIS OR ID (Due to tinea of feet)

FUNGUS INFECTION

CONTACT DERMATITIS (Shoes)

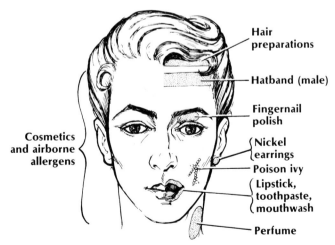

Hair
preparations

Hatband (male)

Fingernail
polish

Nickel
earrings

Poison ivy

Lipstick,
toothpaste,
mouthwash

Perfume

Cosmetics
and airborne
allergens

CONTACT DERMATITIS

RASH, LOCAL

pretibial myxedema, necrobiosis lipoidica diabeticorum, diabetic ulcers, and the flushed face of Cushing's syndrome and carcinoid.

Approach to the Diagnosis

The approach to the diagnosis is similar to that of the general rash (see p. 439) A list of useful diagnostic procedures are presented in Appendix I.

RED EYE ▪

Most textbooks consider the causes of red eye as conjunctivitis, iritis, or glaucoma, but it may be the result of taking the night plane from Los Angeles to New York. If these are all the causes you can remember you will be sadly mistaken in some cases. Most of the causes can be quickly recalled by simply considering the **anatomy** of the eye, because

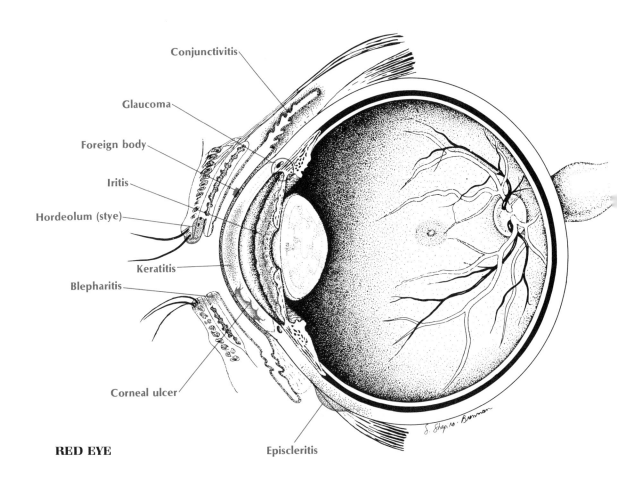

Conjunctivitis

Glaucoma

Foreign body

Iritis

Hordeolum (stye)

Keratitis

Blepharitis

Corneal ulcer

Episcleritis

RED EYE

trauma or inflammation are the usual etiologies.

Beginning with the **eyelids** one recalls blepharitis and hordeolum. The **conjunctiva** suggests conjunctivitis. The **cornea** may be involved by a foreign body or keratitis; corneal ulcers should also be looked for. Proceeding to deeper layers, the physician should consider iritis, and scleritis or injury to these structures. Finally, between the cornea and iris is the **canal of Schlemm,** which recalls glaucoma. The **vascular supply** suggests a cavernous sinus thrombosis.

Another method that will bring to mind even more of the possibilities is to use the mnemonic **FOREIGN.** The word and the first letter signify foreign bodies. The **O** suggests otolaryngological conditions such as upper respiratory infections. The **R** brings to mind refractive errors and astigmatism. The **E** suggests the exanthema and the conjunctivitis of measles. It will also help recall episcleritis and scleritis. **I** should signify iritis, conjunctivitis, and other inflammatory lesions. The **G** suggests glaucoma. Finally, the **N** should indicate neoplasms of the orbit.

Approach to the Diagnosis

Pinning down the diagnosis of a red eye is usually not difficult because most causes will be evident to the naked eye. However, a careful search for a foreign body with a magnifying glass and a corneal abrasion using fluorescene will be necessary in some cases. The association of other signs and symptoms will be invaluable. Diffuse erythema of the eye usually indicates trauma, conjunctivitis, or scleritis, whereas circumcorneal injection suggests iritis or glaucoma. A dilated pupil suggests glaucoma whereas a constricted or distorted pupil suggests iritis. A slit lamp will differentiate keratitis and obscure foreign bodies. Tonometry is useful in differentiating

glaucoma from other conditions. A smear and culture will help differentiate infectious conjunctivitis from allergic conjunctivitis, but the latter is usually bilateral whereas the former is usually unilateral. Other laboratory tests are listed in Appendix I.

SKIN PIGMENTATION AND OTHER PIGMENTARY CHANGES ■

To recall the causes of a diffuse pigmentation of the skin, one might simply visualize various organs of the body where a cause may originate. The **adrenal gland** brings to mind Addison's disease; the **liver** suggests hemochromatosis; the **thyroid** suggests hyperthyroidism; the **uterus** suggests pregnancy (more likely to cause chloasma); and the **ovaries** suggest the chloasma of menopause. The liver is also the cause of jaundice (see p. 346). The skin itself is the site of melanotic carcinoma, which in occasional cases causes a deeply pigmented skin, and tinea versicolor, which produces patchy yellow-brown pigmented area over the trunk. Any dermatitis that takes a long time to heal may cause a patchy pigmentation.

Other causes of patchy pigmentation are the *cafe´ au lait* spots of neurofibromatosis, stasis dermatitis from chronic thrombophlebitis and varicose veins, the pigmentation of the dorsal surfaces of the hands and face in pellagra, carcinoid syndrome, porphyria, and Gaucher's disease. Ochronosis produces a bluish-blackish or brownish pigment of the sclera, ears, skin, and nails. Vitiligo (idiopathic type) suggests a patchy pigmentation but is really a depigmentation.

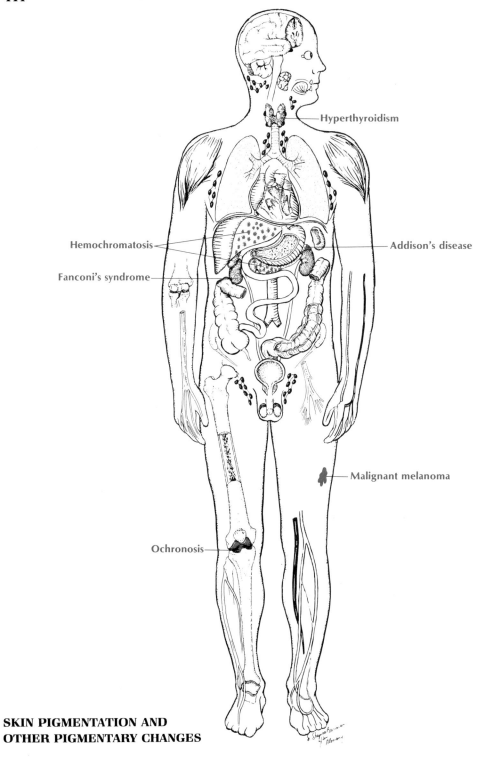

Hyperthyroidism

Hemochromatosis

Addison's disease

Fanconi's syndrome

Malignant melanoma

Ochronosis

**SKIN PIGMENTATION AND
OTHER PIGMENTARY CHANGES**

Approach to the Diagnosis

The workup for diffuse pigmentation involves ruling out hemochromatosis, hepatobiliary disease, and Addison's disease with appropriate tests for these disorders (see Appendix II) and using the expertise of a dermatologist in the cases of patchy pigmentation.

SKIN ULCERS ■

The differential diagnosis of skin ulcers may be approached with **anatomy** as the basic science, particularly if the ulcer is on one of the legs. Beginning with the skin itself and applying the mnemonic **MINT,** one can recall the following:

M—Malformations and sickle cell anemia come to mind.

I—Infection, syphilis, chancroid, lymphogranuloma, actinomycosis, and tularemia are suggested, as well as other infections.

N—Neoplasms suggest basal cell and squamous cell carcinomas.

T—Trauma suggests third-degree burns, unsutured lacerations, and pressure sores (bedsores).

Now visualize the structure beneath the skin. The **arteries** suggest arteriosclerosis and diabetic ulcers; the **veins** prompt the recall of varicose ulcers or postphlebitic ulcers; the **nerves** suggest trophic ulcers of tabes dorsalis, syringomyelia, and peripheral neuropathy; and the **bone** suggests osteomyelitis (*e.g.,* staphylococcal, tuberculosis) which penetrates the skin.

In contrast to the method described above, a somewhat more complete differential diagnosis may be developed with the mnemonic **VINDICATE.**

V—Vascular suggests peripheral arteriosclerosis, diabetic ulcers, and varicose ulcers.

I—Infections suggest syphilis, chancroid, yaws, and tularemia.

N—Neoplasm suggests carcinomas, sarcomas, and mycosis fungoides, and so forth.

D—Degenerative suggests ulcers associated with degenerative and deficiency diseases, such as peripheral neuropathy, syringomyelia, muscle atrophy, and peroneal muscular atrophy.

I—Intoxication suggests the ulcer of chronic dermatitis.

C—Congenital recalls the ulcers of sickle cell anemias.

A—Autoimmune brings to mind the ulcers of periarteritis nodosa, pyoderma gangrenosum (associated with ulcerative colitis), and Stevens–Johnson syndrome.

T—Trauma identifies ulcers of burns, radiation secondary to unhealed lacerations, and decubitus ulcers.

E—Endocrine suggests diabetic ulcers.

I—Infections can be further elucidated by working from the smallest organism to the largest. Beginning with **viruses** herpes simplex and lymphogranuloma are suggested. **Bacteria** reminds one of tuberculosis, tularemia, leprosy, and cutaneous diphtheria. **Spirochetes** suggest syphilis and yaws. **Parasites** identify leishmaniasis and amebiasis cutis. The rest are **fungal** and include actinomycosis, blastomycosis, sportrichosis, and cryptococcosis.

Approach to the Diagnosis

The approach to the diagnosis of a skin ulcer involves an assessment of the vascular supply to the area, a neurological examination, and a good history (especially important is venereal disease). The laboratory can support the diagnosis with a smear and culture, skin tests for tuberculosis and fungi, and serological tests.

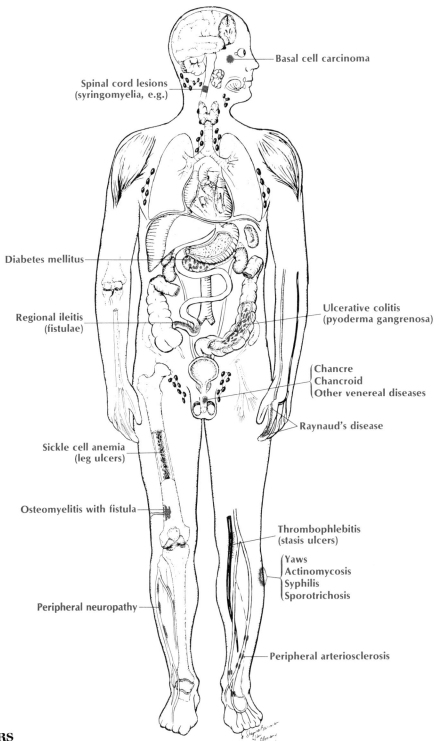

Basal cell carcinoma

Spinal cord lesions
(syringomyelia, e.g.)

Diabetes mellitus

Regional ileitis
(fistulae)

Ulcerative colitis
(pyoderma gangrenosa)

Chancre
Chancroid
Other venereal diseases

Raynaud's disease

Sickle cell anemia
(leg ulcers)

Osteomyelitis with fistula

Thrombophlebitis
(stasis ulcers)

Yaws
Actinomycosis
Syphilis
Sporotrichosis

Peripheral neuropathy

Peripheral arteriosclerosis

SKIN ULCERS

An x-ray film of the bone may identify the cause. A biopsy may be necessary. Roentgenogram and laboratory survey of other organs may be necessary if a systemic disease (e.g., collagen disease or ulcerative colitis) is suspected.

SKULL DEFORMITIES

The best method to recall the causes of skull deformities is to think of the mnemonic **VINDICATE**.

V—Vascular suggests Cooley's anemia with its characteristic enlargement of the head and cheek bones with a small bridge of the nose.

I—Infection includes syphilis, in which the head assumes the shape of a hotcross bun.

N—Neurologic disease suggests microcephaly (small, underdeveloped brain) and hydrocephaly, which may be due to several causes; the most important from a treatable standpoint are subdural hematomas, brain abscesses, and neoplasms. Cerebral palsy should be included here too.

D—Deficiency disease includes rickets, in which the head is elongated, square, and flattened at the vertex.

I—Idiopathic disease recalls Paget's disease. There is symmetrical enlargement and occasionally a triangular shape because the bones of the face do not enlarge. In facial hemiatrophy one side of the head is smaller than the other side.

C—Congenital disorders include scaphocephaly (elongated from front to back), oxycephaly or tower skull, hypertelorism (increased breadth of the skull and eyes far apart), mongolism, and arachnodactyly.

A—Achondrodysplasia features a large head with depression of the nose and prognathism.

T—Trauma includes any trauma to the skull causing edema (caput succedeneum), hematomas, and fractures.

E—Endocrine disorders such as acromegaly and myxedema cause a large head. Acromegaly is usually easily distinguishable by the protruding jaw.

Approach to the Diagnosis

Obviously the most important things in the workup of this symptom are a good neurological examination and a skull x-ray film. Other studies will be dictated by the findings of the above. A blood count and morphological study are worthwhile if Cooley's anemia is suspected and a Wassermann test or FTA–ABS if congenital syphilis is suspected.

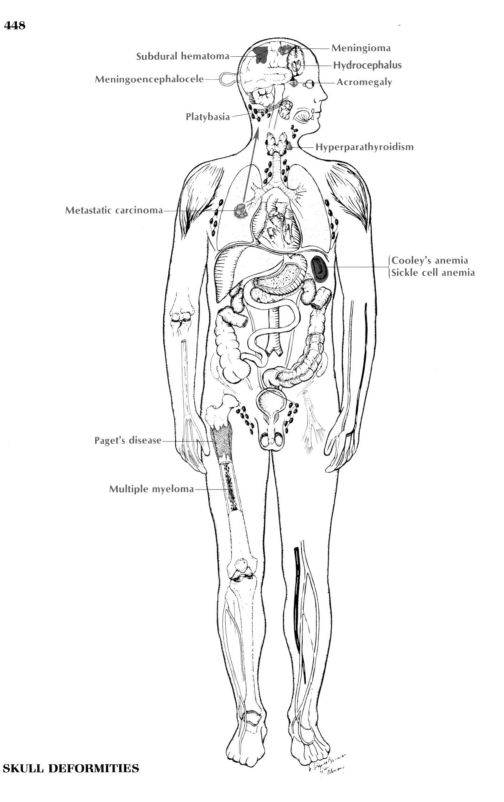

Subdural hematoma

Meningioma

Meningoencephalocele

Hydrocephalus

Acromegaly

Platybasia

Hyperparathyroidism

Metastatic carcinoma

Cooley's anemia
Sickle cell anemia

Paget's disease

Multiple myeloma

SKULL DEFORMITIES

SMOOTH TONGUE AND OTHER CHANGES ■

There was a time when the first thing a physician did was to look at the tongue. The art of examining the tongue is all but lost, even though over 30 diseases can be diagnosed by looking at the tongue. Recalling these may be best accomplished with the mnemonic **VINDICATE.** No attempt to cover all of them will be made, but the important ones are considered here.

V—Vascular diseases that may be diagnosed by looking at the tongue include the cyanosis of congestive heart failure, lung diseases, and polycythemia. The sublingual veins are also distended in these conditions.

I—Inflammatory diseases that cause tongue changes are streptococcal pharyngitis (strawberry tongue), tuberculosis (ulcers or furring of the tongue), chronic gastritis (coated gray), measles (furry tongue), appendicitis and peritonitis (moist and furry to dry and brown), typhoid (dense white fur), poliomyelitis (atrophy), syphilis (smooth or fissured tongue), herpes (ulcers), and moniliasis (white patches to white fur).

N—Neoplasms suggest carcinoma of the tongue (ulceration), leukoplakia (white plaques), diffuse lymphoma (small vesicles and a large tongue), fibroma (pediculated lesion on tongue), hemangioma (port-wine stain), and lingual warts.

D—Deficiency diseases include pernicious anemia (smooth tongue), iron deficiency anemia (smooth tongue), vitamin A deficiency, sprue, pellagra, and riboflavin deficiency (red and smooth).

I—Intoxication suggests bromism (tremulous tongue with excessive salivation), alcoholism (tremulous, white furry tongue),

mercury poisoning (ulcers), and lead poisoning (atrophy).

C—Congenital disorders include mongolism (large, coarsely papillated tongue), geographic tongue, and cerebral palsy.

A—Autoimmune diseases include amyloidosis (swollen tongue), erythema multiforme (swollen tongue with ulcers and blisters), angioneurotic edema, and multiple sclerosis (tremulous with fibrillary twitching).

T—Trauma to the tongue is important to look for in cases of undiagnosed epilepsy.

E—Endocrine disorders include acromegaly (swollen tongue), myxedema (large tongue), lingual thyroid, and thyroglossal cysts.

Approach to the Diagnosis

The workup of these lesions will include biopsy, culture, and further tests for the disease that are suggested in Appendix II.

SPINE DEFORMITIES ■

Deformities of the spine are basically of four types: scoliosis (lateral curvature of the spine), lordosis (lumbar concavity of the spine), kyphosis (thoracic convexity of the spine or "hunchback"), and kyphoscoliosis (curvature with a "hunchback"). The differential diagnosis of all of these is essentially the same and may be best recalled by the mnemonic **VINDICATE.**

V—Vascular suggests a large aortic aneurysm that may damage the vertebrae by compression, but this category is used with the prime purpose of recalling the spinal deformities associated with various congenital heart diseases (*e.g.,* tetralogy of Fallot).

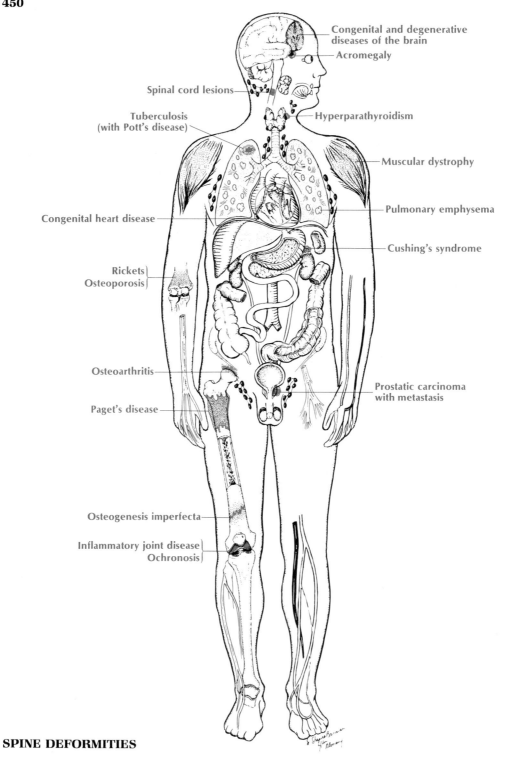

Congenital and degenerative diseases of the brain

Acromegaly

Spinal cord lesions

Hyperparathyroidism

Tuberculosis (with Pott's disease)

Muscular dystrophy

Pulmonary emphysema

Congenital heart disease

Cushing's syndrome

Rickets
Osteoporosis

Osteoarthritis

Prostatic carcinoma with metastasis

Paget's disease

Osteogenesis imperfecta

Inflammatory joint disease
Ochronosis

SPINE DEFORMITIES

I—Inflammatory recalls osteomyelitis and tuberculosis of the spine; one should also remember infectious diseases of the nervous system like poliomyelitis.

N—Neoplasms include metastatic tumors, myeloma, Hodgkin's disease, and primary tumors of the spinal cord.

D—Degenerative and **deficiency** diseases include degenerative disc disease, osteoarthritis, and spondylosis along the spine. In this category should be mentioned the kyphosis associated with pulmonary emphysema and fibrosis. Vitamin D deficiency will cause kyphoscoliosis.

I—Intoxication includes the kyphosis associated with pneumoconiosis and the osteoporosis from menopause or long-term corticosteroid therapy.

C—Congenital is perhaps the largest category, including congenital scoliosis, kyphoscoliosis, Hurler's disease, hemivertebrae, muscular dystrophy, Friedreich's ataxia, achondroplasia, and spondylolisthesis.

A—Autoimmune disease suggests rheumatoid spondylitis with the characteristic "poker spine."

T—Trauma indicates fractures, ruptured discs, and spinal cord injuries, all of which may leave a residual deformity of the spine.

E—Endocrine diseases remind one of the kyphosis associated with menopausal osteoporosis and osteomalacia of hyperparathyroidism. Acromegaly may also cause a kyphosis from the osteoarthritis and osteoporosis.

Approach to the Diagnosis

Obviously a good family history and a thorough physical and neurological examination are essential. The busy physician who has not the time for a neurological exam should refer the patient to a neurologist or orthopedist. An x-ray film of the spine will often demonstrate the lesion, but a bone scan, myelography, and bone biopsy may be necessary. The bone scan has become especially useful in diagnosing early rheumatoid spondylitis.

STOOL COLOR CHANGES ■

What may be black and white and red all over? The answer is not the newspaper but the pathological changes in the stool. A **black stool** is usually melena (see p. 189), but do not be fooled by iron ingestion or the bismuth in a commonly used antacid. A **white** or **light-colored stool** is most commonly found following the ingestion of a barium test meal, but the clay-colored stool of obstructive jaundice suggests the most important disease to be considered. The stool is light yellow to foamy in celiac disease. In mucous colitis a large cast of white mucus (sometimes 6 to 10 inches long) may be described as a white "stool." A **red stool** signifies blood from the lower bowel (see p. 201) in most cases, but ingestions of red beets is not an uncommon cause.

The riddle mentioned above forms a key to remembering the causes of aberrations in stool color. Another method is to apply biochemistry. The normal color of the stool is due to the pigment urobilinogen. Color changes may result from a decrease in or absence of this pigment (obstructive jaundice), from an increase in (hemolytic anemias) or the addition of another pigment (hemoglobin in melena), and finally, from the addition of another substance such as mucus in mucous colitis, fat in celiac disease, and bismuth in antacid ingestion.

Approach to the Diagnosis

The workup for changes in stool color includes most of the tests for either melena (see p. 480) or jaundice (see p. 485). The workup of celiac disease can be found in Appendix II.

(Text continues on p. 454)

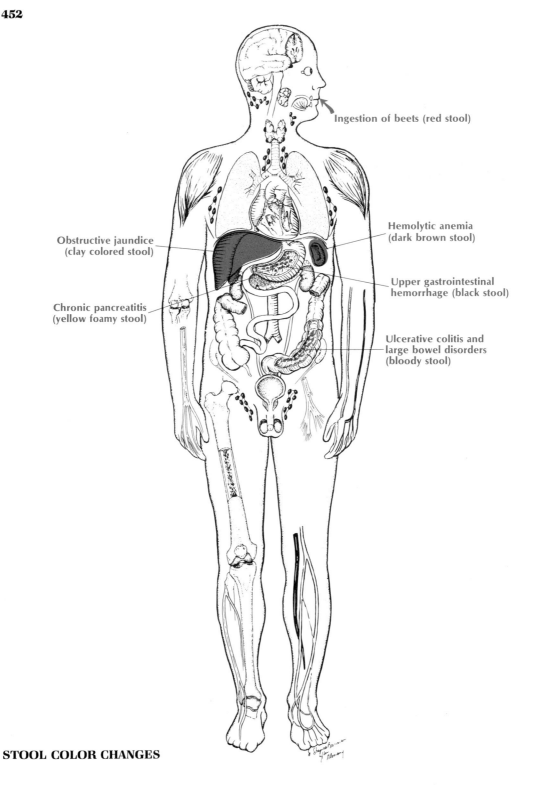

Ingestion of beets (red stool)

Hemolytic anemia
(dark brown stool)

Obstructive jaundice
(clay colored stool)

Upper gastrointestinal
hemorrhage (black stool)

Chronic pancreatitis
(yellow foamy stool)

Ulcerative colitis and
large bowel disorders
(bloody stool)

STOOL COLOR CHANGES

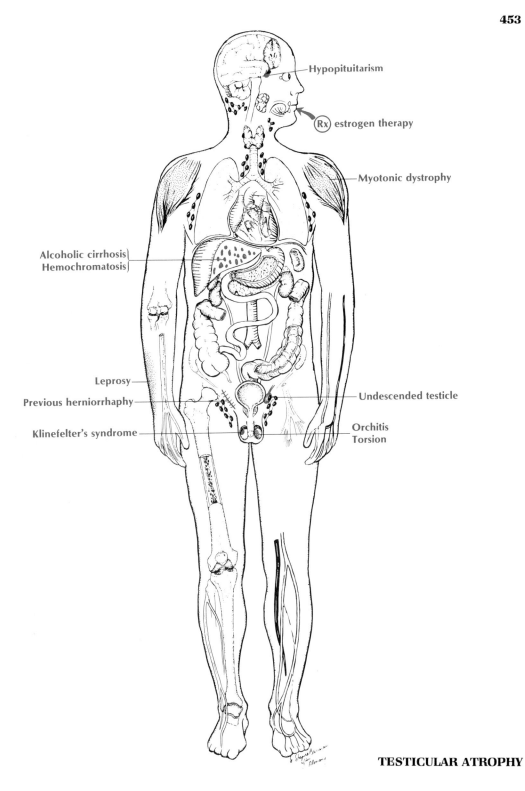

Hypopituitarism

Rx estrogen therapy

Myotonic dystrophy

Alcoholic cirrhosis
Hemochromatosis

Leprosy

Previous herniorrhaphy

Klinefelter's syndrome

Undescended testicle

Orchitis
Torsion

TESTICULAR ATROPHY

TESTICULAR ATROPHY ■

The causes of this sign can best be recalled by using the mnemonic **VINDICATE.**

V—Vascular conditions bring to mind varicoceles, which cause atrophy on the side of the dilated veins.

I—Inflammation recalls the atrophy following mumps, orchitis, and other causes of epidydimo-orchitis.

N—Neoplasms suggest the atrophy that occurs in the estrogen treatment of prostatic carcinoma.

D—Degenerative suggests the atrophy resulting from aging.

I—Intoxication should remind one of the atrophy resulting from chronic alcoholism, Laennec's cirrhosis, and hemochromatosis. X-ray exposure may also produce atrophy.

C—Congenital recalls undescended testes and torsion.

A—Autoimmune and **allergic** suggest nothing.

T—Trauma reminds one of the atrophy following vasectomy and accidental ligation of the blood supply during hernia repair.

E—Endocrine suggests the atrophy of hypopituitarism, Klinefelter's syndrome, and other eunuchoidal states.

Approach to the Diagnosis

The workup of testicular atrophy may require a chromatin analysis, serum testosterone, FSH and LH levels, and biopsy, but referral to an endocrinologist is the best way to get this accomplished with accuracy.

URINE COLOR CHANGES ■

Apart from hematuria, a **red urine** may signify hemoglobinuria or myoglobinuria, suggesting the various hemolytic anemias, the march hemoglobinuria, paroxysmal "cold" hemoglobinuria and noctural hemoglobinuria, and the Crush syndrome. A red urine is also found in acute porphyria, especially the erythropoetic type. Ingestions of beets and purple cabbage may cause a red urine. Pyridium, a urinary tract anesthetic, will turn the urine reddish-orange. A **dark yellow-brown** urine usually signifies jaundice (see p. 346), but the chartreuse yellow from riboflavin ingestion should be remembered; urobilinogen may make the urine yellow. A **brown or smoky urine** may be found in nephritis and is usually due to hemoglobinuria or red cells discolored by an acid pH. A malignant melanoma may present with a brown urine. **Black urine** is characteristic of alkaptonuria but this usually occurs on standing (as the urine turns from acid to alkaline). Melanuria will also turn black on standing but may even be voided black. The **green urine** of pseudomonas infections and the blue-green urine of methylene blue dye should be remembered.

How can these causes of urine discoloration be remembered? One method is to group them into endogenous and exogenous causes (*e.g.*, beets, pyridium, and methylene blue). The endogenous causes are invariably related to the metabolism of a body pigment. Hemoglobin metabolism will suggest porphyria and hemoglobinuria, whereas melanin metabolism will suggest melanuria and alkaptonuria. The other method is to apply the mnemonic **VINDICATE.** I suggest that the reader use this as an exercise.

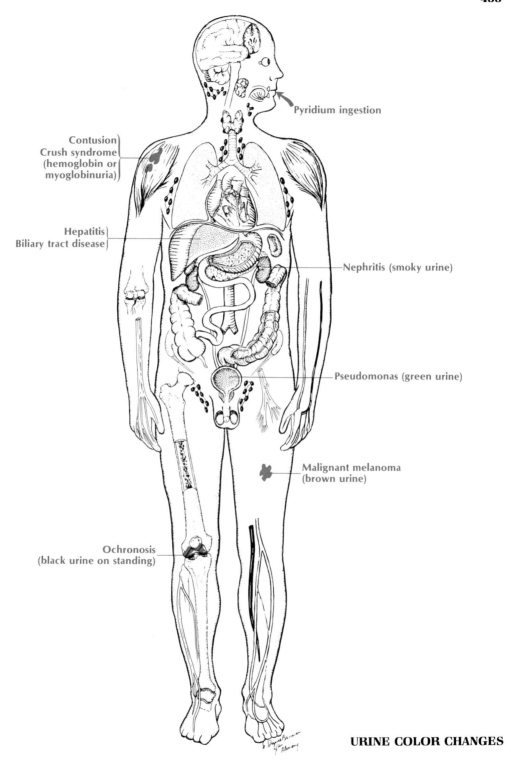

Pyridium ingestion

Contusion
Crush syndrome
(hemoglobin or
myoglobinuria)

Hepatitis
Biliary tract disease

Nephritis (smoky urine)

Pseudomonas (green urine)

Malignant melanoma
(brown urine)

Ochronosis
(black urine on standing)

URINE COLOR CHANGES

THE LABORATORY WORKUP OF SYMPTOMS

Appendix I

ABDOMINAL MASS

1. cbc sedimentation rate
2. Amylase and lipase
3. SMA–24
4. Glucose tolerance test
5. Liver function tests
6. Gastric analysis
7. Pregnancy test
8. Stool for occult blood
9. Stool for ova and parasites
10. Serum protein electrophoresis
11. Bone marrow examination
12. Catheterize for residual urine
13. Flat plate of abdomen
14. Upper GI series
15. Small bowel series
16. Barium enema
17. IVP and cystogram
18. Cholecystogram
19. Liver and spleen scan
20. Ultrasonography
21. CT scan
22. Aortography
23. Esophagoscopy
24. Gastroscopy
25. Duodenoscopy
26. Sigmoidoscopy
27. Colonoscopy
28. Cystoscopy
29. Culdoscopy
30. Peritoneoscopy
31. Liver biopsy
32. Node biopsy
33. Exploratory laparotomy
34. Lymphangiogram
35. Peritoneal tap

ABDOMINAL PAIN ■

1. cbc
2. Urinalysis
3. Sedimentation rate
4. SMA–24
5. Wassermann
6. ECG
7. Chest roentgenogram and flat plate of abdomen
8. PPD, intermediate
9. Amylase
10. Lipase
11. 2-hour postprandial blood sugar
12. Transaminase series
13. Lactic dehydrogenase (LDH) series, MBCPK series
14. Urine culture and sensitivity, colony count
15. Save all urine and examine for stones
16. Vaginal culture (pelvic inflammatory disease) for GC and chlamydia
17. Stool culture
18. Liver function studies
19. Uric acid
20. Calcium, phosphates, alkaline phosphatase (renal calculus)
21. Pregnancy test (ruptured ectopic pregnancy)
22. Blood lead level
23. Urine porphobilinogen and porphyrins
24. Wassermann
25. Stool for occult blood
26. Stool for ova and parasites
27. Gastric analysis, duodenal analysis
28. Spinal tap (spinal cord tumor)
29. Serum protein electrophoresis
30. Flat plate, upright and lateral decubiti of abdomen
31. Cholecystogram or ultrasonogram
32. Intravenous pyelogram
33. Upper GI series
34. Barium enema
35. Small bowel series
36. Roentgenogram of lumbosacral spine
37. Myelogram
38. Aortography (dissecting aneurysm)
39. Liver scan, CT scan, ultrasonography
40. Esophagoscopy
41. Gastroscopy, duodenoscopy with ERCP
42. Sigmoidoscopy
43. Cystoscopy
44. Culdoscopy
45. Peritoneoscopy
46. ECG and exercise tolerance test
47. Bernstein test (esophagitis)
48. Catheterize for residual urine
49. Peritoneal tap
50. Lymph node biopsy (Hodgkin's disease)
51. Double enema (intestinal obstruction)
52. Exploratory laparotomy

ANAL MASS ■

1. cbc and differential
2. Urinalysis
3. Sedimentation rate
4. Frei test
5. Tuberculin test
6. VDRL
7. Biopsy and excision
8. I & D and culture exudate
9. Sigmoidoscopy
10. Barium enema
11. Culdoscopy
12. Cystoscopy
13. Exploratory surgery
14. Stool examination and culture

ANEMIA ■

1. cbc
2. Urinalysis
3. Sedimentation rate

4. SMA–24
5. Wassermann
6. ECG
7. Chest roentgenogram and flat plate of abdomen
8. PPD, intermediate
9. Red cell count, indices
10. Reticulocyte count
11. Wright's stain of peripheral blood for cell morphology
12. Serum ferritin or iron and iron-binding capacity
13. Gastric analysis
14. Stools for occult blood and chromium-tagged red cells
15. Stools for ova and parasites
16. Serum bilirubin
17. Urine and fecal urobilinogen
18. Blood cell fragility
19. Coombs' test
20. Radioactive chromium-tagged red cell survival
21. Ham's test
22. Sickle cell preparation
23. Platelet count
24. Repeated WBC and differential and smears for atypical cells
25. Blood lead level
26. Plasma hemoglobin, haptoglobin, and methemalbumin
27. Coagulation studies (see Purpura, this table)
28. Hemoglobin electrophoresis
29. Donath–Landsteiner test
30. T3, T4, T7, TSH
31. Urine 17–ketosteroids and 17–hydroxysteroids or serum cortisol
32. Serum protein electrophoresis
33. ANA test
34. Blood smear for parasites
35. Blood cultures
36. Febrile agglutinins
37. Urine formiminoglutamic acid
38. Serum carotene, D-xylose absorption
39. Serum B_{12} assay, serum folic acid
40. Skull and long bones, reticuloendothelial (RE) scan, bone scan
41. Upper GI series and small bowel follow-through
42. Barium enema
43. Sigmoidoscopy
44. Esophagoscopy
45. Gastroscopy
46. Bone marrow aspiration or biopsy
47. Lymph node biopsy
48. Liver biopsy
49. Duodenal aspiration for parasites (strongyloides)
50. Liver–spleen scan
51. Schilling test

ANOREXIA ■

1. cbc and differential
2. Urine
3. Sedimentation rate
4. Fever chart
5. SMA–24
6. Serum amylase and lipase
7. Thyroid function studies
8. Liver function studies
9. Carcino-embryonic antigen (CEA)
10. D-xylose absorption test
11. Schilling test
12. Chest roentgenogram
13. Upper GI series
14. Esophagram
15. Small bowel series
16. Barium enema
17. Cholecystogram
18. Liver scan
19. Pancreatic scan
20. CT scan (abdomen)
21. Ultrasonography
22. Esophagoscopy
23. Gastroscopy
24. Duodenoscopy

25. Liver biopsy
26. Small intestine biopsy
27. Gastric biopsy
28. Venous pressure and circulation time
29. ECG
30. Exploratory laparotomy

ANURIA ■

1. cbc and differential
2. Sedimentation rate
3. SMA–24
4. Serum protein eletrophoresis
5. ASO titer
6. Serum haptoglobins
7. Urinalysis
8. Catheterize for residual urine
9. Urine cultures
10. Blood cultures
11. Monitor blood pressure
12. Serum complement
13. Serum electrolytes
14. Serum calcium and phosphates
15. Renal function tests
16. Flat plate of abdomen
17. Retrograde pyelography
18. Cystoscopy
19. Renal biopsy
20. CT scan
21. Ultrasonogram
22. Fluid or diuretic challenge

ARM PAIN ■

1. cbc and differential
2. Urine
3. Sedimentation rate
4. SMA–24
5. VDRL
6. Synovial fluid analysis

7. Serial SGOT, LDH, CPK, MBCPK
8. R-A test
9. Roentgenogram of arm and joints
10. Roentgenogram of cervical spine
11. Chest roentgenogram
12. EMG, NCV
13. ECG, serial
14. GXT
15. Myelography, CT scan
16. Arteriography
17. Phlebography
18. Lymphangiography
19. Bone scans
20. Nerve blocks
21. Muscle biopsy
22. Coronary angiography
23. Stellate ganglion block
24. Injection of trigger points with lidocaine
25. Exploratory surgery

AURAL DISCHARGE ■

1. cbc and differential
2. Sedimentation rate
3. Smear and culture
4. Routine bacteria, AFB, and fungi culture
5. Tuberculin test
6. VDRL
7. Roentgenogram of skull, mastoids, and petrous bones
8. Biopsy
9. Blood cultures
10. CT scan

AUSCULTATORY SIGNS OF PULMONARY DISEASE ■

1. cbc and differential
2. Urinalysis
3. Sedimentation rate

4. Tuberculin test
5. VDRL
6. SMA–24
7. ECG
8. Sputum examination
9. Sputum smear and culture for bacteria, AFB, fungi, and parasites
10. Sputum cytology
11. Sputum for eosinophils
12. Serology for fungi
13. ANA test
14. Heterophil antibody titer
15. Skin tests for fungi, lung scans
16. Chest roentgenogram with special views
17. Tomography
18. Bronchogram
19. Barium swallow
20. Bronchoscopy
21. Lung biopsy
22. Lymph node biopsy
23. Kveim test
24. Roentgenogram of hands
25. Bone marrow examination
26. R-A test
27. Serum protein electrophoresis
28. CT scan of mediastinum
29. Pulmonary function tests
30. Blood cultures
31. Metastatic survey
32. Thoracentesis

11. Roentgenogram of chest
12. Bone scan
13. Mammography
14. Breast biopsy
15. Lymphangiography
16. Arteriography
17. Phlebography

BACK MASS

1. cbc and differential
2. Urinalysis
3. Sedimentation rate
4. VDRL
5. Tuberculin test
6. SMA–24
7. I & D and culture
8. Serum protein electrophoresis
9. Roentgenogram of spine
10. Roentgenogram of chest
11. Bone scan
12. Ultrasonography
13. CT scan
14. Biopsy
15. Exploratory surgery
16. Myelography

AXILLARY MASS

1. cbc and differential
2. Urinalysis
3. Sedimentation rate
4. SMA–24
5. Tuberculin test
6. VDRL
7. I & D and culture of exudate
8. Lymph node biopsy
9. Skin biopsy
10. Exploratory surgery

BACK PAIN

1. cbc
2. Urine
3. Urine for Bence–Jones protein
4. Serum protein electrophoresis (multiple myeloma)
5. Calcium, phosphorus, alkaline phosphatase (metastatic carcinoma)
6. Sedimentation rate
7. Latex flocculation (rheumatoid spondylitis)
8. Serum amylase and lipase

9. Urine culture and sensitivity
10. Acid phosphatase
11. Spinal fluid examination and culture
12. Wassermann
13. Roentgenogram of thoracolumbar or lumbosacral spine
14. Chest roentgenogram
15. Roentgenogram of long bones and skull
16. Myelogram, CT scan
17. Barium enema
18. Intravenous pyelogram
19. Aortogram
20. Upper GI series
21. Gallbladder series
22. ECG
23. Blood pressure in lower extremities (dissecting aneurysm)
24. Sigmoidoscopy
25. Cystoscopy
26. Culdoscopy
27. Nerve block
28. Procaine infiltration at site of pain
29. PPD, intermediate
30. Thermography
31. EMG
32. Bone scan and sacroiliac scan (rheumatoid spondylitis, Paget's)
33. HLA B27 antigen

BALDNESS

1. cbc and differential
2. Sedimentation rate
3. ANA test
4. Ultraviolet examination
5. Scrapings for fungi
6. Thyroid function studies
7. Serum testosterone
8. Urine 17-ketosteroids
9. Chest roentgenogram
10. Skull roentgenogram
11. Skin biopsy

BLEEDING UNDER THE SKIN

See Purpura

BLURRED VISION AND BLINDNESS

1. cbc and differential
2. Sedimentation rate
3. SMA–24
4. Wassermann
5. Tuberculin test
6. Histoplasmin test
7. Serology for histoplasmosis
8. Serology for toxoplasmosis
9. Kveim test
10. Chest roentgenogram
11. Roentgenogram of orbit
12. Roentgenogram of skull
13. CT scan
14. Arteriography
15. Spinal tap
16. EEG
17. Tonometry
18. Visual fields
19. Pituitary function studies

BRADYCARDIA

1. cbc and differential
2. Thyroid function tests
3. SMA–24
4. Serum electrolytes
5. Digitalis levels
6. Wassermann
7. Tuberculin test
8. ANA test
9. R-A test

10. Chest roentgenogram
11. Barium swallow with cardiac series
12. ECG
13. Holter monitoring
14. Echocardiography
15. Hiss bundle study
16. Muscle biopsy
17. Rectal biopsy
18. Coronary angiography
19. Angiocardiography

BREAST DISCHARGE

1. cbc and differential
2. Sedimentation rate
3. Urinalysis
4. VDRL
5. Tuberculin test
6. Smear and culture of exudate
7. SMA–24
8. Cytology of exudate
9. Aspiration and cytology of cysts
10. Mammography
11. Biopsy
12. Exploratory surgery
13. Serum prolactin
14. Skull roentgenogram, CT scan of brain
15. Lymph node biopsy
16. Ultrasonography

BREAST MASS OR SWELLING

1. cbc and differential
2. Sedimentation rate
3. Culture of discharge
4. Serum estradiol levels
5. Serum prolactin
6. Urine of 17-ketosteroids

7. Mammography, ultrasonography
8. Aspiration
9. Analysis of cystic fluid
10. Biopsy
11. Skull roentgenogram (pituitary tumor)
12. CT scan of brain

BREAST PAIN

1. cbc and differential
2. Sedimentation rate
3. SMA–24
4. Tuberculin test
5. Culture of discharge
6. Serum estradiol
7. Serum prolactin
8. Chest roentgenogram
9. Lung scan
10. Mammography
11. Skull roentgenogram
12. ECG
13. Venous pressure and circulation time
14. Biopsy
15. Discontinue drugs if possible

CARDIAC ARRHYTHMIAS

1. cbc and differential
2. Urinalysis
3. Sedimentation rate
4. ASO titer
5. ANA test
6. R-A test
7. Serum electrolytes
8. Thyroid function studies
9. Blood gas analysis
10. Blood alcohol level
11. Chest roentgenogram
12. ECG

13. Pulmonary function studies
14. GXT
15. Echocardiography
16. Coronary arteriography
17. Angiocardiography
18. Trial of therapy
19. Holter monitoring
20. Tuberculin test

CARDIOMEGALY

1. cbc and differential
2. Urinalysis
3. Sedimentation rate
4. VDRL, SMA–24
5. Tuberculin test
6. ANA test
7. Serum protein electrophoresis
8. T3, T4, T7, TSH
9. Lipoprotein electrophoresis
10. R-A test
11. ECG and GXT
12. Roentgenogram of chest with obliques and a barium swallow
13. Angiocardiography
14. Echocardiography
15. Cardiac catheterization studies
16. Coronary angiography
17. Phonocardiogram
18. Liver biopsy
19. Muscle biopsy
20. Skin biopsy
21. Venous pressure and circulation time
22. Radioactive isotope scans of myocardium (*e.g.*, thallium)
23. Urine thiamine after load

CHEST PAIN

1. Transaminase series
2. Lactic dehydrogenase series and fractionation

3. CPK series, MB-CPK
4. Serum amylase
5. Echocardiography
6. Wassermann (aortic aneurysm)
7. Spinal fluid examination
8. Serum bilirubin (cholecystitis)
9. LE preparations and ANA test
10. Sickle cell preparation
11. Chest roentgenogram, posteroanterior and laterals
12. Flat plate of abdomen
13. Roentgenogram of cervical and thoracic spine
14. Upper GI series, including esophagram
15. Cholecystogram
16. Bernstein test
17. CT scan of mediastinum
18. Myelography
19. Aortogram
20. Lung scan
21. ECG
22. GXT
23. Bronchoscopy
24. Esophagoscopy
25. Gastroscopy
26. Therapeutic trial with nitroglycerin
27. Local lidocaine infiltration
28. Nerve block
29. Arterial blood gases
30. Thallium-201 scintigraphy

CHEST WALL MASS

1. cbc and differential
2. RAI uptake and scan
3. Sedimentatioin rate
4. VDRL
5. Tuberculin test
6. SMA–24
7. Serum protein electrophoresis
8. I & D and culture
9. Biopsy of lesion
10. Chest roentgenogram and tomography
11. Bone scans

12. Barium swallow
13. Angiocardiography
14. Mammography
15. Ultrasonography
16. CT scans
17. Mediastinoscopy

CHEYNE–STOKES RESPIRATIONS ■

See Decreased Respirations

CHILLS ■

1. cbc and differential
2. Sedimentation rate
3. Nose and throat cultures
4. Sputum smear
5. Sputum cultures
6. Tuberculin test
7. Urine cultures
8. Blood cultures
9. Liver function tests
10. Bone marrow smear and cultures
11. Stool for ova and parasites
12. Blood smear for parasites
13. Febrile agglutinins
14. ASO titer
15. Brucellin antibody titer
16. Leptospirosis titer
17. ANA test
18. Serum protein electrophoresis
19. Sickle cell preparation
20. CSF smear and culture
21. Urine for etiocholanolone
22. Fibrindex
23. Nitroblue tetrazolium test
24. Histoplasmin skin test
25. Coccidiodin skin test
26. Trichinella skin test

27. Frei test
28. Chest roentgenogram
29. Flat plate of the abdomen
30. IVP
31. Cholecystogram
32. Roentgenogram of bones
33. Upper GI series
34. Roentgenogram of teeth
35. Lymph node biopsy
36. Temperature chart
37. Muscle biopsy
38. Kveim test
39. Exploratory laparotomy

CHOREA ■

1. cbc and differential
2. Sedimentation rate
3. SMA–24
4. Serum electrolytes
5. Calcium and phosphorus
6. Serum magnesium and manganese level
7. Serum lead level
8. Wassermann
9. ASO titer or steptozyme test
10. Urinalysis
11. Serum copper and ceruloplasmin
12. Skull roentgenogram
13. Chest roentgenogram
14. ECG
15. EEG
16. Spinal tap

CLUBBING AND PULMONARY OSTEOARTHROPATHY ■

1. cbc and differential
2. Urinalysis
3. SMA–24
4. Tuberculin test

5. VDRL
6. Sedimentation rate
7. Blood gas analysis
8. Pulmonary function tests
9. Sputum examination
10. Sputum smear and culture
11. Sputum cytology
12. Sputum for AFB smear and culture
13. Chest roentgenogram
14. Tomography
15. ECG
16. Cardiac catheterization
17. Angiography
18. Lung scans
19. Perfusion–ventilation scans
20. Histoplasmin skin test
21. Coccidiodin skin test
22. Blastomycin skin test
23. Serology for histoplasmosis and other fungi
24. Blood cultures
25. Bronchoscopy
26. Lung biopsy
27. Exploratory surgery

CONSTIPATION

1. cbc and differential
2. Sedimentation rate
3. Glucose tolerance test
4. Stool for occult blood
5. Stool for ova and parasites
6. Serum electrolytes
7. Urine porphobilinogen
8. Thyroid function tests
9. Liver function tests
10. Gastric analysis
11. Schilling test
12. Drug screen
13. ANA test
14. Flat plate of abdomen
15. Barium enema

16. Upper GI series
17. Cholecystogram
18. Proctoscopy
19. Colonoscopy
20. Exploratory laparotomy

CONSTRICTED PUPILS

1. cbc and differential
2. Sedimentation rate
3. SMA–24
4. Wassermann test
5. Tuberculin test
6. Histoplasmin test
7. Toxoplasma serology
8. Roentgenogram of skull
9. Roentgenogram of orbits
10. Roentgenogram of cervical spine
11. Roentgenogram of chest
12. CT scans
13. Arteriography
14. Epinephrine test
15. Cocaine test
16. Slit-lamp examination
17. Tonometry
18. Visual field
19. Mecholyl test
20. Starch test
21. Spinal tap
22. Myelography

CONVULSIONS

1. cbc
2. Stat FBS, and BUN
3. Stat serum calcium
4. Electrolytes
5. SMA–24
6. Drug screen

7. ABG
8. VDRL
9. Wake and sleep EEG
10. ECG
11. Holter monitoring
12. 24-hour EEG monitoring
13. CT scan
14. Spinal tap
15. PET study
16. MRI
17. Urine porphobilinogen

7. Sputum analysis
8. Sputum smear and culture
9. Test for methemoglobinemia
10. Chest roentgenogram
11. Lung scan
12. Angiography
13. Angiocardiography
14. Venous pressure and circulation time
15. ECG
16. Pulmonary function tests
17. Bronchoscopy and lung biopsy
18. Echocardiography

COUGH

1. cbc
2. Sedimentation rate
3. SMA–24
4. Sputum smear and culture
5. Chest roentgenogram
6. Pulmonary function tests
7. ABG
8. Bronchoscopy
9. Lung biopsy
10. Sputum for cytology
11. Lung scan
12. Sputum for eosinophils
13. RAST
14. Sweat test
15. Alpha-1 trypsin assay

DANDRUFF

See Baldness

DEAFNESS AND TINNITUS

1. cbc and differential
2. Sedimentation rate
3. Culture of discharge
4. Nose and throat culture
5. Wassermann
6. Protein electrophoresis
7. SMA–24
8. Thyroid function studies
9. Skull roentgenogram
10. Roentgenogram of petrous bones
11. Roentgenogram of mastoids
12. CT scan
13. Posterior fossa myelography
14. Myelogram
15. Arteriogram
16. Audiograms
17. Calorics, ENG
18. Microscopic examination of the drum
19. Eustachian tube insufflation test for drum mobility

CYANOSIS

1. cbc and differential
2. Sedimentation test
3. SMA–24
4. Arterial blood gases
5. Tuberculin test
6. Drug screen

20. Allergy skin tests
21. Spinal tap

13. Arteriography
14. Pulmonary function studies

DELUSIONS

1. cbc and differential
2. Sedimentation rate
3. Wassermann
4. Spinal fluid examination
5. Thyroid function test
6. Serum cortisol
7. Blood alcohol level
8. Blood lead level
9. Blood bromide level
10. Drug screen
11. Serum B_{12}
12. EEG
13. CT scan
14. Brain biopsy
15. Arteriography
16. Trial of B vitamins
17. Gamma cysternography

DEPRESSION AND ANXIETY

1. cbc and differential
2. Urine
3. SMA–24
4. Urine porphobilinogen
5. Thyroid function studies
6. Urine 17–ketosteroids
7. Urine 17–hydroxysteroids
8. Serum cortisol
9. Wassermann
10. Skull roentgenogram
11. EEG
12. CT scan
13. Spinal tap
14. Drug screen
15. Vaginal smear for estrogen function
16. Serum FSH
17. Dexamethasone suppression test

DECREASED RESPIRATIONS

1. cbc and urine
2. Sedimentation rate
3. Drug screen
4. Arterial blood gases
5. Serum electrolytes
6. Wassermann
7. Chest roentgenogram
8. Skull roentgenogram
9. CT scan
10. Spinal tap
11. EEG
12. ECG

DIARRHEA

1. cbc
2. Sedimentation rate
3. SMA–24
4. Warm stool examination
5. Stool culture
6. Cathartic stool examination
7. Sigmoidoscopy
8. GI and small bowel series
9. Barium enema
10. Duodenal aspiration
11. Lactose tolerance test
12. D-xylose absorption test

13. Urine 5-HIAA
14. Mucosal biopsy
15. Colonoscopy and biopsy

DILATED PUPILS

1. cbc and differential
2. Sedimentation rate
3. Wassermann
4. SMA–24
5. Urinalysis
6. Roentgenogram
7. EEG
8. CT scans
9. Spinal tap
10. Arteriography
11. Tonometry
12. Visual field examination
13. Mecholyl test for Adie's pupil
14. Uveitis workup
15. Slit-lamp examination

DOUBLE VISION

1. cbc and urine
2. Sedimentation rate
3. VDRL and FTA–ABS
4. Tuberculin test
5. Glucose tolerance test
6. Tensilon test
7. Serum protein electrophoresis
8. SMA–24
9. Roentgenogram of skull and orbits
10. Roentgenogram of sinuses
11. EEG
12. CT scans
13. Spinal tap
14. Arteriography

15. Visual fields
16. Tonometry
17. Refraction
18. Histamine test
19. Serum growth hormone
20. Serum ACTH, cortisol
21. Serum LH and FSH
22. Blood cultures

DYSMENORRHEA

1. cbc and urine
2. Sedimentation rate
3. Papanicolaou smear
4. Cervical smear
5. Cervical culture
6. Serum estradiol
7. Serum progesterone
8. Serum FSH and LH
9. Salpingography
10. Cystoscopy
11. Sigmoidoscopy
12. Culdoscopy
13. Peritoneoscopy
14. Endometrial biopsy
15. Cervical biopsy
16. D & C
17. Exploratory laparotomy
18. Trial of progesterone therapy

DYSPAREUNIA

1. cbc and differential
2. Sedimentation rate
3. Vaginal smear
4. Vaginal cultures (bacterial, fungi, and so forth)
5. Papanicolaou smear

6. Tuberculin test
7. Urinalysis and culture
8. Ultrasonography
9. Peritoneoscopy
10. Cystoscopy
11. Sigmoidoscopy
12. MMPI

DYSPHAGIA

1. cbc
2. Urinalysis
3. Sedimentation rate
4. SMA–24
5. Wassermann
6. ECG
7. Chest roentgenogram and flat plate of abdomen
8. PPD, intermediate
9. cbc, indices, Wright's stain of peripheral blood (Plummer–Vinson syndrome)
10. T3, T4, T7, RAI update and scan
11. Spinal fluid examination
12. Upper GI series and esophagram
13. Roentgenogram of cervical spine
14. Aortogram
15. CT scan of mediastinum
16. Tensilon test (myasthenia gravis)
17. Esophagoscopy
18. Gastroscopy
19. Attempt to pass Levin tube (esophageal atresia)
20. Mecholyl test (achalasia of esophagus)
21. Esophageal manometry

DYSPNEA

1. cbc
2. Urinalysis
3. Sedimentation rate

4. SMA–24
5. Wassermann
6. ECG
7. Chest roentgenogram and flat plate of abdomen
8. PPD, intermediate
9. Sputum culture and sensitivity
10. Sputum analysis (eosinophils, and so forth)
11. T3, T4, T7
12. Electrolytes
13. Arterial blood gases
14. Test for methemoglobinemia
15. Urine for salicylates
16. Transaminase and LDH (lactic dehydrogenase), CPK
17. Chest roentgenogram
18. Bronchogram (foreign body)
19. Esophagram
20. Fluoroscopy
21. Pulmonary function studies (emphysema, and so forth)
22. Therapeutic trial of sublingual Isuprel (bronchial asthma)
23. Trial of diuretic (congestive heart failure)
24. Venous pressure and circulation time
25. Bronchoscopy (foreign body)
26. Lung scan, phlebography (pulmonary embolism)
27. Pulmonary angiography

DYSURIA

1. cbc and differential
2. Urinalysis
3. Urine culture
4. Colony count
5. Urethral smear and culture
6. Smear of prostatic fluid
7. Vaginal smear and culture routine and chlamydia
8. IVP

9. Cystogram
10. Cystoscopy
11. Catheterize for residual urine
12. Culdoscopy
13. Peritoneoscopy
14. Cystometric studies
15. Roentgenogram
16. Ultrasonogram

EARACHE

1. cbc and differential
2. Sedimentation rate
3. Wassermann
4. Smear and culture
5. Throat culture
6. SMA–24
7. Roentgenogram of mastoids
8. Roentgenogram of petrous bones
9. Roentgenogram of skull
10. Roentgenogram of temporomandibular joints
11. Roentgenogram of teeth
12. Roentgenogram of sinuses
13. CT scan
14. Impedance tympanography
15. Laminography
16. Nasopharyngoscopy
17. Audiogram
18. Caloric tests
19. Spinal fluid examination
20. EEG
21. ENG
22. Nerve blocks

EDEMA

1. cbc and urine
2. Sedimentation rate
3. Na, K, Cl, CO_2

4. Serum protein and albumin/globulin ratio
5. 24-hour urine protein and serum cholesterol
6. Addis count (nephritis)
7. Liver function tests (see Jaundice, this table)
8. Blood volume (congestive heart failure)
9. Stools for ova and parasites (*Taenia solium*, and so forth)
10. T3, T4, T7, TSH
11. Eosinophil count (trichinosis)
12. 24-hour urine 17–ketosteroids and 17–hydroxysteroids
13. Renal function tests
14. Chest roentgenogram
15. Flat plate of abdomen (ovarian tumor)
16. Roentgenogram of long bones (metastatic carcinoma)
17. Venous pressure and circulation time
18. Muscle biopsy (trichinosis, and so forth)
19. Lymph node biopsy (Hodgkin's disease)
20. Lymphangiogram
21. Liver scan
22. CT scan
23. Phlebography

ENURESIS

1. cbc and differential
2. SMA–24
3. Sedimentation rate
4. Tuberculin test
5. Serum electrolytes
6. Catheterize for residual urine
7. Urinalysis
8. Urine cultures and colony counts
9. IV pyelogram and voiding cystogram
10. Cystoscopy
11. Cystometric tests
12. Psychometric tests
13. EEG

EPISTAXIS

1. cbc
2. Urinalysis
3. Sedimentation rate
4. SMA–24
5. Wassermann
6. ECG
7. Chest roentgenogram and flat plate of abdomen
8. PPD, intermediate
9. Prothrombin time
10. Partial thromboplastin time
11. Bleeding time
12. Platelet count
13. Rumpel–Leede test
14. Nasal smear for eosinophils (allergic rhinitis, asthma)
15. Liver function tests (cirrhosis)
16. ASO titer
17. Roentgenogram for paranasal sinuses
18. Nasopharyngoscopy
19. Pulmonary function tests
20. Venous pressure and circulation time
21. Arterial blood gas analysis

EXCESSIVE SWEATING

1. cbc and differential
2. Sedimentation rate
3. CRP
4. Wassermann
5. SMA–24
6. Glucose tolerance test
7. R–A test
8. Thyroid function tests
9. 24-hour urine catecholamine
10. Serum insulin levels
11. Tolbutamide tolerance test
12. Urine cultures
13. Blood cultures
14. Urinalysis
15. Liver function tests
16. Chest roentgenogram
17. Flat plate of the abdomen
18. Psychometric tests
19. Chart temperature

EXOPHTHALMOS

1. cbc and differential
2. Sedimentation rate
3. Urinalysis
4. VDRL
5. Tuberculin test
6. SMA–24
7. ANA test
8. R-A test
9. Serum protein electrophoresis
10. T3, T4, T7, RAI uptake and scan
11. Roentgenogram of skull and orbits
12. Roentgenogram of sinuses
13. CT scan
14. Arteriography
15. Ultrasonography
16. EEG
17. ECG
18. Blood cultures
19. Bone marrow exam
20. Liver–spleen scan
21. Spinal tap
22. Nasopharyngoscopy
23. Thyroid-stimulating immunoglobulins

EXTREMITY DEFORMITIES

1. cbc and differential
2. Sedimentation rate
3. Calcium and phosphorus
4. Alkaline phosphatase
5. Acid phosphatase
6. Wassermann
7. Tuberculin test

8. Bone marrow examination
9. Roentgenogram of bones
10. Bone scans
11. Bone biopsy
12. Chromosome analysis

EXTREMITY MASS

1. cbc and differential
2. Sedimentation rate
3. Urinalysis
4. Tuberculin skin test
5. VDRL
6. R-A test
7. ANA
8. Serum protein electrophoresis
9. Synovial fluid analysis
10. Bone marrow examination
11. Tumor survey
12. Roentgenogram of extremity
13. Roentgenogram of joints
14. Bone scan
15. Ultrasonography
16. CT scans
17. Arteriography
18. Phlebography
19. Lymphangiography
20. Skin biopsy
21. Muscle biopsy
22. Bone biopsy
23. Exploratory surgery

EYE PAIN

1. cbc and differential
2. Sedimentation rate
3. SMA–24
4. Wassermann
5. Smear and culture of exudate
6. Thyroid function tests
7. Roentgenogram of skull and orbits

8. Roentgenogram of sinuses
9. CT scan
10. Allergy for skin tests
11. Arteriography
12. Nerve blocks
13. Tonometry
14. Tuberculin test
15. Visual field examination
16. Histamine test
17. Gonioscopy
18. Slit-lamp examination
19. Temporal artery biopsy

FACIAL PAIN

1. cbc and differential
2. Sedimentation rate
3. SMA–24
4. Nose and throat culture
5. Spinal fluid examination
6. Wassermann
7. Roentgenogram of sinuses
8. Roentgenogram of teeth
9. Roentgenogram of temporomandibular joint
10. Roentgenogram of skull
11. CT scan
12. Roentgenogram of cervical spine
13. Angiography
14. Nasopharyngoscopy
15. Histamine test
16. Nerve blocks
17. EEG
18. Tonometry
19. Therapeutic trial of ergotamine

FACIAL PARALYSIS

1. cbc and differential
2. Sedimentation rate
3. Urinalysis

4. VDRL
5. Tuberculin test
6. SMA–24
7. Serum protein electrophoresis
8. Cultures of ear discharge
9. Audiogram and calorics
10. Roentgenogram of skull, mastoids, and petrous bones
11. CT scan
12. Posterior fossa myelography
13. Spinal tap, sialography
14. Electromyography
15. Tensilon test

FASCICULATIONS

1. cbc and differential
2. Sedimentation rate
3. Urinalysis
4. VDRL
5. Tuberculin test
6. Blood lead level
7. T3, T4, T7, TSH
8. Serum protein electrophoresis
9. Glucose tolerance test
10. ANA test
11. R-A test
12. Roentgenogram of spine
13. Spinal tap
14. Myelography
15. Aortography
16. Electromyography, NCV
17. Serum electrolytes
18. Ca, PO4, alkaline phosphatase
19. Serum magnesium levels
20. Family history
21. Tensilon test

FATIGUE

1. cbc
2. Urinalysis
3. Sedimentation rate

4. SMA–24
5. Wassermann
6. ECG (for patients over 40)
7. Chest roentgenogram and flat plate of abdomen
8. Sedimentation rate
9. PPD, intermediate
10. Na, K, Cl, CO2
11. 36-hour fast (hypoglycemia)
12. Thyroid function tests
13. 24-hour urine 17–ketosteroids and 17–hydroxysteroids
14. 24-hour urine aldosterone
15. Liver function tests (see Jaundice, this table)
16. Febrile agglutinins
17. Brucellin antibody titer
18. Heterophil antibody titer
19. LE preparations and ANA test
20. Calcium, phosphorus, alkaline phosphatase
21. Bone scan
22. Response to vitamins and corrective diet
23. Exploratory laparotomy
24. Psychometric tests
25. Lymph node biopsy
26. Tensilon test
27. Arterial blood gases

FEVER OF UNKNOWN ORIGIN

1. cbc
2. Urinalysis
3. Sedimentation rate
4. SMA–24   cmp
5. Wassermann   Syphilis
6. ECG
7. Chest roentgenogram and flat plate of abdomen
8. PPD, intermediate   TB
9. Nose and throat culture
10. Routine sputum culture

11. Sputum for acid-fast bacilli smear and culture (or gastric washings)
12. Urine cultures
13. Blood cultures
14. Bone marrow smear and culture
15. Stool for ova and parasites
16. Blood smear for parasites and spirochetes
17. Febrile agglutinins *Hemolytic Anemia*
18. Heterophil antibody titer *mono*
19. ASO titer *Strep A*
20. Brucellin antibody titer
21. Cold agglutinins
22. Latex flocculation
23. LE preparations and ANA test
24. Serum protein electrophoresis
25. Acute and convalescent-phase sera for viral studies
26. Sickle cell preparation
27. Urine for porphobilinogen
28. Cerebrospinal fluid examination and culture
29. Liver function tests (see Jaundice, this appendix)
30. Urine for etiocholanolone
31. Fibrindex (Mediterranean fever)
32. Nitroblue tetrazolium (NBT) test (for chronic granulomas)
33. Chest roentgenogram
34. Flat plate of abdomen
35. Upper GI series
36. Intravenous pyelogram (hypernephroma)
37. Roentgenogram of long bones (metastatic carcinoma)
38. Roentgenogram of teeth
39. Roentgenogram of hands (sarcoidosis)
40. PPD, intermediate
41. Histoplasmin skin test
42. Coccidioidin skin test
43. Blastomycin skin test
44. Trichinella skin test
45. Brucellergen skin test
46. Frei test
47. Amebic hemagglutinin inhibition test
48. Lymph node biopsy
49. Kveim test
50. Liver biopsy
51. Muscle biopsy
52. Exploratory laparotomy
53. Ultrasonography
54. CT scan of abdomen
55. Bone scan
56. Lung scan

FLATULENCE, EXCESSIVE GAS, AND BORBORYGMI ■

1. cbc and differential
2. Sedimentation rate
3. SMA–24
4. Amylase and lipase
5. Serum electrolytes
6. Stool for occult blood
7. Stool for ova and parasites
8. Stool for fat and trypsin
9. D-xylose uptake
10. Lactose tolerance test
11. Glucose tolerance test
12. Liver function tests
13. Stool culture
14. Serum protein electrophoresis
15. Urine 5-HIAA
16. Blood lead level
17. Gastric analysis
18. Bernstein test
19. Flat plate of abdomen
20. Cholecystogram
21. Esophagram
22. Upper GI series, small bowel series
23. Barium enema
24. Proctoscopy
25. Esophagoscopy
26. Gastroscopy
27. Colonoscopy
28. Liver biopsy
29. Exploratory laparotomy
30. Analysis of flatus

FLANK PAIN

1. cbc and differential
2. Sedimentation rate
3. Urinalysis
4. Urine culture routine and AFB
5. Blood cultures
6. SMA–24
7. Protein electrophoresis
8. Liver function studies
9. Roentgenogram of spine, chest
10. IVP
11. Myelography
12. Cystoscopy and retrograde pyelography
13. Cholecystogram
14. Bone scans
15. CT scan of abdomen
16. Ultrasonography
17. Arteriography
18. ECG
19. Tuberculin test
20. Exploratory surgery

FLASHES OF LIGHT

1. cbc and differential
2. Sedimentation rate
3. Urinalysis
4. VDRL
5. Tuberculin test
6. Histoplasmin skin test and serology
7. Toxoplasma serology
8. Kveim test
9. Roentgenogram of skull and orbits
10. Roentgenogram of hands
11. CT scan
12. Visual field examination
13. Tonometry
14. Refraction
15. Slit-lamp examination
16. Histamine test

17. EEG
18. Spinal tap
19. Trial of anticonvulsants

FLUSHED FACE

1. cbc and differential
2. Blood smear
3. Urinalysis
4. VDRL
5. Tuberculin test
6. Blood gases
7. Blood volume
8. Venous pressure and circulation time
9. Pulmonary function tests
10. ECG
11. Urine 5-HIAA
12. Serum LH, FSH, and estradiol
13. Plasma cortisol before and after ACTH
14. Skull roentgenogram
15. Chest roentgenogram
16. Histamine test
17. IVP

FOOT, HEEL, AND TOE PAIN

1. cbc with differential
2. Urine
3. Sedimentation rate
4. SMA–24
5. VDRL
6. R-A test
7. Synovial fluid analysis
8. Roentgenogram of foot and ankles
9. Roentgenogram of lumbosacral spine
10. Phlebography, arteriography
11. Lymphangiography
12. EMG
13. Bone scan

14. Nerve blocks
15. Injection of trigger points with lidocaine
16. Injection of joints and plantar fascia with lidocaine
17. Biopsy, exploratory surgery
18. Myelography

8. Trial of estrogen replacement therapy
9. Chromosomal analysis
10. Vaginal smear and culture
11. Vaginal cytology
12. D & C and biopsy
13. Referral to psychiatrist or therapist

FREQUENCY OF URINATION ■

1. cbc and differential
2. Urinalysis
3. Urine culture and colony count
4. Sedimentation rate
5. SMA–24
6. Prostatic massage and examination of exudate
7. Catheterize for residual urine
8. Fishberg concentration test
9. IVP and cystogram (voiding)
10. Roentgenogram of skull, CT scan
11. Cystoscopy
12. Serum, ACTH, LH, FSH
13. Visual fields
14. Response to pitressin
15. Hickey–Hare test
16. Creatinine clearance
17. Cystometric studies
18. Venous pressure and circulation time

GAIT DISTURBANCES ■

1. cbc and differential
2. Sedimentation rate
3. Urinalysis
4. VDRL
5. FTA–ABS
6. Tuberculin test
7. SMA–24
8. Serum protein electrophoresis
9. Schilling test
10. Urine porphobilinogen
11. Blood lead levels
12. Glucose tolerance test
13. 24-hour urine creatinine and creatine
14. ANA test
15. R-A test
16. Roentgenogram of extremities
17. Roentgenogram of spine
18. Roentgenogram of skull
19. CT scan
20. Myelography
21. Arteriography
22. MRI

FRIGIDITY ■

1. Careful pelvic examination with rectovaginal
2. Psychometric testing
3. Serum FSH, LH, and estradiol
4. Ultrasonogram
5. Laparoscopy
6. Exploratory laparotomy
7. Trial of birth control

GIGANTISM ■

1. cbc and differential
2. Urinalysis
3. Serum Ca, PO4, and alkaline phosphatase
4. Serum growth hormone
5. Serum LH and FSH

6. Serum cortisol
7. Urine 17–ketosteroids
8. Urine 17–hydroxycorticosteroids
9. Skull roentgenogram with tomography of sella
10. Roentgenogram of epiphysis
11. CT scan
12. Chromosomal analysis
13. Testicular biopsy

7. VDRL
8. Frei test
9. Urine culture, urethral smear and culture
10. Roentgenogram of hip
11. Roentgenogram of lumbosacral spine
12. Arteriography
13. Phlebography
14. Lymphangiography
15. Myelography
16. Bone scan
17. Joint aspiration
18. Lymph node biopsy
19. Bone biopsy
20. Exploratory surgery

GROIN MASS

1. cbc and differential
2. Sedimentation rate
3. SMA–24
4. Tuberculin test
5. Mono spot test
6. Wassermann
7. Nitrobule tetrazolium test
8. Protein electrophoresis
9. Kveim test
10. Roentgenogram of hips
11. Roentgenogram of spine
12. Phlebography
13. Lymphangiogram
14. Arteriography
15. Small bowel series
16. Biopsy
17. Exploratory surgery

HALITOSIS

1. cbc and differential
2. Sedimentation rate
3. Wassermann
4. Tuberculin test
5. Liver function tests
6. Gastric analysis
7. Stool for blood and parasites
8. Chest roentgenogram
9. Acid barium swallow and upper GI series
10. Roentgenogram of teeth
11. Roentgenogram of sinuses
12. Bronchogram
13. Esophagoscopy and gastroscopy
14. Bronchoscopy
15. Nasopharyngoscopy

GROIN PAIN

1. cbc and differential
2. Sedimentation rate
3. Urine
4. SMA–24
5. ANA test
6. Tuberculin test

HALLUCINATIONS

1. cbc and differential
2. Urinalysis
3. Blood lead level

4. Serum bromide level
5. Drug screen
6. SMA–24
7. Family history
8. Drug history
9. Skull roentgenogram
10. EEG with sleep
11. CT scans
12. Spinal tap
13. ANA test
14. FTA–ABS
15. Arteriography
16. Psychometric testing
17. Urine porphobilinogen

HAND AND FINGER PAIN ■

1. cbc and differential
2. Urine
3. Sedimentation rate
4. VDRL
5. SMA–24
6. R-A test
7. ANA test
8. Serum protein electrophoresis
9. Sia water test
10. Blood cultures
11. Immunoelectrophoresis
12. Roentgenogram of hands
13. Roentgenogram of elbow and shoulder
14. Roentgenogram of cervical spine
15. Roentgenogram of chest
16. Myelography
17. Arteriography
18. Phlebography
19. EMG, NCV
20. Cold response test
21. Skin biopsy
22. Muscle biopsy
23. Nerve block
24. Carpal tunnel block

25. Culture of exudates
26. Exploratory surgery

HEADACHE ■

1. cbc
2. Urinalysis
3. Sedimentation rate
4. SMA–24
5. Roentgenogram of T-M joints
6. ECG (for patients over age 40)
7. Chest roentgenogram and flat plate of abdomen
8. PPD, intermediate
9. Wassermann
10. Spinal fluid examination and culture
11. Febrile agglutinins
12. CRP (C-reactive protein)
13. Nose and throat culture
14. 24-hour urine catecholamines
15. Skull roentgenogram
16. Roentgenogram of paranasal sinuses and mastoids
17. Roentgenogram of teeth
18. Roentgenogram of cervical spine
19. Angiography
20. CT scan
21. EEG
22. Histamine provocative test (migraine and histamine cephalgia)
23. Therapeutic trial of ergotamine
24. Visual fields (pituitary tumor)
25. Audiogram and caloric testing (acoustic neuroma)
26. Tonometry
27. Irrigation of sinuses
28. MRI
29. Allergic skin tests
30. Block of cervical nerves
31. Block of trigeminal nerve
32. Block of nerve roots of various teeth
33. Elimination diet

HEAD MASS ■

1. cbc and differential
2. Sedimentation rate
3. Urinalysis
4. Tuberculin test
5. VDRL
6. Sickle cell preparation
7. Serum parathyroid hormone
8. Serum protein electrophoresis
9. I & D and culture
10. Hemoglobin electrophoresis
11. Chest roentgenogram
12. Roentgenogram of skull
13. Bone scan
14. Skeletal survey
15. CT scan
16. EEG, spinal tap
17. Arteriography
18. Skin biopsy
19. Bone biopsy
20. Exploratory surgery

HEARTBURN ■

1. cbc and differential
2. Sedimentation rate
3. Stool for occult blood
4. Gastric analysis
5. Liver function studies
6. Pancreatic function studies
7. Upper GI series
8. Esophagram
9. Acid barium swallow
10. Cholecystogram
11. Bernstein test
12. Esophagoscopy
13. Gastroscopy
14. Manometry
15. ECG and GXT
16. Trial of nitroglycerin
17. Biopsy

HEMATEMESIS AND MELENA ■

1. cbc
2. Urinalysis
3. Sedimentation rate
4. SMA–24
5. Wassermann
6. ECG (for patients over age 40)
7. Chest roentgenogram and flat plate of abdomen
8. PPD, intermediate
9. Stools for occult blood
10. Gastric analysis
11. Prothrombin time
12. Coagulation time and partial thromboplastin time
13. Platelet count
14. Bleeding time
15. BSP and other liver function test (see Jaundice, this table)
16. Upper GI series and esophagram
17. Barium enema
18. Small intestinal series
19. Arteriography
20. Liver scan
21. Sigmoidoscopy and colonoscopy
22. Esophagoscopy
23. Gastroscopy
24. Levine tube to see if blood is coming from stomach
25. Fluorescein dye string test
26. Exploratory laparotomy and liver biopsy
27. Nuclear scanning with technetium labeled rbc's

HEMATURIA AND PYURIA ■

1. cbc
2. Urinalysis
3. Sedimentation rate
4. SMA–24
5. Wassermann

6. ECG (for patients over age 40)
7. Chest roentgenogram and flat plate of abdomen
8. PPD, intermediate
9. Repeated urinalysis
10. Strain urine for stones
11. Uric acid
12. Calcium, phosphorus, alkaline phosphatase
13. Urine culture and sensitivity
14. Urine for acid-fast bacilli smear and culture
15. Serum complement
16. ASO titer
17. Addis count
18. 24-hour urine protein
19. Fishberg concentration test
20. Blood cultures
21. Blood smear for malarial parasites
22. Plasma haptoglobins and methemalbumin
23. Red cell fragility test, reticulocyte count, and serum bilirubin
24. Coombs' test
25. Prothrombin time (liver disease)
26. Coagulation time (hemophilia)
27. Bleeding time
28. Platelet count
29. ANA
30. Nose and throat culture (glomerulonephritis)
31. Urine myoglobin
32. Flat plate of abdomen
33. Intravenous pyelogram
34. Retrograde pyelogram
35. Roentgenograms of long bones (metastatic carcinoma)
36. Aortogram (embolism)
37. CT scan
38. Catheterize for residual urine
39. Cystoscopy
40. Three-glass test
41. Muscle biopsy (periarteritis nodosa)
42. Ultrasonograms
43. Renal biopsy
44. Exploration of kidney

HEMOPTYSIS

1. cbc and differential
2. Sedimentation rate
3. SMA–24
4. Sputum smear
5. Sputum cultures
6. Tuberculin test
7. Papanicolaou smears
8. Sputum analysis
9. Coagulation studies
10. Roentgenogram of chest
11. Bronchography
12. Esophagram
13. Tomography
14. Apical lordotic views
15. Lung scan
16. Spirometry
17. ECG
18. Bronchoscopy
19. Venous pressure and circulation time
20. Echocardiography
21. Scalene node biopsy
22. Pleural biopsy
23. Lung biopsy
24. Coccidioidin skin test
25. Histoplasmin skin test
26. Blastomycin skin test

HEPATOMEGALY

1. cbc and differential
2. Sedimentation rate
3. Urinalysis
4. SMA–24
5. ANA test
6. BSP
7. Blood smears
8. Blood cultures
9. Stool examination
10. Serum haptoglobins

11. Serum protein electrophoresis
12. Amylase, lipase
13. Bone marrow examination
14. Serum iron and iron binding capacity
15. Flat plate of abdomen
16. Gallbladder series
17. ERCP
18. GI series and barium enema
19. Endoscopy
20. Liver biopsy
21. CT scans
22. Liver scans
23. Liver–spleen scan
24. Ultrasonography
25. Splenoportogram
26. Peritoneoscopy
27. Venous pressure and circulation time
28. Exploratory laparotomy

HICCOUGHS

1. cbc and differential
2. Urinalysis
3. Sedimentation rate
4. SMA–24
5. VDRL
6. Tuberculin test
7. ANA
8. Serum protein electrophoresis
9. Chest roentgenogram
10. Esophagram and GI series
11. Roentgenogram of cervical spine
12. Cholecystogram
13. Fluoroscopy
14. Esophagoscopy and gastroscopy
15. ECG
16. Echocardiography
17. Ultrasonography
18. CT scan
19. Exploratory surgery
20. Psychometric tests

HOARSENESS

1. cbc and differential
2. Sedimentation rate
3. SMA–24
4. Thyroid function tests
5. Wassermann
6. Blood lead level
7. Tuberculin test
8. R-A test
9. Roentgenogram of neck
10. Roentgenogram of chest
11. Roentgenogram of cervical spine
12. Roentgenogram of skull and sinuses
13. CT scan
14. Thyroid scan
15. Spinal tap
16. Tensilon test
17. Arteriography
18. Laryngoscopy
19. Bronchoscopy
20. Allergy skin testing

HYPERTENSION

1. cbc
2. Urinalysis
3. Sedimentation rate
4. SMA–24
5. Wassermann
6. ECG (for patients over age 40)
7. Chest roentgenogram and flat plate of abdomen
8. PPD, intermediate
9. Blood electrolytes
10. Total eosinophil count
11. 12-hour Addis count
12. Fishberg concentration test
13. 24-hour urine protein
14. 24-hour urine potassium
15. 24-hour urine catecholamines

16. 24-hour urine aldosterone and plasma and renal vein renin
17. Dexamethasone suppression test
18. Urine culture
19. Morning urines for acid-fast bacilli smear and culture
20. Intravenous pyelogram with 1–, 2–, 3– minute shots
21. Retrograde pyelogram
22. Renal scan
23. Renal angiography
24. Perirenal air insufflation
25. Direct recording of arterial pressure
26. Differential sodium excretion test
27. Histamine or Regitine test
28. Renal biopsy
29. Exploratory laparotomy
30. Angiotensin infusion test
31. CT scan of abdomen

HYPOMENORRHEA AND AMENORRHEA

1. cbc and differential
2. Blood smear
3. Sedimentation rate
4. Vaginal smear for estrogen function
5. Serum prolactin
6. Serum estradiol and FSH
7. Serum progesterone
8. Urine 17–ketosteroids
9. Urine 17–hydroxysteroids
10. Urine FSH
11. Thyroid function tests
12. Papanicolaou smear
13. Endometrial biopsy
14. Trial of progesterone therapy
15. Skull roentgenogram
16. Culdoscopy
17. Uterosalpingogram
18. Peritoneoscopy
19. Exploratory laparotomy

HYPOTENSION AND SHOCK

1. cbc and differential
2. Type and crossmatch
3. Stat. FBS, BUN
4. Monitor I & O, vital signs and cardiac rhythm
5. Sedimentation rate
6. SMA–24
7. Tuberculin test
8. Swan–Ganz monitoring
9. Blood volume
10. Serial electrolytes and STAT
11. Stool for occult blood
12. Insert Levin tube to test for blood in GI tract
13. Serum amylase and lipase
14. Serial ECGs
15. Serial CPK, LDH, SGOT, MB–CPK
16. Lung scan
17. Blood gases STAT
18. Chest roentgenogram and flat plate of abdomen
19. Plasma cortisol
20. Blood cultures
21. Gastroscopy and other endoscopic procedures
22. T3–T4–T7, TSH
23. Drug screen

HYPOTHERMIA

1. cbc and differential
2. Blood smear
3. Urinalysis and culture
4. Foley catheter to drainage
5. Monitor urine output
6. Blood gases STAT
7. Electrolytes STAT
8. SMA–24
9. STAT FBS and BUN

10. STAT T3, T4, T7, TSH
11. STAT blood cultures
12. STAT ECG
13. Serial ECGs and cardiac enzymes
14. Serum cortisol
15. Skull roentgenogram
16. EEG
17. Spinal tap
18. CT scan
19. Drug screen
20. Lung scan
21. Circulation time

INCONTINENCE ■

1. cbc and differential
2. Sedimentation rate
3. Urinalysis
4. Urine culture and colony count
5. Catheterization for residual urine
6. Cystometric studies
7. Cystoscopy
8. IVP
9. VDRL
10. Tuberculin test
11. SMA–24
12. Roentgenogram of spine
13. Pad test
14. Myelography
15. Skull roentgenogram
16. Sigmoidoscopy
17. Stool examination
18. Electromyography
19. Serum protein electrophoresis
20. EEG
21. CT scan

IMPOTENCY ■

1. cbc and differential
2. Urinalysis
3. Urine culture and colony count

4. VDRL
5. Tuberculin test
6. Prostatic massage and examination of exudate
7. ANA test
8. T3, T4, T7, TSH
9. Plasma cortisol
10. Serum FSH, LH
11. Serum testosterone
12. Roentgenogram of spine
13. Skull roentgenogram
14. Spinal tap
15. Psychometric testing
16. CT scan
17. Myelography
18. Chromosome analysis
19. Sperm count
20. Testicular biopsy
21. Nocturnal penile tumescent study
22. Penile blood pressure
23. Cystometric study

INDIGESTION ■

1. cbc differential
2. Sedimentation rate
3. Urinalysis
4. SMA–24
5. VDRL
6. Tuberculin test
7. ANA
8. Electrolytes
9. Serum protein electrophoresis
10. ECG
11. Cardiac enzymes
12. Stool examination for occult blood, ovum, and parasites
13. Gastric analysis
14. Serum lipase and amylase
15. Esophagram
16. Upper GI series
17. Small bowel series
18. Cholecystogram
19. IVP

20. Barium enema
21. Chest roentgenogram
22. Esophagoscopy
23. Gastroscopy
24. Duodenoscopy
25. Duodenal analysis
26. Ultrasonography
27. CT scan of abdomen
28. Liver scan
29. Liver biopsy
30. Exploratory laparotomy

INFERTILITY

1. cbc and differential
2. Sedimentation rate
3. Urinalysis
4. Urine culture and colony count
5. Vaginal smear and culture
6. Vaginal cytology
7. KOH and Saline preparation of vaginal fluid
8. VDRL
9. Tuberculin test
10. T3, T4, T7, TSH
11. Serum LH, FSH
12. Serum progesterone
13. Serum estradiol
14. Skull roentgenogram
15. Tubal insufflation
16. Hysterosalpingogram
17. Laparoscopy
18. Exploratory laparotomy
19. Semen analysis
20. Urethral smear and culture
21. Prostatic massage and examination of exudate
22. Temperature chart
23. Spin–Barkeit test of cervical mucus
24. Testicular biopsy
25. Trial of clomiphene
26. Psychometric testing
27. Psychiatric evaluation

INSOMNIA

1. cbc and differential
2. Blood smear for parasites
3. Serum iron and IBC
4. Sedimentation rate
5. Drug screen
6. Urinalysis
7. VDRL
8. FTA–ABS
9. Tuberculin test
10. Febrile agglutinins
11. SMA–24
12. Liver function tests
13. T3, T4, T7, TSH
14. Blood gases
15. Pulmonary function tests
16. ECG and GXT
17. Circulation time
18. Chest roentgenogram
19. Esophagram and upper GI roentgenogram series
20. Endoscopy
21. EEG
22. Skull roentgenogram, CT scan
23. Spinal tap
24. Psychometric testing
25. Psychiatric evaluation

JAUNDICE

1. cbc
2. Urinalysis
3. Sedimentation rate
4. Wassermann
5. ECG (for patients over age 40)
6. Chest roentgenogram and flat plate of abdomen
7. PPD, intermediate
8. Serum haptoglobins
9. SMA–24
10. Serum bilirubin

11. Urine bilirubin and urobilinogen
12. Stool for urobilinogen
13. Alkaline phosphatase
14. Total cholesterol and esters
15. Serum protein electrophoresis
16. Prothrombin time and coagulation profile
17. Reticulocyte count and red cell fragility
18. Coombs' test
19. Blood ammonia level
20. ANA
21. Serum amylase and lipase
22. Stool for occult blood and parasites
23. Heterophil antibody titer
24. Eosinophil count (chlorpromazine sensitivity)
25. Febrile agglutinins
26. Brucellin antibody titer
27. Guinea pig inoculation of blood (Weil's disease)
28. Blood smear for parasites
29. Blood cultures
30. Hepatitis associated antigen (HAA)
31. CEA
32. Gamma-glutamyl transpeptidase (GGT)
33. Cholecystogram or cholangiogram after jaundice subsides
34. Upper GI series
35. Barium enema
36. Lymphangiogram
37. Liver biopsy
38. Rectal biopsy
39. Sigmoidoscopy and colonoscopy
40. Gastroscopy, duodenoscopy with ERCP
41. Lymph node biopsy
42. Occupational history
43. Duodenal analysis
44. Peritoneoscopy
45. Exploratory laparotomy
46. Steroid whitewash
47. Transhepatic cholangiography
48. Serum for mitochondrial antibodies
49. Serum for alpha fetoprotein
50. Ultrasonography
51. CT scan of abdomen

JAW SWELLING ■

1. cbc and differential
2. Sedimentation rate
3. Tuberculin test
4. VDRL
5. I & D, culture of exudate for bacteria, fungi, and AFB
6. Serologic tests for fungi
7. Ca, PO4, and alkaline phosphatase
8. Roentgenogram of jaw
9. Roentgenogram of teeth
10. Sialography
11. Biopsy
12. Mumps skin test
13. Histoplasmin skin test
14. Coccidiodin skin test
15. Kveim test

JOINT PAIN OR SWELLING ■

1. cbc
2. Urinalysis
3. Sedimentation rate
4. SMA–24
5. Wassermann
6. ECG
7. Chest roentgenogram, flat plate of abdomen
8. PPD, intermediate
9. ASO titer
10. C-reactive protein (CRP)
11. Latex flocculation for rheumatoid arthritis
12. Blood cultures
13. Cervical or urethral smears and cultures for gonococci
14. Sickle cell preparation
15. LE preparations and ANA
16. Blood uric acid

17. Febrile agglutinins
18. Heterophil antibody titer
19. Brucellin antibody titer
20. Eosinophil count (trichinosis, periarteritis)
21. Synovianalysis (for mucin clot, cell count, uric acid crystals, and so forth)
22. Synovial fluid culture and sensitivity for bacteria, fungi, spirochetes
23. Coagulation profile (hemophilia)
24. Serum protein electrophoresis
25. Chest roentgenogram
26. Roentgenogram of joint involved
27. Roentgenogram of additional joints
28. Lymphangiogram
29. Arthrogram
30. Synovial biopsy
31. Muscle biopsy (periarteritis nodosa)
32. Therapeutic trial with colchicine
33. Therapeutic trial with salicylates
34. Arthroscopy
35. Bone scans

LEG PAIN

1. cbc and differential
2. SMA–24
3. Sedimentation rate
4. R-A test
5. Serum protein electrophoresis
6. Glucose tolerance test
7. Impedance plethysmography
8. Coagulation profile
9. Roentgenogram of extremity and spine
10. Roentgenogram of joints
11. Phlebography
12. Arteriography
13. Lymphangiography
14. Myelography and CT scan
15. Bone scan
16. Oscillometry

17. Thermography
18. Ultrasound flow study
19. Nerve blocks
20. Electromyography

LYMPHADENOPATHY

1. cbc and differential
2. Sedimentation rate
3. Nose and throat culture
4. Sputum for acid-fast smear and culture
5. Blood cultures
6. Heterophil antibody titer
7. Brucellin antibody titer
8. Febrile agglutinins
9. Wassermann
10. Bone marrow examination
11. Nitroblue tetrazolium (NBT) test for chronic granulomas
12. Chest roentgenogram
13. Bone scan (metastatic carcinoma)
14. Roentgenogram of hands (sarcoidosis)
15. Lymphangiogram
16. Lymph node biopsy
17. PPD, intermediate
18. Skin tests for fungi (histoplasmosis, and so forth)
19. Brucellergen skin test
20. Kveim test

MEMORY LOSS AND DEMENTIA

1. cbc and differential
2. Sedimentatioin rate
3. Blood smear
4. Schilling test

5. Urinalysis
6. Drug screen
7. SMA–24
8. R-A test
9. ANA test
10. VDRL
11. Serial electrolytes
12. FTA–ABS
13. T3, T4, T7, TSH
14. Serum protein electrophoresis
15. Skull roentgenogram
16. EEG
17. CT scan
18. Spinal tap
19. Skeletal survey
20. Psychometric testing
21. Nuclear flow study (RISA)

MISCELLANEOUS SITES OF BLEEDING ◼

1. cbc and differential
2. Sedimentation rate
3. Urinalysis
4. VDRL and SMA–24
5. Tuberculin test
6. Coagulation studies
7. Serum protein electrophoresis and im-munoelectrophoresis
8. Blood smear
9. Sickle cell prep
10. Bone marrow examination
11. ANA test
12. Blood cultures
13. Liver-spleen scan
14. Soft tissue roentgenogram
15. Biopsy of tissue involved
16. Exploratory surgery
17. Arteriography
18. Bone scans
19. Lymph node biopsy
20. CT scan

MURMURS ◼

1. cbc and differential
2. Sedimentation rate
3. Blood smear
4. CRP
5. Streptozyme test
6. Nose and throat culture
7. Blood cultures
8. ANA test
9. VDRL
10. FTA–ABS
11. SMA–24
12. Tuberculin test
13. T3, T4, T7, TSH
14. ECG
15. Echocardiography
16. Phonocardiography
17. Cardiac catheterization
18. Angiocardiography
19. Serum iron and IBC
20. Venous pressure and circulation time
21. R-A test
22. Bone marrow exam and culture

MUSCULAR ATROPHY ◼

1. cbc and differential
2. Sedimentation rate
3. Thyroid function tests
4. Blood lead level
5. Glucose tolerance test
6. Liver function tests
7. ANA test
8. R–A test
9. SMA–24
10. Wassermann
11. Roentgenogram of spine and long bones
12. Spinal tap
13. Myelography
14. EMG

15. Arteriography of extremity
16. Muscle biopsy

MYOCLONUS

1. cbc and differential
2. Sedimentation rate
3. Urinalysis
4. VDRL
5. FTA–ABS
6. ANA test
7. Serum copper and ceruloplasmin
8. SMA–24
9. T3, T4, T7, TSH
10. Skull roentgenogram
11. CT scan
12. EEG, awake and sleep
13. Spinal tap
14. Drug screen
15. Drug history
16. Psychometric tests

NAIL CHANGES

1. cbc and differential
2. Blood smear for morphology
3. Serum iron and iron-building capacity
4. Urinalysis
5. Sedimentation rate
6. SMA–24
7. VDRL
8. Tuberculin test
9. Blood gases
10. Pulmonary function tests
11. T3, T4, T7
12. Bone marrow examination
13. Chest roentgenogram
14. Cardiac catheterization
15. Angiocardiography
16. Bronchoscopy

17. Bronchograms
18. Lymph node biopsy
19. Mediastinoscopy
20. Tomography
21. Skull roentgenogram
22. CT scan
23. Serum parathyroid hormone assay
24. Phosphate reabsorption test

NASAL DISCHARGE

1. cbc and differential
2. Sedimentation rate
3. Urinalysis
4. Tuberculin test
5. VDRL
6. FTA–ABS
7. ANA test
8. Smear and culture for bacteria, fungi, and AFB
9. Smear for eosinophils
10. Allergy skin testing
11. Chest roentgenogram
12. Roentgenogram of sinuses
13. Skull roentgenogram
14. CT scan, spinal tap
15. Nasopharyngoscopy
16. Histamine test
17. Biopsy

NECK MASS

1. cbc and differential
2. Sedimentation rate
3. Serum protein electrophoresis
4. SMA–24
5. Sputum culture
6. Tuberculin test
7. Nose and throat culture
8. Roentgenogram of cervical spine

9. Roentgenogram of chest
10. Arteriography
11. Roentgenogram of long bones
12. Venous pressure and circulation time
13. Laryngoscopy and bronchoscopy
14. Gastroscopy, esophagoscopy
15. Biopsy
16. RAI uptake and scan
17. Fine needle aspiration and biopsy
18. CT scan
19. MRI

NECK PAIN ■

1. cbc
2. Sedimentation rate
3. Calcium, phosphorus, alkaline phosphatase (metastatic carcinoma)
4. Serum protein electrophoresis (multiple myeloma)
5. Acid phosphatase
6. Bone marrow examination
7. Wassermann
8. Spinal fluid examination
9. Roentgenogram of cervical spine
10. Chest roentgenogram
11. Skull roentgenogram with special views of foramen magnum
12. Roentgenogram of long bones
13. Myelogram
14. PPD, intermediate
15. Nerve block
16. EMG
17. RAI uptake and scan

NOCTURIA ■

1. cbc and differential
2. Sedimentation rate
3. Urinalysis

4. VDRL
5. Tuberculin test
6. Catheterization for residual urine
7. SMA–24
8. Ca, PO4, alkaline phosphatase
9. Glucose tolerance test
10. T3, T4, T7, TSH
11. Frishberg concentration test
12. Creatinine clearance
13. Monitor I & O
14. Pitressin, test
15. Hickey–Hare test
16. Serial electrolytes
17. IVP and voiding cystogram
18. Cystoscopy
19. Skull roentgenogram
20. Visual fields
21. Plasma renin
22. Urine aldosterone
23. ECG
24. Pulmonary function tests
25. Venous pressure and circulation time

NUCHAL RIGIDITY ■

1. cbc and differential
2. Blood smear
3. Urinalysis and culture
4. Blood cultures
5. Sedimentation rate
6. Nose and throat culture and smear
7. Spinal tap, smear and cultures of CSF
8. SMA–24
9. VDRL
10. FTA–ABS
11. Tuberculin test
12. ANA test
13. Serum protein electrophoresis
14. Chest roentgenogram
15. Skull roentgenogram
16. Roentgenogram of cervical spine
17. CT scan

18. Echoencephalography
19. Arteriography

NYSTAGMUS

1. cbc and differential
2. Urinalysis
3. Sedimentation rate
4. SMA–24
5. VDRL
6. Tuberculin test
7. Audiograms and caloric tests
8. Electronystagmography
9. Roentgenogram of skull, mastoids, and petrous bones
10. Roentgenogram of sinuses
11. CT scan
12. EEG
13. Spinal tap
14. Posterior fossa myelography
15. Roentgenogram of cervical spine
16. Arteriography
17. Drug history
18. Visual fields
19. Refraction

OBESITY

1. cbc and differential
2. Urinalysis
3. Sedimentation rate
4. SMA–24
5. VDRL
6. Tuberculin test
7. Glucose tolerance test
8. 48-hour fast with frequent blood glucose determinations
9. Tolbutamide tolerance test
10. T3, T4, T7, TSH
11. Plasma cortisol with ACTH stimulation

12. Urine 17-ketosteroid and 17-hydroxysteroids
13. Skull roentgenogram
14. CT scan
15. EEG
16. Spinal tap
17. Psychometric tests
18. Plasma and urine osmolality
19. Venous pressure and circulation time
20. Serial electrolytes

ORAL OR LINGUAL MASS

1. cbc and differential
2. Sedimentation rate
3. Urinalysis
4. VDRL
5. Tuberculin test
6. SMA–24
7. I & D culture
8. Throat culture
9. Roentgenogram of teeth
10. Roentgenogram of jaw
11. Roentgenogram of skull
12. Roentgenogram of sinuses
13. Biopsy
14. Laryngoscopy

ORBITAL DISCHARGE

1. cbc and differential
2. Sedimentation rate
3. Urinalysis
4. Smear and culture of discharge
5. VDRL
6. Tuberculin test
7. ANA test
8. Smear for eosinophils
9. Tonometry
10. Refraction

11. T3, T4, T7
12. Visual fields
13. Roentgenogram of skull
14. Roentgenogram of sinuses
15. Ultrasonography
16. CT scan
17. Biopsy
18. Exploratory surgery
19. Mumps skin test
20. Histamine test

ORBITAL MASS

1. cbc and differential
2. Sedimentation rate
3. Urinalysis
4. Tuberculin test
5. Smear and culture of discharge
6. VDRL
7. SMA–24
8. ANA
9. Protein electrophoresis
10. T3, T4, T7, TSH
11. Blood cultures
12. Skull roentgenogram
13. Roentgenogram of sinuses
14. Special views of orbits and optic foramina
15. Arteriography
16. Ultrasonography
17. CT scan
18. Brain scan
19. Spinal tap
20. Nasopharyngoscopy
21. Lymph node biopsy
22. Biopsy of mass
23. Exploratory surgery

PAPILLEDEMA

1. cbc and differential
2. Sedimentation rate
3. Urinalysis

4. Tuberculin test
5. VDRL
6. FTA–ABS
7. Blood cultures
8. Serum protein electrophoresis
9. SMA–24
10. Skull roentgenogram
11. EEG
12. CT scans
13. Echoencephalography
14. Arteriography
15. Visual fields
16. Brain scan
17. Psychometric testing

PARESTHESIAS OF ONE OR MORE EXTREMITIES

1. cbc and differential
2. Sedimentation rate
3. Urinalysis
4. VDRL
5. FTA–ABS
6. Tuberculin test
7. SMA–24
8. Glucose tolerance test
9. Schilling test
10. Blood smear
11. Chest roentgenogram
12. Roentgenogram of cervical spine
13. Roentgenogram of thoracic and lumbar spine
14. Skull roentgenogram
15. CT scan
16. EEG
17. Spinal tap
18. Arteriography
19. Muscle biopsy
20. Electromyography
21. Myelography
22. Blood lead level
23. Urine porphobilinogen

24. Analysis for arsenic
25. Examination for Trousseau's sign

PELVIC MASS

1. cbc and differential
2. Sedimentation rate
3. Urinalysis
4. Tuberculin test
5. VDRL
6. Catheterize for residual urine
7. Enema
8. Vaginal smear and culture
9. Stool examination
10. Stool culture
11. Pregnancy test
12. Culdocentesis
13. Flat plate of abdomen
14. Roentgenogram of spine
15. Barium enema
16. IVP and cystogram
17. Sigmoidoscopy and colonoscopy
18. Cystoscopy
19. Culdoscopy
20. Hysterosalpingography
21. Peritoneoscopy
22. Ultrasonography
23. CT scan
24. Aortography
25. Exploratory surgery

PENILE PAIN

1. cbc and differential
2. Urine
3. Serum calcium and uric acid
4. Urethral smear
5. Urethral culture
6. Urine culture
7. Catheterize for residual urine
8. Prostatic fluid examination

9. Strain urine for stones
10. IVP and voiding cystogram
11. Retrograde pyelography
12. Roentgenogram of the spine
13. Special diagnostic procedures: cystoscopy, urethral sounding, proctoscopy, peritoneoscopy

PERIORBITAL AND FACIAL EDEMA

1. cbc and differential
2. Sedimentation rate
3. Urinalysis
4. Tuberculin test
5. VDRL
6. SMA–24
7. Serum protein electrophoresis
8. ANA
9. Streptozyme test
10. R-A test
11. Nose and throat culture
12. Serological test for trichinella
13. T3, T4, T7, TSH
14. Skull roentgenogram
15. Roentgenogram of sinuses
16. Spinal tap
17. Blood cultures
18. Pulmonary function tests
19. Plasma renin
20. Urine aldosterone levels
21. Serial electrolytes
22. Muscle biopsy
23. Skin biopsy
24. Venous pressure and circulation time

PHOTOPHOBIA

1. cbc and differential
2. Blood smear
3. Urinalysis

4. Sedimentation rate
5. Febrile agglutinins
6. R–A test
7. Blood cultures
8. SMA–24
9. VDRL
10. Tuberculin test
11. Serum protein electrophoresis
12. Chest roentgenogram
13. Skull roentgenogram
14. EEG
15. CT scan
16. Spinal tap
17. Arteriography
18. Visual fields
19. Tonometry
20. Refraction
21. Slit-lamp examination
22. Kveim test
23. Histoplasmin skin test and serology
24. Toxoplasmosis serology
25. Glucose tolerance test
26. Histamine test

POLYDIPSIA

1. cbc and differential
2. Urinalysis
3. Fishberg concentration test
4. Glucose tolerance test
5. SMA–24
6. Tubular phosphate reabsorption test
7. Serum parathyroid hormone assay
8. T3, T4, T7
9. RAI uptake and scan
10. Serial electrolytes
11. Skull roentgenogram
12. CT scan
13. EEG
14. Spinal tap
15. Monitoring of I & O

16. Psychometric tests
17. Plasma renin
18. Urine aldosterone
19. Response to pitressin
20. Hickey–Hare test

POLYURIA

1. cbc and differential
2. Sedimentation rate
3. Urinalysis
4. Fishberg concentration test
5. Creatinine clearance
6. Monitor I & O
7. SMA–24
8. Ca, PO4, alkaline phosphatase
9. Tubular phosphate reabsorption test
10. Serum parathyroid hormone assay
11. Glucose tolerance test
12. T3, T4, T7
13. PSP test
14. ANA test
15. Hickey–Hare test
16. Response to Pitressin
17. Skull roentgenogram
18. CT scan, EEG
19. Spinal tap
20. Psychometric tests
21. Skeletal survey

POPLITEAL SWELLING

1. cbc and differential
2. Sedimentation rate
3. Urinalysis
4. SMA–24
5. VDRL
6. Tuberculin test

7. Aspiration and culture
8. Synovial fluid analysis
9. Roentgenogram of knee
10. Arthrogram
11. Arteriography
12. Phlebography
13. Lymphangiogram
14. Bone scans
15. Ultrasonography
16. CT scans
17. Exploration and biopsy

4. Tuberculin test
5. Acid phosphatase
6. Alkaline phosphatase
7. Prostatic massage and smear
8. Culture of exudate
9. Urine culture
10. Catheterize for residual urine
11. Cystogram
12. Cystoscopy
13. Biopsy
14. Skeletal survey
15. Bone scan

PRIAPISM

1. cbc and differential
2. Blood smear
3. Bone marrow examination
4. Coagulation studies
5. Urinalysis
6. FTA–ABS
7. Urine culture and colony count
8. Prostatic massage and examination of discharge
9. Culture of prostatic fluid
10. Cystoscopy
11. IVP and voiding cystogram
12. Anoscopy
13. Sigmoidoscopy
14. Drug screen
15. Roentgenogram of spine
16. Spinal tap
17. Myelography

PRURITIS

1. cbc and differential
2. Blood smear
3. Sedimentation rate
4. Bone marrow examination
5. SMA–24
6. Protein electrophoresis
7. Glucose tolerance test
8. Serum bile salt analysis
9. Roentgenogram of chest
10. Roentgenogram of abdomen
11. Skeletal survey
12. Liver scan
13. Skin biopsy
14. Liver biopsy
15. Node biopsy

PTOSIS

1. cbc and differential
2. Urinalysis
3. Sedimentation rate
4. VDRL
5. Tuberculin test

PROSTATIC MASS

1. cbc and differential
2. Sedimentation rate
3. Urinalysis

6. SMA–24
7. ANA test
8. Lymph node biopsy
9. Kveim test
10. Glucose tolerance test
11. Tensilon test
12. Roentgenogram of skull and orbits
13. CT scan
14. Roentgenogram of chest
15. Roentgenogram of cervical spine
16. Spinal tap
17. Arteriography
18. Histamine test

PURPURA

1. cbc
2. Sedimentation rate
3. Coagulation time and partial thrombo-plastin time
4. Bleeding time
5. Prothrombin time
6. Platelet count
7. Rumpel–Leede test
8. Thromboplastin generation test
9. Bone marrow examination
10. LE preparations and ANA test
11. Blood cultures
12. Coombs' test
13. Heterophil antibody titer
14. Cold agglutinins
15. Chest roentgenogram
16. Long bone survey
17. Flat plate of abdomen for size of spleen
18. Response to corticosteroids
19. Skin biopsy (Ehlers–Danlos syndrome)
20. Muscle biopsy
21. Liver biopsy
22. Liver–spleen scan
23. Bone scan

PYURIA

See Hematuria

RASH, GENERAL AND LOCAL

1. cbc and differential
2. Blood smear
3. Platelet count
4. Rumple–Leede test
5. Other coagulation tests
6. Urinalysis, culture of discharge
7. Blood cultures
8. VDRL
9. FTA–ABS
10. KOH preparation
11. Tuberculin test
12. ANA skin test
13. Weil–Felix reaction
14. Serology for Rocky Mountain spotted fever
15. Febrile agglutinins
16. Brucellin antibody titer
17. Serum for viral studies
18. Serology for fungi
19. Serum for HAA
20. Skin testing
21. IgE antibody study
22. Bone marrow examination
23. Dark field examination of lesions and blood
24. Mono spot test
25. Streptozyme test
26. Blood smear for parasites
27. Stool for ova and parasites
28. Skin biopsy
29. Muscle biopsy
30. Roentgenogram of chest
31. Skeletal survey
32. Lymph node biopsy

33. Wood's lamp examination
34. Skin tests for fungi

RECTAL DISCHARGE

1. cbc and differential
2. Urinalysis
3. Sedimentation rate
4. Tuberculin test
5. VDRL
6. Smear and culture of exudate
7. Frei test
8. Anoscopy
9. Sigmoidoscopy
10. Barium enema
11. Small bowel series
12. Cystogram
13. Cystoscopy
14. Vaginoscopy
15. Stool for ova and parasites
16. Biopsy of lesions
17. Exploratory surgery

RECTAL BLEEDING

1. cbc and differential
2. Urinalysis
3. Sedimentation rate
4. SMA–24
5. VDRL
6. Frei test
7. Proctoscopy and colonoscopy
8. Barium enema
9. Rectal biopsy
10. Stool for ova and parasites
11. Small bowel series
12. Arteriography

RECTAL MASS

1. cbc and differential
2. Sedimentation rate
3. Stool for occult blood
4. Stool for ova and parasites
5. SMA–24
6. Tuberculin test
7. VDRL
8. Lipoprotein electrophoresis
9. Barium enema
10. Cystogram
11. Sigmoidoscopy
12. Colonoscopy
13. Biopsy
14. I & D and culture of exudate
15. Ultrasonography, CT scan of abdomen
16. CEA

RECTAL PAIN

1. cbc and differential
2. Urinalysis
3. Sedimentation rate
4. SMA–24
5. VDRL
6. Frei test
7. Urine culture
8. Urethral smear and culture
9. Prostatic massage and examination of exudate
10. Barium enema
11. IVP and cystogram
12. Roentgenogram of lumbosacral spine
13. Sigmoidoscopy
14. Anoscopy
15. Colonoscopy
16. Cystoscopy
17. Culdoscopy
18. Rectal biopsy

19. Papanicolaou smears
20. Stool examination and culture
21. Vaginal smear and culture
22. Pregnancy test

RED EYE

1. cbc and differential
2. Urinalysis
3. Sedimentation rate
4. SMA–24
5. Smear and culture of discharge
6. Nose and throat culture
7. Culture of urethral discharge
8. VDRL
9. Tuberculin test
10. Skin tests for histoplasmosis and other fungi
11. Serology for toxoplasmosis and histoplasmosis
12. Smear for eosinophils
13. Roentgenogram of sinuses
14. Roentgenogram of skull and orbits
15. Slit-lamp examination
16. Tonometry
17. Visual fields
18. Histamine test
19. Allergy skin testing
20. Refraction
21. HLA typing

SHOULDER PAIN

1. cbc and differential
2. R-A test
3. Uric acid

4. Sedimentation rate
5. Wassermann
6. Tuberculin test
7. Protein electrophoresis
8. Calcium, phosphorus, alkaline phosphatase
9. Roentgenogram of shoulder and chest
10. Roentgenogram of cervical spine
11. Myelography
12. Arteriography
13. Lymphangiogram
14. ECG
15. Nerve blocks
16. EMG
17. Bone scan
18. Synovial fluid analysis
19. Injection of bursa with lidocaine
20. Serial CPK, SGOT, LDH

SKIN DISCHARGE

1. cbc and differential
2. Urinalysis
3. Sedimentation rate
4. Tuberculin test
5. VDRL
6. Serum protein electrophoresis
7. Smear and culture of exudate for bacterial, fungi, or parasites
8. Roentgenogram of chest
9. Roentgenogram of bones
10. Biopsy
11. Frei test
12. Skin tests and serology for fungi
13. Muscle biopsy
14. Kveim test
15. NBT test
16. Blood cultures

SKIN PIGMENTATION

1. cbc and differential
2. Urinalysis
3. Serum iron and iron-binding capacity
4. Urine porphyrins and porphobilinogen
5. Urine for homogentisic acid
6. Urine melanin
7. SMA–24
8. Urine bilirubin
9. Urine 5-HIAA
10. Wood's lamp examination of skin
11. KOH preparation
12. Plasma cortisol before and after ACTH
13. Urine 17–ketosteroids
14. Serial electrolytes
15. T3, T4, T7
16. Serum FSH and LH
17. Pregnancy test
18. Liver biopsy

SKIN ULCER

1. cbc and differential
2. Urinalysis
3. Sickle cell preparation
4. VDRL
5. FTA–ABS
6. Tuberculin test
7. Smear for sulfur granules
8. Culture for bacteria and fungi
9. Seriological tests for fungi
10. Wood's lamp examination
11. Roentgenogram of bones
12. Phlebography
13. Arteriography
14. Skin tests for fungi
15. ANA test
16. Dark field examination
17. Gram's stain

18. Lymph node biopsy
19. Biopsy of edge of lesion

SKULL DEFORMITIES

1. cbc and differential and blood smear
2. Sedimentation rate
3. Urinalysis
4. VDRL
5. FTA–ABS
6. Tuberculin test
7. Sickle cell preparation
8. Ca, PO4, and alkaline phosphatase
9. T3, T4, T7, TSH
10. Serum growth hormone
11. Skull roentgenogram
12. CT scan
13. Arteriography
14. EEG
15. Spinal tap
16. Bone biopsy
17. Skeletal survey
18. Neurological examination
19. Chromosome analysis

SMOOTH TONGUE AND OTHER CHANGES

1. cbc and differential
2. Blood smear
3. Bone marrow examination
4. Urinalysis
5. Serum folic acid and B12
6. Schilling test
7. Serum protein electrophoresis
8. SMA–12
9. Congo red test
10. Culture

11. VDRL
12. Tuberculin test
13. Urine vitamin assay after load
14. Skeletal survey
15. Chest roentgenogram
16. Upper GI series
17. Esophagram
18. Endoscopy
19. Lingual biopsy

SNEEZING

1. cbc and differential
2. Blood smear
3. Sedimentation rate
4. Nose and throat culture
5. Nose and throat smear
6. Examination for eosinophils
7. Serum for viral studies
8. SMA–24
9. VDRL
10. Tuberculin test
11. ANA test
12. Serum protein electrophoresis
13. Immunoelectrophoresis for IgE antibodies
14. Roentgenogram of skull and sinuses
15. Roentgenogram of chest
16. Pulmonary function tests
17. Skin tests
18. Nasopharyngoscopy

SORE THROAT

1. cbc and differential
2. Streptozyme test
3. Mono spot test
4. Blood smear examination
5. Throat smear
6. Throat culture
7. Bone marrow examination

8. Acute and convalescent serum for viral studies
9. Thyroid function studies
10. Roentgenogram of sinuses
11. Roentgenogram of teeth
12. Nasopharyngoscopy
13. Laryngoscopy
14. Biopsy
15. Rapid strept agglutination test of throat swab

SPINE DEFORMITIES

1. cbc and differential
2. Blood smear
3. Urinalysis
4. Urine for mucopolysaccharides
5. Urine for amino acids
6. VDRL
7. Tuberculin test
8. Serum protein electrophoresis
9. HLA typing
10. Sedimentation rate
11. Bone marrow examination
12. SMA–12
13. Alkaline and acid phosphatase
14. Roentgenogram of spine
15. Skeletal survey
16. Bone biopsy
17. Serum parathyroid hormone
18. Serum growth hormone
19. Bone scan
20. Myelography
21. R-A test
22. ANA test

SPLENOMEGALY

1. cbc and differential
2. Blood smear for morphology
3. Reticulocyte count

4. Platelet count and clot retraction
5. Radioactive chromium-tagged red cell survival
6. Serum bilirubin
7. Bone marrow examination
8. Blood cultures
9. Febrile agglutinins
10. Heterophil antibody titer
11. Brucellin agglutinins
12. Blood smear for parasites
13. Liver function studies (see Jaundice, this table)
14. Latex flocculation (Felty's disease)
15. ANA test
16. Serum protein electrophoresis
17. Hemoglobin electrophoresis
18. Esophagram (esophageal varices)
19. Roentgenogram of long bones (Gaucher's disease)
20. Flat plate of abdomen for spleen size
21. Lymph node biopsy
22. Liver biopsy
23. Splenic aspirate
24. Splenoportogram and splenic pulp pressure
25. PPD, intermediate, and skin tests for various fungi (see Hemoptysis, this table)
26. Skin biopsy (hemochromatosis)
27. Muscle biopsy
28. Diagnostic ultrasound
29. CT scan
30. Liver–spleen scan

8. Smear and culture for routine bacteria, AFB, and fungi
9. Anaerobic cultures
10. Sputum cytology
11. Sputum smear for eosinophils
12. Gastric washings for AFB
13. Nose and throat culture
14. Chest roentgenogram
15. Tomography
16. Apical lordotics
17. Bronchograms
18. Bronchoscopy and biopsy
19. Scalene node biopsy
20. ECG
21. Venous pressure and circulation time
22. Pulmonary function tests
23. Lung scans
24. Open lung biopsy
25. Coccidiodin skin test
26. Blastomycin skin test
27. Histoplasmin skin test
28. Kveim test
29. Cold agglutinins
30. MG streptococcus agglutinins
31. Febrile agglutinins
32. Serology for fungi
33. Blood cultures
34. Acute and convalescent serum for viral studies

STOOL COLOR CHANGES

1. cbc and differential
2. Blood smear
3. Sedimentation rate
4. Urinalysis
5. Stool for fat and trypsin
6. Stool for occult blood
7. Stool for ova and parasites
8. Stool urobilinogen (stercobilinogen)
9. Barium enema
10. Upper GI series and esophagram
11. Esophagoscopy and gastroscopy

SPUTUM

1. cbc and differential
2. Sedimentation rate
3. Urinalysis
4. SMA–24
5. VDRL
6. Tuberculin test
7. Sputum examination

12. Sigmoidoscopy and colonoscopy
13. D-xylose absorption
14. Urine 5-HIAA

14. Roentgenogram of sinuses
15. Biopsy

STRIDOR AND SNORING

1. cbc and differential
2. Blood smear
3. Nose and throat culture
4. Urinalysis
5. Nasal smear for eosinophils
6. Tensilon test
7. Roentgenogram of sinuses
8. Roentgenogram of chest
9. Nasopharyngoscopy
10. Laryngoscopy and bronchoscopy
11. SMA–24
12. VDRL
13. Tuberculin test
14. Tensilon test
15. Neurological examination
16. EEG with sleep study

SWOLLEN GUMS AND GUM MASS

1. cbc and differential
2. Sedimentation rate
3. Tuberculin test
4. VDRL
5. I & D and culture
6. Blood smear
7. Bone marrow examination
8. History for drugs
9. Platelet count
10. Ca, PO4, and alkaline phosphatase
11. T3, T4, T7
12. Skull roentgenogram
13. Roentgenogram of teeth

SWOLLEN TONGUE

1. cbc and differential
2. Sedimentation rate
3. Urinalysis
4. VDRL
5. Tuberculin test
6. Blood smear
7. Bone marrow examination
8. Coagulation studies
9. Smear and culture of exudate
10. T3, T4, T7, TSH
11. Skull roentgenogram
12. Growth hormone assay
13. Circulation time
14. Schilling test
15. Tests for vitamin deficiency
16. Lingual biopsy

SYNCOPE AND COMA

1. cbc
2. Urine
3. Sedimentation rate
4. FBS
5. BUN creatinine
6. ABG
7. Plasma acetone (diabetes mellitus)
8. Na, K, Cl, CO_2 (emphysema, diabetes mellitus, Addison's disease)
9. Blood bromide level
10. Blood lead level
11. Drug screen
12. Urine porphobilinogens
13. Blood alcohol
14. IV thiamine

SYNOVIAL FLUID ANALYSIS (UNDER JOINT PAIN OR SWELLING)

	White Cell Count (cu mm)	Crystals	Mucin Clot	Culture	Complement
Normal	100–200		Good		
Gonorrhea	50,000 and up		Poor	May be positive	
Gout	Less than 50,000	Uric acid	Fair to poor		
Osteoarthritis	Less than 3000		Good		
Pseudogout	Less than 50,000	Calcium pyrophosphate	Fair to poor		
Rheumatoid Arthritis	Less than 50,000		Poor		↓
Reiter's disease	Less than 20,000		Fair to poor		↑
Lupus Erythematosus	Less than 50,000		Poor		↓

15. Blood cultures (subacute bacterial endocarditis)
16. T3, T4, T7, TSH
17. Blood ammonia level
18. Spinal fluid examination and culture
19. 48-hour fast
20. Skull roentgenogram
21. Chest roentgenogram
22. Arteriography
23. CT scan
24. Ventriculogram
25. ECG, His bundle study
26. EEG with carotid compression (in syncope)
27. Ophthalmodynamometry
28. Visual fields
29. Caloric testing, ENG
30. Audiogram
31. Blood pressure in recumbent and erect positions
32. Carotid sinus massage
33. 24-hour EEG monitoring
34. Echoencephalogram
35. Holter monitoring
36. Carotid scan

TACHYCARDIA

1. cbc, SMA–24
2. T3, T4, T7
3. Blood cultures
4. FBS (hypoglycemia)
5. Febrile agglutinins
6. Sedimentation rate
7. ASO titer (rheumatic fever)
8. CRP
9. 24-hour urine catecholamines
10. Na, K, Cl, CO_2
11. Blood volume
12. Arterial blood gases
13. ECG with carotid sinus massage
14. Temperature q 4 hours
15. Sleeping pulse rate

16. Pulmonary function studies
17. ECG
18. Holter monitoring
19. Chest roentgenogram

TESTICULAR ATROPHY

1. cbc and differential
2. Sedimentation rate
3. Urinalysis and culture
4. VDRL
5. FTA–ABS
6. Glucose tolerance test
7. Tuberculin test
8. Mumps skin test
9. Serum FSH and LH
10. Serum iron and iron-binding capacity
11. Chromosome analysis
12. Skull roentgenogram
13. Skeletal survey
14. Testicular biopsy
15. Liver biopsy

TESTICULAR MASS

1. cbc and differential
2. Sedimentation rate
3. Urethral smear
4. Urethral culture, urine culture
5. Urinalysis
6. Urine chorionic gonadotropin
7. Prostatic fluid smear and culture
8. IVP and cystogram
9. GI series and small bowel follow through
10. Cystoscopy
11. Biopsy
12. Exploratory surgery
13. Mumps skin test and serology
14. Tuberculin test

15. Aspiration
16. VDRL
17. Ultrasonography

TESTICULAR PAIN

1. cbc and differential
2. Sedimentation rate
3. Urethral smear
4. Urethral culture
5. Urinalysis
6. Urine culture
7. Prostatic fluid culture
8. IVP
9. Roentgenogram of spine
10. Cystoscopy
11. Exploratory surgery

TONGUE PAIN

1. cbc and differential
2. Sedimentation rate
3. Serum iron and iron-binding capacity
4. Schilling test
5. Urine tests for vitamins after loading dose
6. Tuberculin test
7. Wassermann
8. Roentgenogram of teeth
9. Biopsy
10. Trial of vitamin therapy

TOOTHACHE

1. cbc and differential
2. Sedimentation rate
3. VDRL

4. Tuberculin test
5. Culture of exudates
6. Calcium, phosphorus, alkaline phosphatase
7. Roentgenogram of teeth
8. Roentgenogram of jaw, skull, and sinuses
9. CT scan
10. Nerve blocks

TORTICOLLIS

1. cbc and differential
2. Urinalysis
3. Sedimentation rate
4. Streptozyme test
5. ANA test
6. SMA–24
7. VDRL
8. Tuberculin test
9. Roentgenogram of cervical spine
10. Roentgenogram of skull
11. EEG
12. CT scan
13. Psychometric testing
14. Serum copper and ceruloplasmin

TREMORS

1. cbc and differential
2. Sedimentation rate
3. Thyroid function studies
4. Blood alcohol level
5. Serum electrolytes
6. Serum calcium and phosphorus
7. Urine copper
8. Serum copper and ceruloplasmin
9. Skull roentgenogram
10. EEG

11. CT scan
12. EMG
13. Drug screen
14. Therapeutic trials

URETHRAL DISCHARGE

1. cbc and differential
2. Urinalysis
3. Urethral smear and culture
4. Urine culture
5. Prostatic massage, smear and culture of exudates
6. VDRL
7. Tuberculin test
8. Frei test
9. Chancroid skin test
10. IVP and cystogram
11. Cystoscopy
12. Smears for cytology
13. Biopsy

URINE COLOR CHANGES

1. cbc and differential
2. Blood smear
3. Urinalysis and culture
4. Urine for porphyrins and porphobilinogens
5. Urine for bilirubin
6. Urine for hemoglobin
7. Urine for homogentisic acid
8. Urine melanin
9. SMA–24
10. Serum haptoglobins
11. Serum methemalbumin
12. Creatinine clearance
13. Renal biopsy
14. Drug history

VAGINAL BLEEDING

1. cbc and differential
2. Sedimentation rate
3. Urinalysis (catheterized specimen)
4. VDRL
5. Tuberculin test
6. Pregnancy test
7. Coagulation tests
8. T3, T4, T7, TSH
9. Blood smear
10. Bone marrow examination
11. ANA
12. DNA
13. Coombs' test
14. Vaginal culture
15. Vaginoscopy
16. Smears for cytology
17. Endometrial biopsy
18. Cervical biopsy
19. Culdoscopy
20. Peritoneoscopy
21. Serum LH & FSH
22. Serum estradiol and progesterone
23. Flat plate of abdomen
24. Ultrasonography
25. D & C and biopsy
26. Hysterosalpingography
27. Culposcopy
28. CT scan of abdomen

VAGINAL DISCHARGE

1. cbc and differential
2. Sedimentation rate
3. VDRL
4. Tuberculin test
5. Urinalysis and culture
6. Vaginal smear and culture
7. Rectal culture
8. Stool culture
9. Fresh wet saline preparation examination
10. KOH prep, examination
11. Culture for fungi and parasites
12. Vaginal and cervical cytology
13. Biopsy of cervix
14. D & C and biopsy
15. Hysterosalpingography
16. Laparoscopy
17. Trial of antibiotics

VERTIGO

1. cbc
2. FBS, glucose tolerance test
3. BUN
4. Na, K, Cl, CO_2
5. Spinal fluid examination
6. Roentgenogram of chest
7. Roentgenogram of skull
8. Roentgenogram of mastoids and internal auditory foramina, tomography
9. Roentgenogram of cervical spine
10. T_3, T_4, FT_4I
11. CT scan
12. Arteriography, myelography
13. ECG
14. EEG
15. Audiogram
16. Caloric tests, Hallpike maneuvers
17. Carotid scans
18. Carotid sinus massage
19. Blood pressure in recumbent and erect positions
20. Inflation of external auditory canal
21. Myringotomy
22. Allergy skin testing
23. Electronystagmography
24. 24-hour BP monitoring
25. ENG
26. Withdraw all medication

VOMITING ■

1. cbc
2. Urinalysis
3. Sedimentation rate
4. SMA–24
5. Wassermann
6. ECG (for patients over age 40)
7. Chest roentgenogram and flat plate of abdomen
8. PPD, intermediate
9. FBS
10. Stools for occult blood
11. Stools for ova and parasites
12. Pregnancy test
13. Amylase
14. Lipase
15. Serum bilirubin (acute cholecystitis)
16. Transaminase and LDH (acute myocardial infarction)
17. Gastric analysis
18. Spinal fluid examination and culture
19. T3, T4, T7, TSH
20. Calcium, phosphorus, alkaline phosphatase (hyperparathyroidism)
21. Na, K, Cl, CO_2
22. Liver function tests
23. Chest roentgenogram
24. Flat plate of abdomen
25. Upper GI series and esophagram
26. Cholecystogram or IV cholangiogram
27. Intravenous pyelogram (renal calculus)
28. Esophagoscopy
29. Gastroscopy
30. ECG
31. EEG (brain tumor, and so forth)
32. Peritoneal tap
33. Culdoscopy
34. Histamine test (migraine)
35. Tonometry
36. Peritoneoscopy
37. Exploratory laparotomy
38. Ultrasonography
39. CT scan of abdomen

VOMITUS ■

1. cbc and urine
2. Sedimentation rate
3. Blood smear
4. VDRL
5. Tuberculin test
6. SMA–24
7. Amylase and lipase
8. Gastric analysis
9. Flat plate of abdomen
10. Esophagram and GI series
11. Gallbladder series
12. IVP
13. Esophagoscopy and gastroscopy and duodenoscopy
14. Arteriography
15. Ultrasonography
16. CT scan
17. Liver scan
18. Exploratory laparotomy
19. Stools for ova and parasites
20. Duodenal analysis

WALKING DIFFICULTY ■

1. cbc and differential
2. Sedimentation rate
3. Urine porphobilinogen
4. Blood lead level
5. Blood alcohol level
6. ANA test
7. R-A test
8. SMA–24
9. Roentgenogram of spine
10. Roentgenogram of skull
11. Roentgenogram of hips and joints
12. Roentgenogram of extremities
13. Bone scan
14. Myelography
15. CT scan

16. Arteriography
17. Phlebography
18. Spinal tap
19. EEG
20. EMG
21. Muscle biopsy
22. Tensilon test
23. Schilling test
24. Glucose tolerance test

28. Gallbladder series
29. IVP
30. Bone scan
31. Liver scan
32. CT scans
33. Urine culture
34. Blood cultures
35. Febrile agglutinins
36. Bone marrow examination
37. Exploratory laparotomy
38. Psychometric testing

WEAKNESS AND FATIGUE

1. cbc and differential
2. Urinalysis
3. Sedimentation rate
4. SMA–24
5. VDRL
6. ECG
7. Tuberculin test
8. ANA
9. R-A test, serum protein electrophoresis
10. Serial electrolytes
11. T3, T4, T7, TSH
12. Liver function tests
13. Venous pressure and circulation time
14. Glucose tolerance test
15. Serum B_{12}
16. Serum parathyroid hormone
17. Serum cortisol
18. Tolbutamide tolerance test
19. Tensilon test, acetylcholine receptor antibody titer
20. Pulmonary function tests
21. Blood gas analysis
22. Chest roentgenogram
23. Skull roentgenogram
24. Roentgenogram of long bones
25. Upper GI series
26. Small bowel series
27. Barium enema

WEAKNESS OR PARALYSIS OF ONE OR MORE EXTREMITIES

1. cbc and differential
2. Urinalysis
3. Sedimentation rate
4. VDRL
5. Tuberculin test
6. ANA test
7. SMA–24
8. Serial electrolytes
9. T3, T4, T7, TSH
10. RAI uptake and scan
11. Tensilon test
12. Glucose tolerance test
13. Urine creatine and creatinine
14. Blood lead level
15. Drug screen
16. Roentgenogram of spine
17. Roentgenogram of skull
18. CT scan, EEG
19. Spinal tap
20. Arteriography
21. Electromyography, NCV
22. Muscle biopsy
23. Urine prophobilinogen
24. Myelography
25. Thermography

WEIGHT LOSS ■

1. cbc
2. Urinalysis
3. Sedimentation rate
4. SMA–24
5. Wassermann
6. ECG (for patients over age 40)
7. Chest roentgenogram and flat plate of abdomen
8. PPD, intermediate
9. 2-hour postprandial blood sugar
10. Fractional urines
11. T3, T4, T7
12. Calcium, phosphorus, alkaline phosphatase (hyperparathyroidism)
13. Electrolytes (Addison's disease)
14. Serum amylase and lipase
15. D-xylose uptake, radioactive triolein uptake (malabsorption syndrome)
16. Urine 5-HIAA
17. Stool for fat and trypsin
18. Stool for ova and parasites
19. Stool for occult blood
20. Liver function tests (see Jaundice, this table)
21. Serum electrophoresis
22. Acid and alkaline phosphatase
23. Sputum for routine and acid-fast bacilli
24. Sputum for Papanicolaou test
25. Gastric analysis (carcinoma of the stomach, pernicious anemia)
26. Febrile agglutinins
27. Heterophil antibody titer
28. Brucellin antibody titer
29. Urine for Bence–Jones protein
30. Chest roentgenogram
31. Long bone series (metastatic malignancy)
32. Upper GI series
33. Barium enema
34. Intravenous pyelogram
35. Lymphangiogram
36. Liver scan
37. Bone scan
38. Sigmoidoscopy
39. Gastroscopy
40. PPD, intermediate, and other skin tests
41. Liver biopsy
42. Bone marrow aspiration
43. Lymph node biopsy
44. Exploratory laparotomy
45. CT scan of abdomen
46. Ultrasonography

THE LABORATORY WORKUP OF DISEASES

Appendix II

A

Abortion, threatened: serum B-CGH, urine CGH and pregnanediol, ultrasonography

Achalasia: barium swallow, Mecholyl test, esophagoscopy, and esophageal manometry

Acoustic neuroma: skull roentgenogram, CT scan, posterior fossa myelogram

Acromegaly: skull roentgenogram, CT scan, serum growth hormone

Actinomycosis: smear for sulfur granules, culture skin lesions

Addison's disease: serum cortisol before and after ACTH, CT scan of abdomen

Adrenogenital syndrome: serum cortisol, hydroxyprogesterone, 11-deoxy cortisol, urine 17-ketosteroids and pregnanetriol, dexamethasone suppression test

Adult respiratory distress syndrome: chest roentgenogram, sputum culture, blood culture, Swan–Ganz catheterization, arterial blood gases (ABG)

Agammaglobulinemia: serum electrophoresis and immunoelectrophoresis, blood type, lymph node biopsy, bone marrow biopsy

Agranulocytosis, idiopathic: cbc, bone marrow examination, spleen scan

Albright's syndrome: roentgenogram of long bones, bone biopsy

Alcaptonuria: urinary homogentisic acid, roentgenogram of spine

Alcoholism: blood alcohol level, liver function tests, liver biopsy

Aldosteronism, primary: electrolytes before and after spironolactone, plasma renin, 24-hour urine aldosterone, CT scan, exploratory laparotomy

Allergic rhinitis: nasal smear for eosinophils, serum IgE antibody, RAST

Alveolar proteinosis: LDH, sputum for PAS-positive material, PSP, lung biopsy

Amebiasis: stool for ova and parasites, rectal biopsy, hemagglutinin inhibition test

Amyloidosis: Congo red test, rectal biopsy, liver biopsy, gingival biopsy, subcutaneous fat aspiration and stain

Angina pectoris: GXT, thallium-201 scintigraphy, coronary angiography, trial of nitroglycerin

Anthrax: smear and culture of lesion, skin biopsy

Aortic aneurysm: ultrasonography, CT scan, aortography

Aortic valvular disease: echocardiogram, CT scan, MRI, cardiac catheterization

Aplastic anemia: bone marrow, lymph node biopsy, immunoelectrophoresis

Ascaris lumbricoides: cathartic stool for ova and parasites, eosinophil count

Asthma: spirometry, sputum for eosinophils, serum IgE antibodies, RAST

Atrial arrhythmias: free thyroxine index, ECG Holter monitoring, His bundle study

Atypical pneumonia, primary: see Mycoplasma pneumonia

Beriberi: transketolose activity coefficient, urine thiamine after load, therapeutic trial

Bilharziasis: stool or urine sediment for eggs, rectal biopsy

Biliary cirrhosis: liver function tests, mitochondrial antibodies, serum bile acids, ERCP, liver biopsy

Blastomycosis: KOH prep, culture, chest roentgenogram

Boeck's sarcoid: chest roentgenogram, transbronchial lung biopsy, lymph node biopsy, Kveim test, liver biopsy

Botulism: culture of food and stool, mouse assay of toxin

Brain tumor: CT scan, magnetic resonance imaging (MRI)

Brill–Symmer's disease: lymph node biopsy

Bromide poisoning: blood bromide level

Bronchiectasis: bronchogram, bronchoscopy

Bronchitis: sputum culture, chest roentgenogram

Bronchopneumonia: sputum smear and culture, chest roentgenogram, cbc

Brucellosis: blood cultures, serologic tests

Bubonic plague: culture of bubo, blood, or sputum; animal inoculation, serologic tests

Buerger's disease: phlebography, arteriography, biopsy of affected vessels

B

Bacillary dysentery: stool smear (for leukocytes) and culture, febrile agglutinins

Balantidiasis: stool for ova and parasites

Banti's syndrome: liver function tests, liver–spleen scan, bone marrow examination, hepatic vein catheterization

Barbiturate poisoning: blood or urine for barbiturates, EEG

Basilar artery insufficiency: 4-vessel cerebral angiography

Bell's palsy: roentgenogram of mastoids and petrous bones, EMG

C

Carbon monoxide poisoning: carboxyhemoglobin determination

Carbon tetrachloride poisoning: liver function tests, infrared spectrometry, liver biopsy, blood carbon tetrachloride

Carcinoid syndrome: serum serotonin, urine 5-HIAA, exploratory laparotomy, bronchoscopy

Carcinoma of the breast: mammography, ultrasound, fine-needle aspiration, biopsy

Carcinoma of the cervix: Papanicolaou smears, cervical biopsy, culposcopy

Carcinoma of the colon: stool for occult blood, sigmoidoscopy, barium enema, colonoscopy, carcinoembryonic antigen (CEA)

Carcinoma of the endometrium: Papanicolaou smear, D&C

Carcinoma of the esophagus: barium swallow, esophagoscopy and biopsy

Carcinoma of the lung: sputum Papanicolaou smears, bronchoscopy and biopsy, needle biopsy, open lung biopsy, scalene node biopsy

Carcinoma of the pancreas: ultrasonography, CT scan of abdomen, liver function tests, ERCP, exploratory laparotomy

Carcinoma of the stomach: GI series, gastroscopy and biopsy, gastric cytology

Cardiac arrhythmias: ECG, Holter monitoring, echocardiography, EPS

Carpal tunnel syndrome: nerve conduction study (NCV)

Celiac disease: D-xylose absorption, mucosal biopsy, urine 5-HIAA, small bowel series

Cellulitis: smear and culture of wound exudates

Cerebellar ataxia: CT scan, MRI

Cerebral abscess: CT scan, MRI

Cerebral aneurysm: CT scan, MRI, arteriography

Cerebral embolism: CT scan, blood culture, echocardiography, carotid scan, 4-vessel cerebral angiography, ECG

Cerebral hemorrhage: CT scan

Cerebral thrombosis: CT scan, carotid scan, digital subtraction angiography, 4-vessel cerebral angiography

Cervical spondylosis: roentgenogram of cervical spine, EMG, MRI or myelography with CT scan simultaneously

Chagas' disease: blood smear and culture, CSF smear and culture, bone marrow or tissue biopsy, animal inoculation, serologic tests

Chancroid: smear and culture of lesion, skin biopsy

Cholangioma: liver function tests, transhepatic cholangiogram, ERCP, CT scan of abdomen, exploratory laparotomy

Cholangitis: liver function tests, transhepatic cholangiogram, ERCP, exploratory laparotomy

Cholecystitis: ultrasonography, cholecystogram, liver function tests

Choledocholithiasis: liver function tests, duodenal drainage, ERCP, transhepatic cholangiogram, ultrasonography

Cholelithiasis: ultrasonography, cholecystogram, liver function tests, ERCP

Cholera: stool smear and culture, dark field microscopy

Choriocarcinoma: urine chorionic gonadotropin, D & C

Cirrhosis: Liver function tests, liver scan, CT scan, liver biopsy

Coarctation of the aorta: chest roentgenogram, clinical evaluation, aortograms rarely required

Coccidiomycosis: smear, animal inoculation, serology, skin test, chest roentgenogram

Congestive heart failure: ECG, chest roentgenograms, spirometry, circulation time, ABG, echocardiography

Coronary insufficiency: see Angina pectoris

Costochondritis (Tietze's syndrome): lidocaine infiltration

Craniopharyngioma: skull roentgenogram, CT scan, MRI

Cretinism: Free thyroxine index, TSH, RAI uptake and scan, roentgenogram for bone age

Crigler–Najjar syndrome: see Gilbert's disease

Cryoglobulinemia: serum protein electrophoresis and immunoelectrophoresis, SIA water test, cold agglutinins, R–A test

Cryptococcosis: spinal fluid smear and culture, sputum or blood cultures

Cat-scratch disease: skin test, lymph node biopsy

Cushing's syndrome: 24-hour urine free cortisol, single-dose overnight dexamethasone suppression test, CT scan of brain or abdomen

Cystic fibrosis: quantitative pilocarpine iontophoresis

Cysticercosis: serologic tests, CT scan, biopsy of subcutaneous cysticerci

Cystinosis: slit-lamp examination, liver biopsy

Cystinuria: serum and urine cystine and arginine, cyanide–nitroprusside test, thin-layer chromatography

Cytomegalic inclusion disease: blood smear for atypical lymphs, CMV–IgM antibody titer

D

Dehydration: intake and output of fluid, electrolytes, BUN/creatinine ratio, serum/urine osmolarity

Dengue: viral isolation from blood, serology tests

Dermatomyositis: ANA, SGOT, LDH, CPK and aldolase, EMG, muscle biopsy

Diabetes insipidus: Hickey–Hare test, serum/urine osmolality, intake and output before and after Pitressin, CT scan

Diabetes mellitus: Glucose tolerance test, cortisone glucose tolerance test

Digitalis intoxication: serum digoxin level, ECG

Diguglielmo's disease: bone marrow, peripheral blood study

Diphtheria: nose and throat culture

Diphyllobothrium latum: stool for ova and parasites, serum B_{12} level

Dissecting aneurysm: chest roentgenogram, CT scan of aorta, aortography

Diverticulitis: sigmoidoscopy, barium enema, colonoscopy, gallium scan, ultrasonography, exploratory laparotomy

Dracunculiasis: noting presence of worms in subcutaneous tissues

Dubin–Johnson syndrome: liver function tests, liver biopsy

Ductus arteriosus, patent: cardiac catheterization, angiocardiography, echocardiography

Duodenal ulcer: see Peptic ulcer

Dwarfism: roentgenogram of bones; endocrine, renal and GI function tests

E

Eaton–Lambert syndrome: EMG, tensilon test, muscle biopsy

Echinococcosis: liver scan, roentgenogram of long bones, Casoni skin test, serologic tests, liver biopsy

Eclampsia: uric acid, renal function tests, renal biopsy

Ectopic pregnancy: serum beta hCG by immunoassay, ultrasonography, laparoscopy, culdocentesis, exploratory laparotomy

Ehlers–Danlos syndrome: capillary fragility test, bleeding time, skin biopsy

Emphysema: pulmonary function tests, arterial blood gases

Empyema: chest roentgenogram, sputum cultures, gallium scan thoracentesis

Encephalitis: viral isolation from brain tissue and spinal fluid, MRI, serologic tests

Encephalomyelitis: viral isolation from brain tissue and spinal fluid, MRI serologic tests

Endocardial fibroelastosis: ECG, chest roentgenogram, echocardiography, angiocardiography

Endocarditis: see Subacute bacterial endocarditis

Epilepsy: wake and sleep EEG, CT scan, pre-eclamptic toxemia (PET) scan, ambulatory EEG monitoring

Erythema multiforme: skin biopsy, patch test

Erythroblastosis fetalis: bilirubin, direct Coombs' test

Esophageal varices: esophagoscopy, spleno-venography

Esophagitis: Bernstein test, esophagoscopy, and biopsy, esophageal manometry

Extradural hematoma: skull roentgeno-gram, CT scan, arteriography

F

Fanconi syndrome: roentgenogram (pelvis, scapula, femur, ribs), urinary amino acids, glucose, electrolytes, serum uric acid, alkaline phosphatase, renal biopsy

Filariasis: blood smear for microfilariae, skin test, complement-fixation test

Folic acid deficiency: serum folic acid, therapeutic trial

Friedlander's pneumonia: sputum smear and culture, blood cultures, lung puncture, serial chest roentgenograms

Friedreich's ataxia: clinical diagnosis

G

Galactosemia: Paigen assay of blood galactose, RBC assay of Gal-1-PUT transferase

Gall stones: see Cholelithiasis

Gargoylism: urinary chondroitin sulfuric acid, serum assay of α-L-iduronidase, tissue culture and enzyme assay

Gastroenteritis: stool for culture, smear, and ova and parasites

Gaucher's disease: assay of leukocytes for beta-glucosidase, bone marrow examination, roentgenogram of long bones

General paresis: blood and spinal fluid FTA–ABS

Giardia lamblia: cathartic stool for ova and parasites, duodenal analysis

Gilles de la Tourette disease: urinary catecholamines

Gigantism: CT scan of brain, serum growth hormone

Gilbert's disease: liver function tests, liver biopsy

Glanders: culture of skin lesion, skin test, serologic tests, animal inoculation

Glanzmann's disease: platelet counts, cloth retraction, prothrombin time, bleeding time, capillary fragility test. See also Thrombocytasthemia

Glomerulonephritis: serum complement, streptozyme test, ANA, renal biopsy

Glossitis: culture, biopsy, therapeutic trial of vitamins and iron

Glycogen storage disease: glucose tolerance test, epinephrine test, liver biopsy and analysis for glucose-6 phosphatase

Goiter: free thyroxine index (FT_4I), RAI uptake and scan, TSH, serum antibodies

Gonorrhea: urethral, rectal, vaginal or throat smear and cultures

Gout: serum uric acid, synovial fluid analysis, roentgenogram of bones and joints

Granuloma inguinale: Wright's stain of scraping from lesion

Grave's disease: see Hyperthyroidism

Guillain–Barre syndrome: EMG, spinal fluid analysis

Gumma: FTA–ABS

H

Haemophilus influenzae: nose, throat and sputum culture or spinal fluid smear and culture

Hamman–Rich syndrome: chest roentgenogram, pulmonary function tests, lung biopsy

Hand–Schuller–Christian disease: roentgenogram of skull, bone biopsy, bone marrow examination

Hansen's disease: see Leprosy

Hartnup disease: urinary amino acids, indican and indolacetic acid; free thyroxine index, TSH

Hashimoto's disease: FT_4I, TSH, serum thyroglobulin antibodies

Haverhill fever: agglutination titer, aspiration of affected joint or abscess for streptobacillus moniliformis

Hay fever: see Allergic rhinitis

Heart failure: see Congestive heart failure

Helminth infections: stool for ova and parasites, serologic tests, skin tests, liver function tests

Hemangioblastoma: CT scan

Hemochromatosis: serum ferritin, serum iron and IBC, liver or skin biopsy

Hemoglobin C disease: blood smear for target cells, hemoglobin electrophoresis

Hemoglobinuria, paroxysmal cold: cbc, Coomb's test, Donath–Landsteiner test, FTA–ABS, serum haptoglobins

Hemoglobinuria, paroxysmal nocturnal: cbc, Ham test, sucrose hemolysis test

Hemolytic anemia: serum haptoglobins, radioactive-chromium tagged red cell survival, urine and fecal urobilinogen, Coomb's test, blood smear

Hemophilia: coagulation profile, thromboplastin generation test

Hepatitis: liver function tests, hepatitis profile, IgM anti-HAV, HBs Ag, IgM anti-HBc, liver biopsy

Hepatitis, chronic active: HBs Ag, liver function tests, ANA, liver biopsy

Hepatolenticular degeneration: see Wilson's disease

Hepatoma: liver scan, CT scan, alpha fetoprotein, liver biopsy, arteriography

Hernia, diaphragmatic: see Hiatal hernia

Herniated disc: EMG, thermography, CT scan, myelography, discography

Herpangina: serologic tests, viral isolation

Herpes genitalis: examination of skin scrapings (Tzanck test), culture, serologic tests

Herpes simplex: serologic tests, viral isolation, Tzanck test

Herpes zoster: Tzanck test, serologic tests

Hiatal hernia: Berstein test, esophogram, esophagoscopy and biopsy, esophageal manometry, therapeutic trial

Hirschsprung's disease: Rectal or colon biopsy

Histamine cephalgia: test trial of histamine subcutaneously

Histoplasmosis: sputum culture, bone marrow culture, animal inoculation, skin test, serologic tests, chest roentgenogram

Hodgkin's disease: lymph node biopsy, bone marrow, lymphangiogram, CT scan, liver/spleen scan, exploratory laparotomy

Huntington's chorea: clinical diagnosis, genetic markers, CT scan

Hurler's syndrome: see Gargoylism

Hydronephrosis: IVP, ultrasonogram

Hyperaldosteronism: see Aldosteronism

Hypercholesterolemia, familial: lipoprotein electrophoresis, lipid profile

Hyperlipemia, idiopathic: lipoprotein electrophoresis, ultracentrifugation

Hypernephroma: intravenous or retrograde pyelogram, CT scan angiography

Hyperparathyroidism: serum calcium, phosphorus, alkaline phosphatase, urine calcium, serum PTH, 1,25-$(OH)_2D$, phosphate reabsorption test, exploratory surgery

Hypersplenism: cbc, blood smear, red cell survival, spleen–liver ratio, bone marrow, epinephrine test, exploratory laparotomy

Hypertension, essential: see page 482 (or Hypertension, Appendix I)

Hyperthyroidism: Free T_3, FT_4I

Hypoparathyroidism: serum calcium and

phosphorus, 24-hour urine calcium, skull roentgenogram, phosphate reabsorption, therapeutic trial

Hypopituitarism: serum cortisol, serum thyroxine, serum ACTH, TSH, FSH, LH, CT scan, MRI

Hypotension, idiopathic postural: clinical observation, response to Pitressin, tests to rule out causes of secondary hypotension

Hypothyroidism: FT$_4$I, TSH, therapeutic trial

Hypovitaminosis: see specific vitamin deficiencies

I

Ileitis: see Regional enteritis

Inappropriate ADH secretion: plasma and urine osmolality, spot urinary sodium

Infectious mononucleosis: monospot test, heterophil antibody titer, smear for atypical lymphocytes, liver function tests, repeat tests

Influenza, viral: nasopharyngeal washing, complement fixation tests

Insulinoma: see Islet cell tumor

Intestinal obstruction: flat plate of the abdomen with lateral dicubiti, double enema, ultrasonography, CT scan, GI series with hypaque, exploratory laparotomy

Iron deficiency anemia: serum ferritin, serum iron and iron-binding capacity, free erythrocyte protoporphyrins (FEP), bone marrow

Islet cell tumor: glucose tolerance test, 72-hour fast, plasma insulin, tolbutamide tolerance test, pancreatic arteriography, exploratory laparotomy

K

Kala–azar: blood smear, bone marrow or splenic aspirate for parasites, culture, serologic tests (ELISA)

Klinefelter's syndrome: sex chromatin pattern, testicular biopsy, serum FSH and LH

Kwashiorkor: serum albumin, cbc

L

Lactase deficiency: lactose tolerance test, mucosal biopsy, hydrogen breath test

Laennec's cirrhosis: see Cirrhosis of the liver

Larva migrans, visceral: eosinophil count, serum globulin, skin testing, serologic tests, liver biopsy

Laryngitis: nose and throat culture, washings for viral studies

Lead intoxication: serum and urine lead content, urine for ALA, coproporphyrin, FEEP, test dose of EDTA, roentgenogram of long bones

Leishmaniasis: cbc, blood and bone marrow smears for parasites, biopsy

Leprosy: Wade's scraped incision procedure, culture of lesion, biopsy of skin nerves, roentgenogram of hands and feet, histamine test, lepromin skin test

Leptospirosis: see Weil's disease

Letterer–Siwe disease: roentgenogram of bones, bone marrow, lymph node biopsy

Leukemia: blood smear, bone marrow, uric acid, serum B$_{12}$ concentration and iron binding capacity

Lipoid pneumonia: chest roentgenogram, sputum examination, biopsy

Listeriosis: blood or spinal fluid culture, serum agglutination titer, bone marrow biopsy

Liver abscess: liver scan with technetium or Gallium, liver aspiration and biopsy, CT scan, amebic hemagglutinin inhibition titer, cathartic stool for ova and parasites

Loeffler's syndrome: eosinophil count, sputum for eosinophils, stool for ova and parasites

Lung abscess: chest roentgenogram, tomography, CT scan, sputum culture, bronchoscopy, sputum cytology, needle aspiration and biopsy and culture

Lupoid hepatitis: see Hepatitis, chronic active

Lupus erythematosus: ANA, anti-ds DNA antibody titer, Coomb's test, lupus erythematosus (LE) prep, coagulation profile, biopsy of skin, muscle, lymph node or kidney

Lymphangitis: cbc, sedimentation rate

Lymphoblastoma: lymph node biopsy, cbc, bone marrow examination

Lymphogranuloma inguinale: Lygranum test, Giemsa stained smear, serologic tests, tissue or node biopsy

Lymphogranuloma venereum: Frei test, serologic tests, lymph node biopsy

Lymphoma: see Hodgkin's disease

Lymphosarcoma: CT scan, roentgenograms of chest and abdomen, lymphangiography

M

McArdle's syndrome: liver biopsy, enzyme assay of muscle phosphorylase, muscle biopsy, urine myoglobin

Macroglobulinemia: serum electrophoresis and immunoelectrophoresis, ultracentrifugation, Sia water test, bone marrow

Malabsorption syndrome: D-xylose absorption test, urine 5-HIAA, mucosal biopsy, small bowel series

Malaria: blood smear for parasites, bone marrow

Marfan's syndrome: roentgenogram of long bones and ribs, slit-lamp examination of eyes, IVP, urinary hydroxyproline, CT scan of aorta

Marie–Strumpell spondylitis: roentgenogram of lumbosacral spine, bone scan, HLA typing

Mastocytosis: skin biopsy, Darier's sign, long bone roentgenogram, bone marrow biopsy

Mastoiditis: roentgenogram of mastoids, CT scan

Measles: smear of nasal secretions for giant cells, serologic tests

Meckel's diverticulum: technetium scan, exploratory laparotomy

Mediastinitis: CT scan of chest, mediastinoscopy, exploratory surgery

Medullary sponge kidney: IVP, CT scan

Medulloblastoma: CT scan, MRI

Megaloblastic anemia: see Pernicious anemia

Meig's syndrome: thoracentesis, culdoscopy, laparoscopy, exploratory laparotomy, ultrasonography

Melanoma: serum or urinary melanin, biopsy

Meniere's disease: CT scan, posterior fossa myelography, audiogram, caloric tests, ENG

Meningioma: CT scan, MRI, roentgenogram of skull or spine, myelography

Meningitis: spinal fluid examination, smear and culture, serum for viral serologic studies, blood cultures

Meningococcemia: blood cultures, spinal fluid examination, smear and culture, Gram's stain of punctured petechiae

Menopause syndrome: serum LH, FSH, serum estradiol, vaginal smear for estrogen effects, therapeutic trial

Mental retardation: CT scan, EEG, psychometric testing, skull roentgenogram, PKU, FT_4I, TSH, urinary amino acids

Methemoglobinemia: erythrocyte methemoglobin, ABG blood diaphorase I

Migraine: nitroglycerin test, histamine test

Mikulicz's disease: cbc, bone marrow, tuberculin test, biopsy of lesion, ANA, lymph node biopsy

Milk–alkali syndrome: serum calcium, phosphorus, alkaline phosphatase, urinary calcium and phosphates

Milroy's disease: clinical diagnosis

Mitral insufficiency or stenosis: ECG, chest roentgenogram, echocardiogram, phonocardiogram, cardiac catheterization

Mongolism: chromosome study, urinary beta-amino-isobutyric acid

Moniliasis: vaginal smear or culture, skin scrapings with KOH prep, biopsy

Mononucleosis, infectious: see Infectious mononucleosis

Mucormycosis: nose and throat culture, biopsy

Mucoviscidosis: see Cystic fibrosis of the pancreas

Multiple myeloma: serum protein, electrophoresis and immunoelectrophoresis, 24-hour urine electrophoresis, bone marrow, roentgenogram of skull and spine

Multiple sclerosis: somatosensory evoked potentials (SSEP), VEP, spinal fluid globulin and myelin basic protein, MRI

Mumps: skin test, serologic tests

Muscular dystrophy: EMG, muscle biopsy, urine creatine, chromosome analysis, serum enzymes (CPK, and so forth)

Myasthenia gravis: EMG, Tensilon test, acetylcholine receptor antibody titer

Mycoplasma pneumonia: cold agglutinins, MG streptococcal agglutinins, culture

Mycosis fungoides: skin biopsy

Myeloid metaplasia, agnogenic: red cell morphology, cbc, bone marrow, leukocyte alkaline phosphatase, urine and serum erythropoietin

Myelophthisic anemia: cbc, bone marrow, bone scan, lymph node biopsy

Myocardial infarction: serial enzymes (MBCPK, and so forth) serial ECGs serum myoglobin, Thallium-201 scintigraphy, pyrophosphate imaging, echocardiogram

Myocarditis/myocardiopathy: echocardiography, endomyocardial biopsy

Myotonia atrophica: EMG, urine creatinine and creatine, muscle biopsy

Myxoma, cardiac: echocardiography, angiocardiography

N

Narcolepsy: sleep study, EEG

Nematodes: gastric analysis, muscle biopsy, eosinophil count, skin test, serologic tests, stools for ova and parasites, duodenal aspiration for ova and parasites, GI series, rectal swab with scotch tape

Nephritis: see Glomerulonephritis

Nephrocalcinosis: serum PTH, serum calcium, phosphorus and alkaline phosphatase, IVP, renal biopsy

Nephrotic syndrome: urinalysis, serum complement, sedimentation rate, serum protein electrophoresis, renal function tests, ANA, renal biopsy

Neurinoma, acoustic: see Acoustic neuroma

Neuritis, peripheral: see Neuropathy

Neuroblastoma: urinary VMA and HVA, CT scan, bone marrow, exploratory laparotomy

Neurofibromatosis: biopsy, skeletal survey, CT scan, spinal fluid analysis, myelogram

Neuropathy: glucose tolerance test, blood lead level, urine porphobilinogen, blood and urine arsenic levels, urine N-methyl-nicotinamide, ANA serum B_{12} and folic acid, spinal fluid examination, nerve conduction velocity (NCV), EMG, serum transketolase activity coefficient, nerve biopsy

Neurosyphilis: blood and spinal fluid FTA–ABS

Niacin deficiency: see Pellagra

Niemann–Pick disease: demonstration of sphingomyelin in reticuloendothelial cells, bone marrow biopsy, tissue biopsy, skeletal survey

Nocardiosis: sputum smear and culture, spinal fluid examination, smear and culture

Nonketotic hyperosmolar coma: blood sugar, plasma osmolality

Normal pressure hydrocephalus: CT scan, nuclear flow study (RISA)

Nutritional neuropathy: see Neuropathy

O

Ochronosis: urinalysis (Benedict's solution, isolation of homogentisic acid), roentgenogram of spine

Oppenheim's disease: EMG, muscle biospy

Optic atrophy: CT scan of brain and orbits, visual fields, spinal tap, serum B_{12}, roentgenogram of skull and optic foramina

Osteitis deformans: serum calcium, phosphorus, alkaline phosphatase, skeletal survey, bone scan, bone biopsy, urine hydroxyproline

Osteoarthritis: roentgenogram of spine and joints, exclusion of other forms of arthritis

Osteogenic sarcoma: alkaline and acid phosphatase, roentgenogram of bone, bone scan, bone biopsy

Osteomalacia: serum calcium phosphorus, alkaline phosphatase, roentgenogram of long bones, response to vitamin D and calcium

Osteomyelitis: sediment action rate, blood culture, culture of bone biopsy, roentgenogram of bone, bone scan, teichoic acid antibody titer

Osteopetrosis: bone marrow, roentgenogram of bones, bone biopsy

Osteoporosis: serum, calcium, phosphorus, alkaline phosphatase, bone biopsy, roentgenogram of spine, quantitative computerized tomography

Otitis media: nasopharyngeal or aural smear and culture, cbc, sedimentation rate

P

Paget's disease: see Osteitis deformans

Pancreatic carcinoma: see Carcinoma of the pancreas

Pancreatitis, acute: serum amylase and lipase, BS, serum calcium paracentesis, flat plate of abdomen, 2-hour urinary amylase

Pancreatitis, chronic: serum and urinary amylase and lipase before and after secretin, glucose tolerance test, duodenal analysis for bicarbonate and enzyme concentration, CAT scan, ERCP, fecal fat, triolein I^{131} uptake

Panniculitis: bone marrow, skin and subcutaneous tissue biopsy

Paralysis agitans: clinical diagnosis

Pellagra: urine N-methylnicotinamide, urine niacin after loading dose

Pemphigus: skin biopsy, Tzanck test

Peptic ulcer: upper GI series, stool for occult blood, gastroscopy and duodenoscopy, gastric analysis

Periarteritis nodosa: ANA, eosinophil count, cbc, urinalysis, muscle, skin, subcutaneous tissue and testicular biopsy, nerve biopsy

Pericarditis: ECG, echocardiography, chest roentgenogram, angiocardiography, pericardial tap

Periodic paralysis, familial: serum potassium, ECG, EMG, response to glucose

Peritonitis: cbc, flat plate of abdomen, CT scan, ultrasonography, peritoneal tap, exploratory laparotomy

Pernicious anemia: cbc, blood smear, serum B_{12} and folic acid, Schilling test, gastric analysis with histamine bone marrow

Pertussis: cbc, nasopharyngeal smear and culture

Petit mal: sleep EEG, CT scan

Peutz–Jeghers syndrome: small bowel series, exploratory laparotomy

Pharyngitis: nose and throat culture, rapid agglutination test of throat swab (Abbott test pack strep A), streptozyme test

Phenylpyruvic oligophrenia: urine for PKU and phenylalanine, Guthrie test, serum phenylalanine

Pheochromocytoma: plasma and urine catecholamines, 24-hour urine VMA, CT scan

Phlebitis: see Thrombophlebitis

Phlebotomus fever: serologic tests

Pickwickian syndrome: pulmonary function tests, ABG, sleep study

Pinealoma: CT scan

Pinworms: scotch tape swab of perianal area with microscopic examination for eggs

Pituitary adenoma: CT scan, serum TSH, ACTH, LH and FSH, FT$_4$I, serum cortisol

Plague: see Bubonic plague

Platyhelminthes: stool for ova and parasites, serologic tests, skin tests, urine sediment for eggs, eosinophil count

Pleurisy: chest roentgenogram, thorocentesis, pleural biopsy, bronchoscopy

Pleurodynia, epidemic: serologic tests, stool and throat cultures for Coxsackie B virus

Pneumococcal pneumonia: see Pneumonia

Pneumoconiosis: chest roentgenogram, pulmonary function tests, ABG, sputum smear, lung biopsy, lung scan, scalene node biopsy

Pneumonia: stat sputum smear, culture, blood cultures, chest roentgenogram

Pneumothorax: chest roentgenogram

Poliomyelitis: viral isolation from stool, serologic tests

Polyarteritis: see Periarteritis

Polycystic ovary: see Stein–Leventhal syndrome

Polycythemia vera: cbc, platelet count, uric acid, ABG, pulmonary function tests, serum erythropoietin

Polyneuritis: see Neuropathy

Porphyria: urine porphyrins and porphobilinogen

Portal cirrhosis: see Cirrhosis of the liver

Pott's disease: roentgenogram of the spine, aspiration and culture of synovial fluid, synovial or bone biopsy, PPD

Preeclampsia: see Eclampsia

Pregnancy: blood or urine test for pregnancy

Prostatic carcinoma: serum acid and alkaline phosphatase, skeletal survey, bone scan, biopsy of prostate

Protein–losing enteropathy: I^{131} poly-

vinylpyrrolidone test, serum protein electrophoresis

Pseudohypoparathyroidism: serum calcium, phosphorus, alkaline phosphatase, urine calcium, Ellsworth–Howard test, parathyroid tissue biopsy

Pseudotumor cerebri: CT scan, MRI, spinal tap

Psittacosis: chest roentgenogram, serologic tests, virus isolation

Pulmonary embolism: see Pulmonary infarction

Pulmonary emphysema: see Emphysema

Pulmonary hypertension, idiopathic: ABG, pulmonary function tests, cardiac catheterization, pulmonary angiography

Pulmonary infarction: ABG, lung scan, pulmonary angiography, impedance plethysmography

Pyelonephritis: urine culture, colony count, IVP, cystoscopy, renal biopsy

Pyloric stenosis: GI series, gastroscopy

Pyridoxine deficiency: serum iron and iron-binding capacity, blood pyridoxine, urine pyridoxic acid

Q

Q fever: serologic tests

R

Rabies: autopsy of infected animals, isolation of virus from saliva, serum and csf antibody titer, fluorescent antibody stain of corneal or skin cells

Rat–bite fever: culture of lesion, aspiration

and culture of regional lymph node, animal inoculation, serologic tests

Raynaud's disease: ANA, LE prep, immunoelectrophoresis, cold agglutinins, cryoglobulins, skin or muscle biopsy

Regional enteritis: sedimentation rate, small bowel series, sigmoidoscopy or colonoscopy and biopsy, surgical exploration

Reiter's disease: HLA typing, bone scan

Relapsing fever: peripheral blood smear for Borrelia, animal inoculation, serologic tests, total leukocytes, spinal tap

Renal calculus: IVP, CT scan, cystoscopy and retrograde pyelography

Renal tubular acidosis: serum electrolytes, calcium, phosphorus, alkaline phosphatase, urine calcium, phosphates and bicarbonate, urine *p*H after ammonium chloride load

Reticuloendotheliosis: roentgenogram, cbc, tissue cholesterol content, biopsy of skeletal lesion, bone marrow or lymph nodes

Reticulum cell sarcoma: alkaline phosphatase, lymph node biopsy, roentgenogram of chest, skeletal survey, GI series, IVP, cytologic examination of pleural or ascitic fluid

Rheumatic fever: streptozyme test, CRP, sedimentation rate, ECG, echocardiography, serial ASO titers

Rheumatoid arthritis: R-A test, sedimentation rate, ANA, roentgenogram of joints

Riboflavin deficiency: activity coefficient of erythrocyte glutathione reductase

Rickets: serum calcium, phosphorus, alkaline phosphatase, urine calcium, roentgenogram of bones, serum PTH, serum 25-OHD, bone biopsy

Rickettsialpox: serologic tests

Rocky Mountain spotted fever: specific serologic tests, Weil–Felix test, fluorescent antibody staining of skin lesions

Rubella: viral isolation, latex agglutination card assay, other serologic tests

Rubeola: see Measles

S

Saddle embolus of aorta: oscillometry, Doppler flow study, aortography

Salicylate intoxication: serum or urine salicylates

Salmonellosis: stool culture, febrile agglutinins

Salpingitis: vaginal smear and culture, ultrasonography, laparoscopy, exploratory surgery

Sarcoidosis: see Boeck's sarcoid

Scalenus anticus syndrome: roentgenogram of cervical spine, arteriography, thermography

Scarlet fever: nose and throat culture, streptozyme test, Schultz—Charlton reaction

Schilder's disease: EEG, CT scan, MRI, spinal tap, brain biopsy

Schistosomiasis: stool or urine for ova, rectal biopsy, liver biopsy, serologic tests

Schonlein–Henoch purpura: urinalysis, platelet count, coagulation profile, bleeding time, capillary fragility

Schuller–Christian disease: see Hand–Schuller–Christian disease

Scleroderma: ANA, R-A test, skin biopsy, esophagram, malabsorption workup

Scurvy: serum ascorbic acid, capillary fragility, roentgenogram of bones, therapeutic trial

Seminoma: urine HPG, ultrasonography, exploratory surgery

Septicemia: blood cultures

Sexual precocity: skull roentgenogram, CT scan, urine 17-ketosteroids and 17-hydroxysteroids, plasma cortisol, metapyrapone test, exploratory surgery

Shigellosis: stool examination for leukocytes, stool culture

Sickle cell anemia: cbc, blood smear, sickle cell preparation, hemoglobin electrophoresis

Silicosis: chest roentgenogram, pulmonary function tests, ABG, lung biopsy

Silo–Filler's disease: chest roentgenogram, clinical observations

Simmond's disease: see Hypopituitarism

Sinusitis: roentgenogram of sinuses, nose and throat culture

Sjogren's syndrome: Schirmer test for tear production, ANA, R-A titer, HLA typing, thyroglobulin antibody titer, anti-SS-B (La) antibody titer

Smallpox: smear of vesicular fluid for virus particles, viral isolation, serologic test

Spherocytosis, hereditary: cbc, blood smear, red cell fragility test, reticulocyte count, serum haptoglobins, bilirubin

Spinal cord tumor: roentgenogram of spine, CT scan of spine, myelogram, MRI

Spinal stenosis: CT scan, myelography

Sporotrichosis: culture of exudates from ulcer, serologic tests, skin tests

Staphylococcal pneumonia: sputum smear and culture, chest roentgenogram

Steatorrhea: see Celiac disease

Stein–Leventhal syndrome: culdoscopy, laparoscopy, serum LH, urine 17 ketosteroids, exploratory surgery and biopsy of ovaries

Stevens–Johnson syndrome: streptozyme test, nose and throat culture

Still's disease: R-A test, sedimentation rate, CRP, synovianalysis

Streptococcal pharyngitis: see Pharyngitis

Strongyloidiasis: stool or duodenal aspirate for ova and parasites

Sturge–Weber syndrome: skull roentgenogram, CT scan

Subacute bacterial endocarditis: blood culture, bone marrow cultures, echocardiography, R-A test, teichoic acid antibody titer (TA–AB)

Subarachnoid hemorrhage: CT scan of brain, spinal tap, arteriography

Subdiaphragmatic abscess: chest roentgenogram, gallium scan, CT scan, needle aspiration, exploratory surgery

Subdural hematoma: CT scan, arteriography

Subphrenic abscess: see Subdiaphragmatic abscess

Sulfhemoglobinemia: shaking of venous blood in test tube, spectroscopic examination of blood

Syphilis: blood and spinal fluid VDRL or FTA–ABS, dark-field microscopy

Syringomyelia: CT scan, myelography, MRI

T

Tabes dorsalis: blood and spinal fluid FTA–ABS

Takayasu disease: CT scan of aorta, aortography, serum protein electrophoresis

Tapeworm infections: stool for ova and parasites, serology

Tay–Sachs disease: cortical biopsy

Temporal arteritis: sedimentation rate, biopsy of temporal artery

Tetanus: clinical diagnosis, positive culture does not establish diagnosis

Thalassemia: cbc, blood smear, reticulocyte count, serum haptoglobins, serum bilirubin, hemoglobin electrophoresis

Thromboangitis obliterans: see Buerger's disease

Thrombocythemia (thrombasthenia): platelet count, bleeding time, clotting time, clot retraction, capillary fragility

Thrombocytopenic purpura, idiopathic: coagulation profile, platelet count, bone marrow, liver/spleen scan capillary fragility

Thrombophlebitis: impedance plethysmography, fibrinogen I 125 scan, venography, thermography

Thymoma: chest roentgenogram, CT scan of mediastinum, mediastinoscopy, exploratory thoracotomy

Thyroiditis, subacute: FT$_4$I, RAI uptake and scan, sedimentation rate, antithyroid autoantibodies

Thyroid nodule: RAI uptake and scan, fine-needle aspiration, biopsy, FT$_4$I, ultrasonography, trial of thyroid suppression therapy

Tonsillitis: see Pharyngitis

Torulosis: see Cryptococcosis

Toxemia of pregnancy: see Eclampsia

Toxoplasmosis: indirect fluorescent antibody (IFA) titer, passive hemagglutination test (PHA), skin test

Trachoma: smear of conjunctival scrapings, culture for chlamydia, tears for microimmunofluorescent antibodies

Transfusion reaction: serum hemoglobin, haptoglobins and methemalbumin

Transient ischemic attack (TIA): carotid scan, digital subtraction angiography, CT scan, 4-vessel cerebral angiography

Trichinosis: eosinophil count, skin test, serologic tests, muscle biopsy

Trypanosomiasis: smears of blood, CSF, lymph node aspirate for parasites, animal inoculation

Tuberculosis: smear and culture of sputum and gastric washings, guinea pig inoculation, skin test, chest roentgenogram

Tuberosclerosis: skull roentgenogram, CT scan, skin biopsy, cortical biopsy

Tularemia: smear and culture of ulcer, lymph nodes or nasopharynx, Foshay's skin test, serologic tests

Turner's syndrome: buccal smear for chromatins (Barr bodies), chromosome analysis

Typhoid fever: culture of stool, blood or bone marrow, febrile agglutinins

Typhus, epidemic: serologic tests, Weil–Felix test

Typhus scrub: isolation from blood, serologic tests, Weil–Felix reaction

U

Ulcer: see Peptic ulcer

Ulcerative colitis: barium enema, sigmoidoscopy or colonoscopy and biopsy

Urethritis: urethral smear and culture, vaginal smear and culture, urine culture, chlamydia culture, cystoscopy

Urticaria: RAST allergic skin testing, elimination diet

V

Varicella: serologic tests

Varicose veins: phlebography, thermography

Variola: see Smallpox

Ventricular septal defects: ECG, echocardiogram, cardiac catheterization

Visceral larva migrans: blood typing, serologic tests, biopsy

Vitamin A deficiency: serum vitamin A or carotene, skin biopsy

Vitamin B deficiency: see Beriberi

Vitamin C deficiency: see Scurvy

Vitamin D deficiency: see Rickets

Vitamin K deficiency: coagulation profile including prothrombin time

Von Gierke's disease: see Glycogen storage disease

Von Willebrand's disease: coagulation profile, thromboplastin-generation test, factor VIII assay

W

Waterhouse–Friderichsen syndrome: blood cultures, spinal fluid examination, nose and throat culture, plasma cortisol

Wegener's granulomatosis: roentgenogram of nose, sinuses, chest, urinalysis, renal biopsy, lung biopsy, nasal biopsy

Weil's disease: dark field examination of blood, guinea pig inoculation, serologic tests, spinal tap

Wernicke's encephalopathy: response to IV thiamine

Whipple's disease: small bowel series, lymph node biopsy, jejunal biopsy, malabsorption tests

Whooping cough: see Pertussis

Wilson's disease: urine copper and amino acids, serum copper and ceruloplasmin, liver biopsy, slit-lamp examination of cornea, uric acid

Y

Yaws: dark field examination, serologic tests

Yellow fever: viral isolation, serologic tests, liver biopsy

Z

Zollinger–Ellison syndrome: 12-hour quantitative and MAO gastric analysis, serum gastrin, GI series, gastroscopy, exploratory laparotomy

Index

Numbers followed by an *f* indicate a figure; *t* following a page number indicates tabular material. Page numbers in **boldface** indicate lists of diagnostic tests for a specific symptom or disease.